This book is due for return on or before the last date shown below.

OXFORD MEDICAL PUBLICATIONS

Physiological Measurements with Radionuclides in Clinical Practice

To our wives, Rosemary and Toby, and children, Gil, Simon, Robert and Alice. Also to Professor Peter Lavender for his support, encouragement, and scientific vision.

Physiological Measurements with Radionuclides in Clinical Practice

A. M. Peters

Professor of Diagnostic Radiology,
Imperial College School of Medicine,
London

and

M. J. Myers

Consultant Clinical Scientist,
Hammersmith Hospitals NHS Trust,
London

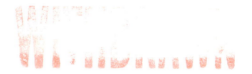

OXFORD   NEW YORK   TOKYO
OXFORD UNIVERSITY PRESS
1998

Oxford University Press, Great Clarendon Street, Oxford OX2 6DP

Oxford New York
Athens Auckland Bangkok Bogota Bombay Buenos Aires
Calcutta Cape Town Dar es Salaam Delhi Florence Hong Kong
Istanbul Karachi Kuala Lumpur Madras Madrid Melbourne
Mexico City Nairobi Paris Singapore Taipei Tokyo Toronto Warsaw

and associated companies in
Berlin Ibadan

Oxford is a trade mark of Oxford University Press

Published in the United States
by Oxford University Press Inc., New York

A catalogue record for this book is available from the British Library

Library of Congress Cataloging in Publication Data

Peters, A. Michael.
Physiological measurements with radionuclides in clinical practice
/ A.M. Peters and M. Myers.
(Oxford medical publications)
Includes bibliographical references.
1. Radioisotope scanning. 2. Patient monitoring. I. Myers, M. (Melvyn)
II. Title. III. Series.
[DNLM: 1. Nuclear Medicine–methods. 2. Monitoring. Physiologic–methods.
3. Radiation Monitoring. 4. Radioisotopes WN 440
P481p 1998]
RC78.7. R4P46 1998 616.07'575–dc21 DNLM/DLC
for Library of Congress 97-21585 CIP

ISBN 0 19 261 994 2

Typeset by EXPO Holdings, Malaysia

Printed in Great Britain by Bath Press

Foreword

This book is the most complete account of methods for quantifying data processed in nuclear medicine procedures that I have ever read. At least four general textbooks in nuclear medicine have been published within the last three years, and these contain brief descriptions of selected methods of quantification. In contrast, all the important methods are included in this text, with extensive references. The only previous book of similar content which I have encountered is *Radioisotope techniques in clinical research and diagnosis* by Veall and Vetter (Butterworth, London) but it was published back in 1958. However, this new textbook by Professor Peters and Dr Myers is not a boring encyclopaedia. Radiation dose calculations from internally administered radionuclides are reviewed briefly, but if further detail is needed, more methodology and data are readily available in the MIRD Pamphlets of the Society of Nuclear Medicine and Annals of the ICRP, Publication 53 (Pergamon Press, 1994).

The book begins with a chapter on basic mathematics; this will be helpful for doctors like myself who have forgotten or feel rusty about calculus and other maths manoeuvres. The first five chapters deal with general topics and the last eight cover methods of quantitation for different organ systems in depth. Chapter three reviews all the methods of blood flow measurement. Chapter four provides a terse review of the properties and biodistribution of common radiodiagnostic agents, and this should be especially helpful to basic scientists who wish to know more about clinical studies. Chapter five covers scintillation detectors and methods of processing the data which they generate. The book ends with Questions and Answers for review.

This book will be invaluable to scientists doing research using radioactive tracers, because quantitative methods provide an objective assessment of experimental results. Many computer programs are available 'off the shelf' to process nuclear data. In fact, one must use caution in selecting the right programs which will produce valid conclusions.

How useful will this textbook be for clinical practitioners of nuclear medicine? This is an important question, particularly in America where the impact of 'managed care' is focused on minimizing the costs of medical care. Any diagnostic procedure which does not influence patient management or eventual outcome will not be reimbursed. American readers of this text may notice differences in emphasis from practitioners of nuclear medicine in Europe. However, one cannot practise modern nuclear medicine anywhere without computer quantitative methods. Clinical practitioners will find the chapters on the heart, kidneys, gastrointestinal tract, and lung particularly important. To understand those studies which are clinically useful, I suggest that practitioners carefully study Chapters two and three also.

Whether you are a researcher or practitioner of nuclear medicine, you will appreciate the efforts of the authors and their intimate knowledge of mathematics, physics, physiology, and pathology.

John G. McAfee, MD, FRCP(Can), FACNP
Consultant, Department of Nuclear Medicine, Clinical Center,
The National Institutes of Health, Bethesda, MD, USA
Clinical Professor, Department of Radiology,
The George Washington School of Medicine,
Washington, DC, USA
Emeritus Professor of Radiology, SUNY Health Science Center,
Syracuse, NY, USA
June 1997

Preface

Our aim in this book is to dispel the sense of intimidation felt by many physicians and medical laboratory scientists when faced with quantification in physiology and clinical medicine.

We have tried to do this by treating physiological quantification with a unified approach, moving from basic mathematics to sophisticated measurement techniques without losing a uniform style. This is reinforced by the use throughout the book of the same symbols for the physiological variables addressed, an approach which is not significantly disadvantaged by the use of unfamiliar symbols for some of the variables. For example, whilst most texts in the medical literature would use 'F' for blood flow, we have used 'Q', a historically well-established symbol for blood flow in certain fields, such as pulmonary and microvascular physiology. We have also tried to illustrate a relative mathematical uniformity of techniques for rather diverse measurements. For example, measurements of single kidney glomerular filtration rate using renography, liver blood flow using organic anions and faecal endogenous calcium excretion using radiocalcium all use essentially the same equation.

In a further attempt to make the numerical text easier to read, we have not always applied conventional notation in the equations, for example, when expressing a dependent variable we have frequently not indicated what the variable is a function of [such as C, instead of $C(t)$], firstly because it is usually obvious and secondly because, nearly always in nuclear medicine, dependent variables are functions of time. We apologize if this irritates the pure mathematician.

It may not always be apparent to the reader whether or not a described technique is of any particular relevance to clinical management or clinical research. Although an attempt is usually made in the text to indicate the correct relevance, we make no apology for describing techniques without much clinical relevance since the technique may illustrate an important quantitative concept or may subsequently assume importance with the development of other technology. Thus, when we started to write the book several years ago, there was little activity in functional CT, MRI, or ultrasound. Currently, however, there is much interest in dynamic CT and in the development of intravascular contrast agents for dynamic CT. In order to generate an outflow time-concentration curve (in contrast to a residue curve – see section 2.1) using a radioactive isotope it is necessary to sample blood, but the spatial and temporal resolution of CT will allow generation of high-quality outflow time-attenuation curves by placement of regions of interest over blood vessels. Even ultrasound can produce time-reflectivity curves now using intravenously injected microscopic bubbles.

Many quantitative indices have been described in physiological measurement in nuclear medicine but, in general, these cannot be defined in a physiologically meaningful way, usually have no units and are generally avoided in this text.

Finally, although centred on nuclear medicine, the techniques described in the book have applications much wider than the discipline of nuclear medicine itself. Indeed, many of the techniques use stable markers rather than radioactive isotopes and, conversely, several quantitative nuclear medicine techniques have been developed from stable markers. In this context, there is no essential difference throughout the book in the meanings of 'tracer' and 'indicator'.

London   A.M.P.
1997   M.J.M.

Abbreviations

exclusively or frequently used throughout this book

Variables and constants

t	time (min)
T	mean transit or residence time (min)
M	mass (mg) or amount of radioactivity (MBq)
Q	blood flow (ml/min) or perfusion (ml/min/ml or ml/min/g)
V	volume (ml)
C	concentration (mg/ml or MBq/ml)
Z	clearance (ml/min, ml/min/ml or ml/min/g)
α, β	exponential rate constants or clearance (min^{-1})
E	extraction fraction or extraction efficiency (%)
J	indicator or tracer flux (mg/min or MBq/min)
P	permeability (cm/min)
S	surface area (cm^2)
PS	permeability surface area product (ml/min, ml/min/ml or ml/min/g)
p	pressure (mm Hg)
$\dot{V}$	ventilation (ml/min)
N	count rate (counts/min)
f	fraction
k	fractional rate constant (min^{-1}) or constant
K	transfer constant representing PS product or clearance
H, h	haematocrit
TBV	total blood volume (ml)
CO	cardiac output (ml/min)
λ	partition coefficient
ρ	density (mg/ml)
δ	physical decay constant (min^{-1})
γ	proportionality constant relating amount of radioactivity to count rate recorded by a detector (MBq/counts/min)
Γ	proportionality constant relating concentration of radioactivity in blood to count rate recorded by a detector (MBq/ml/counts/min)
μ	linear attenuation coefficient (cm^{-1})
d	thickness, depth or distance

subscripts

τ	tissue
a	arterial
v	venous
p	capillary or plasma
b	blood
u	urine
i	intravascular or inspired
e	extravascular or expired

alv   alveolar
m   mesenteric or portal
f   free
χ bound
s   steady state
r   regional

Contents

1 Basic mathematics

Introduction

This chapter introduces the reader to the mathematics relevant to physiological quantification in nuclear medicine. It starts from the very basics and is aimed at the mathematically timid. Several rules can be used to guide you through the equations in nuclear medicine. Firstly, however complicated they may look, they almost always contain only two variables, one dependent on the other. Secondly, the complexity of the equations is often the result of the 'constants' present, which can, in any event, often be 'lumped' together. So, look at the equation, and do not allow yourself to be discouraged by the symbols. Deciphering the symbols can be daunting, and this is why an attempt has been made to use the same symbol for a given variable throughout this book. Another useful exercise to adopt when looking at an equation, is to study the *units* of each variable and constant. The units will follow most of the complicated equations in the following chapters often making the equation easier to understand as well as checking its internal consistencies. Many of the units may eventually cancel out and it is self-evident that the remaining units on the left-hand side of an equation must be the same as those on the right. None of the mathematics in this book are more complex than the reader will encounter in this chapter.

1.1 Equations, variables and graphs

An equation is a statement that one set of terms is equal to another. For example,

$$y = bx.$$

The terms may be single variables or may be more complicated, containing several variables and constants. In the example, as with almost all the equations encountered in quantitative nuclear medicine, the equation has only two variables (x and y), one called the dependent variable, which is dependent on the other, the independent variable. Conventionally, y is the dependent variable placed on the left-hand side of the equation and x is the independent variable placed on the right-hand side. We can also express the relationship between x and y by saying y *is a function of* x. In the example, y is a linear function of x and b is a constant, known as the constant of proportionality. A value of y at a given value of x is written $y(x)$. In nuclear medicine, the independent variable, here referred to as x, is often time, t, while the independent variable is often a count or count rate or concentration of radio-activity, $C(t)$. The initial value of $C(t)$, at zero time would be written $C(0)$.

An equation may also be represented as a graph. Conventionally it is plotted with the dependent y values on the vertical axis and the independent x values on the horizontal axis. The above equation, for example, is represented on these axes by a straight line going through the origin (**Fig. 1.1**) and which has a 'slope' or 'gradient' equal to b.

The graph of the equation

$$y = bx + C \tag{1.1}$$

has a positive 'intercept' of $y = C$ when $x = 0$

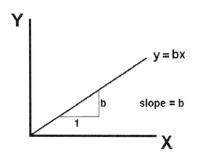

Fig. 1.1 Graph of the equation $y = bx$. This is represented by a straight line going through the origin and having a slope 'b' found by dividing the y increment (b) by the x increment (1).

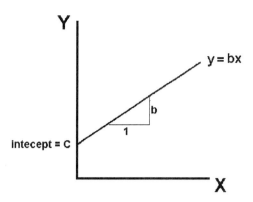

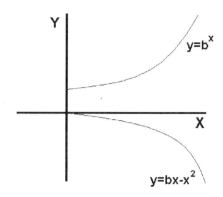

∎ **Fig. 1.2** Graph of the equation $y = bx + C$. This is similar to that shown in the previous figure and has the same slope b but now has an intercept C on the y-axis which is the value of y when $x = 0$.

∎ **Fig. 1.3** Examples when functions do not give a straight line graph. The upper curve represents the power or exponential function $y = b^x$ and the lower curve a combination of a function of x and x^2 as in $y = bx - x^2$.

(**Fig. 1.2**) and the sample slope as above, b. Because the two sides of an equation are equal, anything can be done to the left-hand side of the equation provided exactly the same is done to the right-hand side. Thus, if we double both sides of the equation 1.1 and add a constant 'a' we can write it

$$2y + a = 2bx + 2C + a.$$

Furthermore, one can divide one equation by another because, obviously, the equality between the left and right sides of the resulting equation will be maintained.

For example, if $y_1 = 6x^2$

and $y_2 = 3x$

then $\dfrac{y_1}{y_2} = \dfrac{6x^2}{3x} = 2x.$

Although an equation may contain only two variables, a variable can be represented more than once; e.g.

$$y = bx - x^2, \qquad (1.2)$$

or a variable may be the power to which a constant is raised; e.g.

$$y = b^x. \qquad (1.3)$$

Note that in neither equation 1.2 nor 1.3 is y *linearly* related to x; i.e. neither graph is represented by a straight line or, in other words, both are non-linear equations (**Fig. 1.3**)

When an equation has more than two variables, the relationship between them can be simplified by holding all but two of the variables constant. Consider Ohm's law (voltage = resistance × current or $V = R \times I$) with three variables. Here voltage can be varied at constant resistance to produce a change in current. In this case voltage is the independent variable, current is the dependent variable and the resistance is the constant of proportionality. Alternatively, one can hold the voltage constant and vary the resistance, in which case the resistance is the independent variable, current is the dependent variable and voltage is the constant of proportionality, i.e. $I = V/R$.

To solve y from an equation, it is self-evident that x and any constants have to be known — *one* unknown variable or constant can be solved from *one* equation. If there are two unknowns, two separate and independent equations need to be formulated. Thus, for example, consider

$$y = b - x$$
$$\text{and} \quad y = 2bx. \qquad (1.4)$$

If neither b nor y were known, it would nevertheless be easy to solve the two equations by expressing b in terms of y, or y in terms of b:

Thus, since $y = b - x$ and $y = 2bx$, we can say that

$$b - x = 2bx.$$

There is now one equation and one unknown value, b. So, bringing all terms containing b to the left hand side gives:

$$b - 2bx = x.$$

Taking b outside the brackets gives

$$b(1 - 2x) = x$$

and dividing by $(1 - 2x)$ gives

$$b = \frac{x}{(1 - 2x)}.$$

Having obtained b, we can go back to equation 1.4 to solve y in terms of x, i.e. solve the equation

$$y = \frac{x}{(1 - 2x)} - x = \frac{2x^2}{(1 - 2x)}.$$

If we have two unknowns, we need two independent equations — known as simultaneous equations. If we have three unknowns we would need three equations and so on.

1.2 Simple calculus

1.2.1 Differentiation

The purpose of differentiation is to determine the *rate* at which the variable y changes with respect to the variable x. In graphical terms, the purpose is to determine the slope or gradient of the graph of y versus x at a specific value of x, usually written as $y(x)$. Consider $y = bx$. In this case, b, the gradient, which is equal to $y(x)/x$, is obviously constant and independent of x. However, in the case of

$$y = bx^2$$

the gradient of the graph is continuously changing as x changes, i.e. it is itself a function of x (**Fig. 1.4**). We can calculate the approximate slope of the graph in this case at any value of x by imagining the small change in y (denoted by Δy) resulting from a small change in x (denoted by Δx). Here the slope would be given by $\Delta x/\Delta y$

Thus, if y_1 is the value of y at $x - 0.5\Delta x$ and y_2 the value of y at $x + 0.5\Delta x$,

then $\quad y_1 = b(x - 0.5\Delta x)^2$

$$= b(x^2 - x\Delta x + 0.25[\Delta x]^2)$$

$$= bx^2 - bx\Delta x + 0.25b[\Delta x]^2$$

and $\quad y_2 = b(x + 0.5\Delta x)^2$

$$= b(x^2 + x\Delta x + 0.25[\Delta x]^2)$$

$$= bx^2 + bx\Delta x + 0.25b[\Delta x]^2.$$

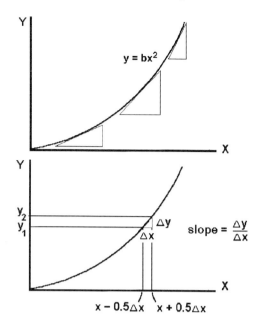

▌ **Fig. 1.4** Illustration of how the slope of a curve (here $y = bx^2$) is defined. The slope increases as the value of x increases as shown in the upper curve. To find the slope at any point on the curve consider the y increment Δy for an increment of Δx about the value of x. The point y_1, corresponds to a value of x equal to $x - 0.5\Delta x$ and the point y_2, corresponds to a value of x equal to $x + 0.5\Delta x$. The y increment is given by the difference Δy equal to $y_2 - y_1$. The slope of the curve is defined as the y increment divided by the x increment $\Delta y/\Delta x$.

Therefore $\quad y_2 - y_1 = bx^2 + bx\Delta x + 0.25b(\Delta x)^2 -$
$$bx^2 + bx\Delta x - 0.25b(\Delta x)^2.$$
$$= 2bx\Delta x.$$

But $\quad\quad y_2 - y_1 = \Delta y,$

therefore $\quad\quad \Delta y = 2bx\Delta x.$

Dividing both sides by Δx gives the slope

$$\frac{\Delta y}{\Delta x} = \frac{2bx\Delta x}{\Delta x} = 2bx.$$

If we specify that $y_2 - y_1$ becomes vanishingly small then y_1 and y_2 could be considered as one and the same point. In mathematical terminology Δy and Δx are replaced by 'dy' and 'dx' and the slope by dy/dx (pronounced 'dee y by dee x'). We can say in the equation above where

$$y = bx^2$$

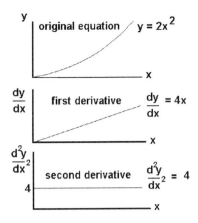

Fig. 1.5 Illustration of the first and second differentials of the function $y = 2x^2$. The upper curve shows the original equation $y = 2x^2$. The middle curve is a plot of the slope of this equation (the 'first differential') and shows that the slope increases linearly with increase in x. The bottom curve is a graph of the slope of the slope of the original function — the second differential. Since the slope of the first differential is constant (equal to 4 in this case) the slope of the slope or the variation in the constant value is naturally zero and is shown by a straight line parallel to the x-axis.

that

$$\frac{dy}{dx} = 2bx.$$

The slope of the curve, equal to $2bx$, is also called the first derivative of bx^2. It will be clear from the last two equations, that in obtaining the first derivative, x has been multiplied by the index 2, whilst the index itself has gone down by one unit. Applying this simple rule, the first derivatives of the following, $7x$, $5x^2$, $6x^3$ and $15x^4$, are, respectively, 7, $10x$, $18x^2$, $60x^3$ and so on (remember that x^0 is 1). In the first of these examples, it can be seen that the slope, or first derivative, dy/dx, is a constant, whilst in the other three it is dependent on x. We can now ask what is the relationship between dy/dx and x?

As can be seen from **Fig. 1.5**, which is a graph of the equation, $y = 2x^2$, the first derivative or slope, $4x$, increases as x increases. At $x = 2$, for example, the slope is 8; at $x = 4$ the slope is 16. We can also derive the *slope of the slope* of a graph, i.e. the slope of the graph of dy/dx versus x. This is called the *second* derivative of y and is denoted by d^2y/dx^2 ('dee two y by dee x squared'). It is obtained by the same rule that was obtained to obtain dy/dx.

Therefore, if

$$\frac{dy}{dx} = 4x$$

then

$$\frac{d(dy/dx)}{dx} = \frac{d^2y}{dx^2} = 4.$$

Consider now a more complex equation, one with more than one term on the right-hand side containing x:

$$y = ax + bx^2.$$

By following the working shown above,

$$y_2 - y_1 = \Delta_y = a\Delta x + 2bx\Delta x$$

and

$$\frac{\Delta y}{\Delta x} = a + 2bx.$$

In other words, the first derivative of y in this case is the sum of the first derivatives of the separate terms on the right. This is illustrated in **Fig. 1.6**, in which at any value x, the gradient, dy/dx of $(ax + bx^2)$ is the sum of the two separate slopes of y versus ax and bx^2, respectively.

Nuclear medicine computer software usually offers the option, 'derivative' (of a time-activity curve), and selection of this option generates a new curve of gradient (i.e. dy/dt) versus time (t).

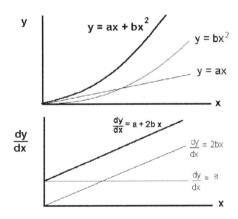

Fig. 1.6 Illustration of the curve $y = ax + bx^2$ and its first differential. The upper curve shows how the relation $y = ax + bx^2$ is made up of two components $y = ax$ and $y = bx^2$. The lower curve is a plot of the slope of $y = ax + bx^2$ and is made up of the slopes of the two components, 'a' and '$2bx$'.

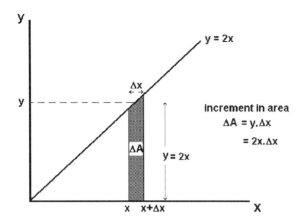

▌ **Fig. 1.7** Illustration of the start of the process of integration. The increase of area ΔA under the curve $y = 2x$ as x increases by an increment of Δx is shown by the shaded area and given by the product height × width or $y \cdot \Delta x$. Since $y = 2x$ the increment in area, $\Delta A = 2x \cdot \Delta x$.

1.2.2 Integration

In practice, whereas differentiation gives the *slope* of a graph y versus x, integration gives the *area* under the graph. Consider the equation $y = 2x$, illustrated graphically in **Fig. 1.7**. As x is increased to $x + dx$ then each small segment of area is written as dA. The area of the small element is $y \cdot dx = 2xdx$

So

$$dA = 2x \cdot dx. \qquad (1.5)$$

An area under a certain section of the curve is formed by summing all these small segments between the start and end of the section and is written in a special way in which summing is represented by the symbol of an elongated s written $\int$. The start of the section is written at the bottom of the $\int$ e.g. $\int_0$ and the end of the section at the top of the symbol e.g. $\int^{\infty}$.

Thus, summing all the small segments of area, dA, from the origin of the graph to a specified value of x is strictly written as $\int_0^x dA$ and called the integral between the limits 0 and x. For our purposes, however, it will be simplified to $\int dA$.

Returning to equation 1.5 and summing or integrating both sides of the equation gives

$$\int dA = \int 2x \cdot dx.$$

Now the result of integrating dA is the total area A i.e. $\int dA = A$. $\qquad (1.6)$

As with differentiation we have to employ a rule to evaluate the right-hand side of the equation. This general rule for integrating an expression (such as x) is to increase the index (here 1) by 1 giving x^2 and dividing the result by the new index (giving $x^2/2$). Thus integrating $2x$ gives $2 \cdot x^2/2$ or x^2, i.e.

$$\int 2x \cdot dx = x^2.$$

When we introduce limits such as integrating between two values of x, say, $x = 2$ and $x = 4$ we write the solution as

$$\int_{x=2}^{x=4} 2x \cdot dx = [x^2]_{x=2}^{x=4}.$$

This is evaluated by replacing x in the square bracket with the top limit, 4, and then subtracting the result of replacing x with the bottom limit, 2 i.e.

$$\int_{x=2}^{x=4} 2x \cdot dx = [x^2]_{x=2}^{x=4} = 4^2 - 2^2 = 12.$$

Thus the area under the graph between the limits of 2 and 4 is 12. The process is illustrated for another equation $y = 2x + 3$ in **Fig. 1.8**.

Since, in practice, we deal with actual areas under a curve either between two values of time or between a value at zero time and infinity, we deal with what is called *definite* integrals. We shall ignore the general case of *indefinite* integrals where a theoretical solution to the integration is obtained that involves a constant.

In personal computer software packages of the spread sheet variety a 'running sum' is available as an operation for columns of data. Running sum is simply a method of obtaining a numerical integration.

1.2.3 Exponential decay and growth

Simple calculus is the mathematics of change and thus useful in dealing quantitatively with changes in volumes or count rates or concentrations of tracer encountered in nuclear medicine. An important physiological application is one where the rate of change, the decay or growth, of an entity is proportional to how much of that entity is present. This type of change is called *exponential decay* or *growth*. For example, the measured rate of decay of an isotope is proportional to the quantity of the

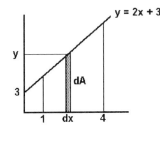

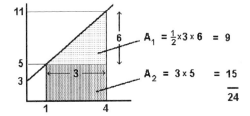

▮ **Fig. 1.8** Illustrating how the process of integration is taken a stage further to include limits of integration by adding all the elements of area such as ΔA between the limits (i.e. x values) of 1 and 4 for the curve $y = 2x + 3$. Geometrically it can be seen in the lower figure that the total area is $A_1 + A_2$, i.e. $9 + 15$ or 24. For the upper curve the same area is given by direct integration.

isotope existing at the time of measurement and is thus termed exponential. To deal with exponential growth and decay some specialized symbols and techniques are required. These, in turn, are related to an important number in mathematics denoted by the symbol e, which is a special number in rather the same way that π is a special number. It is, in fact, the sum of a particular series of numbers

$$e = 1 + 1 + \frac{1}{2} + \frac{1}{6} + \frac{1}{24} + \frac{1}{120} + \frac{1}{720} + \dots \text{ and so on}$$
(1.7)

Although the series goes on to infinity, the terms get smaller so only a limited number of terms needs to be considered to evaluate e. Adding the first seven terms in this series gives $1 + 1 + 0.5 + 0.1667 + 0.0417 + 0.0083 + 0.0014 = 2.7181$, which is very close to the actual value of e, 2.71828 ... (a number going on to an infinite number of decimal places which is obtained when the infinite number of terms is summed). For simplicity it will be written 2.71828.

The above gives the special case of e^1. It can be also be proved that, in general,

$$e^x = 1 + x + \frac{x^2}{2} + \frac{x^3}{6} + \frac{x^4}{24} + \frac{x^5}{120} + \frac{x^6}{720} + \dots$$

(i.e. x is not necessarily 1) and, for a constant, k

$$e^{kx} = 1 + kx + \frac{k^2 x^2}{2} + \frac{k^3 x^3}{6} + \frac{k^4 x^4}{24} + \dots \quad (1.8)$$

The importance of e *is that for the term* e^x, *the* **derivative** *is also* e^x. This property is unique in that **only for the number** 2.71828 will the **value** of 2.71828 to the power of x and the **rate of change** of 2.71828 to the power of x be equal. A hint of this can be seen by looking at the values and slopes for, say, 2^x, e^x (i.e. 2.718^x) and 3^x (**Fig. 1.9**).

A general solution is the following: if

$$e^x = y = 1 + x + \frac{x^2}{2} + \frac{x^3}{6} + \frac{x^4}{24} + \frac{x^5}{120} + \frac{x^6}{720} + \dots$$

then, since each term is differentiated separately,

$$\frac{dy}{dx} = 0 + 1 + \frac{2x}{2} + \frac{3x^2}{6} + \frac{4x^3}{24} + \frac{5x^4}{120} + \dots$$

$$= 1 + x + \frac{x^2}{2} + \frac{x^3}{6} + \frac{x^4}{24} + \dots$$

$$= y.$$

In other words, if $y = e^x$, then

$$\frac{dy}{dx} = y.$$

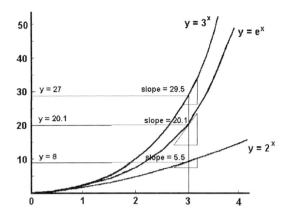

▍ **Fig. 1.9** The figure illustrates the unique properties of the mathematical constant 'e' (equal to 2.781828 ...) by comparing the slopes of the curves 3^x, e^x and 2^x. At an arbitrary point $x = 3$ the y value of 3^x is given by 3^3 or 27 and the slope by 29.7. (Mathematics beyond the scope of this book give the slope of the general curve a^x as $a^x \ln a$. Hence $27 \times \ln 3$ or 29.7). Similarly the y value of 2^x is given by 2^3 or 8 and the slope by 5.5. Only for e^x are the values of y for $x = 3$ ($y = 20.1$) and the value of the slope at $x = 3$ (slope $= 20.1$) equal. This implies that $\frac{\Delta y}{\Delta x} = \frac{dy}{dx} = y$, or the rate of disappearance = amount present which, among other things, is the basis of the isotopic decay relationship.

Similarly, if $y = e^{kx}$

$$= 1 + kx + \frac{k^2 x^2}{2} + \frac{k^3 x^3}{6} + \frac{k^4 x^4}{24} + \ldots$$

(see 1.7)

then $\qquad \frac{dy}{dx} = 0 + k + \frac{2k^2 x}{2} + \frac{3k^3 x^2}{6} + \frac{4k^4 x^3}{24} + \ldots$

$$= k\left(1 + kx + \frac{k^2 x^2}{2} + \frac{k^3 x^3}{6} \cdots\right).$$

In other words

$$\frac{dy}{dx} = ky.$$

Furthermore, by integrating (with respect to x),

$$\int e^x \cdot dx = e^x$$

and integrating,

$$\int e^{kx} \cdot dx = \frac{1}{k} \cdot e^{kx}$$

$$= \frac{y}{k}.$$

So, when differentiating an exponential function involving a constant in the index, the exponential term is *multiplied* by the constant and when integrating it the exponential term is *divided* by the constant.

When $\quad y = Ae^{kx}$

each term on the right of equation 1.8 is multiplied by the constant A, which along with k comes out of the brackets so that

$$\frac{dy}{dx} = kAy$$

and $\quad \int (Ae^{kx}) \cdot dx = \frac{A}{k} e^{kx}.$

In general nuclear medicine equations, exponential change will often be seen as

$$\frac{dM}{dt} = +kM \quad \text{(growth)} \quad \text{or} \quad \frac{dM}{dt} = -kM \quad \text{(decay)}$$

(1.9)

where M is a variable like mass or radioactivity which is a function of time, t, and k is a constant of proportionality. The *positive* sign tells us that an exponential *growth* process is occurring, the *negative* sign that an exponential *decay* occurs.

In general when $\qquad M = Ae^{kt}$

$$dM/dt = Ake^{kt}.$$

(1.10)

By way of checking, integration of equation 1.9 gives

$$\int (dM/dt) \cdot dt = \int (Ake^{kt}) \cdot dt = M = Ae^{kt}. \quad (1.11)$$

(The constant of integration, C, of this indefinite integral will be ignored.)

According to equation 1.11, when $t = 0$, M must be equal to $Ae^{k \cdot 0}$ or Ae^0 or $A \times 1$ or A, so the value of M at $t = 0$, denoted by $M(0)$ is A, i.e, rewriting equation 1.10 the value of M at $t = t$, denoted by $M(t) = M(0) \cdot e^{kt}$. Re-arranging equation 1.11,

$$\frac{M(t)}{M(0)} = e^{kt}.$$

(1.12)

Now $M(t)/M(0)$ is the fraction of the original $M(0)$ remaining at a particular time, so equation 1.12 defines the fractional rate at which M grows. Since the left-hand side of equation 1.12 is a fraction, it is unitless. The right-hand side is therefore unitless. Therefore, since t has units of time, k must have units of the reciprocal of time so that time cancels out. These units are written, for example, as $\sec^{-1}$ or s^{-1} and referred to as 'per second'. The constant k is called the *rate constant* of the change in M with time. Equation 1.9 shows that k defines how *quickly* M grows as a function of time. Equation 1.12 shows how k influences the *fractional change* in M as a function of time.

If $\dfrac{dM}{dt} = -kM$ (an example of decay or disappearance of M)

$$(1.13)$$

then $\dfrac{M(t)}{M(0)} = e^{-kt}.$ $\hspace{2cm}(1.14)$

Equation 1.14 defines the *fractional rate* at which M decays i.e. $M(t)$ is a fraction of the original $M(0)$. The value of k determines the speed of the decay and the larger its value the greater the rate of decay.

Decay is sometimes expressed in terms of a *half-life* often denoted by $T_{1/2}$ or $t_{1/2}$. This is the period of time during which M decreases to $\frac{1}{2}M$.

We can now demonstrate the relationship between the decay constant k and the half-life $t_{1/2}$. This is a very important relationship in nuclear medicine.

If a time $t = t_1$

$$M(1) = M(0) \cdot e^{-kt_1} \hspace{1cm}(1.15)$$

and at time $t = t_2$

$M(2) = M(0) \cdot e^{-kt_2}$ where t_2 is a later time

$$(\text{i.e. } t_2 > t_1) \hspace{1cm}(1.16)$$

and if, in the special case

$$M(2) = \frac{1}{2} \cdot M(1)$$

i.e. at time t_2, M has decreased by one half its value at time t_1, then, dividing equation 1.15 by equation 1.16 gives

$$M(1)/M(2) = 1/\tfrac{1}{2} = 2 = e^{-kt_1}/e^{-kt_2}$$
$$= e^{-k(t_1 - t_2)} \hspace{1cm}(1.17)$$
$$= e^{k(t_2 - t_1)}.$$

We deal with this equation by taking logarithms of both sides of equation 1.17. This is the inverse process of raising a number by an exponent. Thus the logarithm of e^x, defined by $\log_e x$ is x and the logarithm of $e^{k(t_2 - t_1)}$ is $k(t_2 - t_1)$. The logarithm with base e is called the 'natural' logarithm and is denoted by ln, i.e. $\log_e x$ is denoted by $\ln x$. The

logarithm has actual values so $\ln 2 = 0.6931471 \ldots$ (simplified to 0.693) is the inverse process of exponential $e^{0.693} = 2$. Similarly, $\ln 100$ has a value of 4.605, i.e. $e^{4.605} = 100$.

Taking logarithms to the base e of both sides of equation 1.17 gives:

$$\log_e 2 = \ln 2 = \ln \left[e^{k(t_2 - t_1)} \right] = k(t_2 - t_1)$$

We therefore can write

$$k = \frac{\ln 2}{(t_2 - t_1)}.$$

Now because of our set condition that $M(t_2)$ is half of $M(t_1)$, the period $(t_2 - t_1)$ is equal to the *half-life* referred to as $t_{1/2}$, so

$$k = \frac{\ln 2}{t_{1/2}}.$$

This yields the important relationships

$$k = \frac{0.693}{t_{1/2}}$$

and $\hspace{2cm} t_{1/2} = \dfrac{0.693}{k}. \hspace{1cm}(1.18)$

Equation 1.18 confirms that when k is large and the decay fast, $t_{1/2}$ is small and the half-life is short.

1.2.4 The area under an exponential graph

It has already been stated that any equation can be represented graphically. A straight line graph of $y = mx + C$ is illustrated in **Fig. 1.1** and an exponential equation $y = y_0 e^{-kx}$ is illustrated in the left-hand side of **Fig. 1.10** using some actual values, $y_0 = 10$ and $k = 0.115$. We shall now present a method of obtaining the area under this graph.

Areas enclosed by regular shapes are generally easy to calculate. The area under the straight line graph shown in figure 1.1 is simply a triangle and that for the graph of figure 1.2 is the area of a triangle plus the area of a rectangle. For graphs of exponential relationships (such as $10e^{-0.115t}$ illustrated in **Fig. 1.10**) a simple rule can be generated. *The total area under the curve of a decreasing exponential, i.e. between $x = 0$ and $x = \infty$, is simply equal to the value of y at $x = 0$ divided by the rate constant.* This is explained as follows.

For the decreasing exponential

$$y = y_0\, e^{-kx} \qquad (y = y_0 \text{ at } x = 0)$$

the area is found by integrating between defined limits of x (see figure 1.8):

$$\text{Area} = \int_{x=0}^{x=\infty} y \cdot dx = -\frac{y_0}{k}\, e^{-kx} \text{ with the limits 0 and } \infty$$

$$= \left[-\frac{y_0}{k}\, e^{-kx} \right]_{x=0}^{x=\infty}$$

$$= -\frac{y_0}{k}[e^{-kx} - 1].$$

When $x = \infty$, $e^{-kx} = 0$, so

$$\int_0^\infty y \cdot dx = \frac{y_0}{k}. \tag{1.19}$$

Thus the area under the entire curve (between limits $x = 0$ and $x = \infty$) is the intercept y_0 divided by the rate constant k. For the usual time activity curves we encounter in nuclear medicine we can replace x by t and thus $y = y_0 e^{-kt}$.

We can take this further by exploiting the relationship between k and $t_{1/2}$. Since $k = 0.693/t_{1/2}$ equation 1.19 becomes the area under the time activity curve

$$\int_0^\infty y \cdot dt = \frac{y_0}{k} = \frac{t_{1/2} y_0}{0.693} = 1.44\, t_{1/2} y_0.$$

Thus to calculate the total area under a single exponential decaying curve from zero to infinity all that is required is to multiply the initial y intercept by 1.44 times the half-life. It is equivalent to equating the area under the exponential curve to a rectangle of height equal to the initial intercept and a width equal to 1.44 times the half-life as illustrated in the right hand side of **Fig. 1.10**.

Calculating the area under an exponential curve is frequently performed in nuclear medicine, especially under decreasing exponentials (for example, see Sections 7.2.1 and 11.1.2.1 for measurement of cardiac output and glomerular filtration rate, respectively).

1.3 Curve fitting, plotting and stripping

1.3.1 Curve fitting

1.3.1.1 Least squares fitting

When data are acquired experimentally and then used to generate a graph of, say, the concentration of radioactivity (the dependent variable) versus time (the independent variable), it is usually required to 'fit' the discrete points of data to a smooth curve defining the particular equation to which the data are

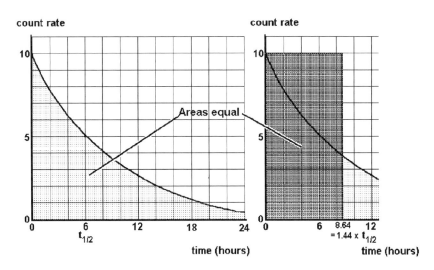

∎ **Fig. 1.10** Calculation of the area under the curve representing exponential decay from zero time to infinite time. The area under the exponential curve is given by that of a rectangle whose height is the initial height of the curve and whose width is equal to 1.44 × the half-time of decay of the exponential. This relationship may be checked by counting the number of squares under the curve and in the rectangle. Both should total about 43.

most likely to be conforming. By obtaining the equation we can determine the concentration in our example at times other than the experimental points. This has a number of uses. One of these is that we can *extrapolate* the curve to provide information about, for example, times not covered by the period of measurement. The extrapolation can be carried out at either end of the curve implying that data can be predicted at times less than or greater than the range of experimental acquisition times. The degree to which extrapolation can be carried out successfully depends on the quality of the fit and, ultimately, on the quantity and quality of the original data. This point is illustrated below. A second use for curve fitting is in *interpolating* data points, essentially filling in missing data. Interpolation is subject to fewer errors than extrapolation since data are available around the interpolated region. A third use is that information, such as rate constants can be derived from the fitted equation and used to define a model of the system such as the compartmental model described in Section 1.4. A fourth use is to provide a curve which can be mathematically manipulated to give more or clearer information. Manipulations include convolution, deconvolution and smoothing.

The process starts by defining the fit that is most likely to conform to the data. This is conventionally taken to be the fit where the discrepancies between the experimental results and the theoretical curve (as defined by the equation) are as small as possible. Mathematically this is expressed as the fit in which the sum of the differences of all experimental data points from the corresponding theoretical points is minimized. Because the differences may be positive or negative and the sum of these would tend to cancel out, they are *squared* before summation to give a sum of positive numbers and thus a sum that is positive. The process, known as *least squares* fitting, defines not only the form of the fitted equation but also the derived constants describing the equation: for example, the gradient b and intercept c for the linear fit and the rate constant α for the exponential fit of the equation. The extent to which the corresponding x and y values fit a straight line is given by a special parameter r the correlation coefficient. The value of r is unity if all of the data points fit exactly (in which case the sum of the squared deviations is zero), or zero if the data points are so randomly scattered around the fit that no correlation whatsoever exists.

An example of the fitting process is as follows. Assume that at 10, 20, 30 and 40 minutes after injection of a radioactive tracer the following count rates are obtained: 500, 400, 300 and 200. The data can unequivocally be said to be best fitted by the equation $y = A - bx$ where $A = 600$ and $b = 10$; i.e. a simple linear fit, since the correlation coefficient is unity. So, although the correlation coefficient for an exponential fit (Section 1.3.1.2 below) is also high, 0.991, the relationship suggested by the given data is most *probably* a linear one. However, it may not, in reality, be linear over a prolonged period. If more data were acquired at, for example, 50, 60, 70 and 80 minutes, to give count rates of 150, 100, 75 and 60 (**Fig. 1.11**) the data could possibly be better fitted to an exponential function since the correlation coefficient for a linear fit is now 0.965, but for an exponential one 0.998. Thus the curve that is best derived from the experimental data will often depend

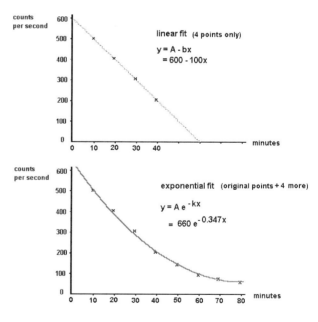

▮ **Fig. 1.11** The figure illustrates the potential for error in trying to fit experimental data when too few data points are available. What appears to be a good linear fit to the first 4 data points is shown to be in error when some additional data points are accumulated. For the complete curve an exponential curve fit is more suitable.

on the amount of time we can spend acquiring the data. 'Late' points in an experiment are often useful in producing a better description of the curve. It is also possible that early points in the curve are not, for practical reasons, available (e.g. if very early blood samples cannot be taken).

1.3.1.2 Exponential fits

The exponential equation $\quad y = e^{-2x}$ can also be expressed as $\quad \ln y = -2x$.

In other words, whereas y shows an exponential relationship with x, $\ln y$ shows a simple linear relationship, and the plot of $\ln y$ against x is a straight line decreasing with a gradient of 2 and going through the origin.

Consider, for example, plotting the decay of a radionuclide. Radionuclide decay is an exponential process; i.e. the rate of loss of activity at any time t is proportional to the level of activity M present at time t, so

$$M(t) = M(0) \cdot e^{-kt}$$

and

$$\ln M(t) = -kt.$$

The plot of $\ln M(t)$ against t is a straight line with a negative gradient equal to the decay constant k.

1.3.2 Plotting data on semi-logarithmic graph paper

If the decay of, for example, technetium-99m is plotted manually on conventional linear graph paper then, for times after about 24 hours (or 4 half-lives) when the activity would have decreased from 100% to less than 6%, any accurate estimate of activity from the plot would be difficult to make.

Manual plotting of such a wide range of values of activity is made easier by employing a special form of graph paper in which the y-axis is *marked* in values of activity but *spaced* according to the log of the activity. Thus having to look up each value of $\ln$ activity is avoided. For so-called semi-logarithmic or log–lin graph paper, the y-axis forms a logarithmic scale and the x-axis intervals are linearly spaced (**Fig. 1.12**). On the logarithmic scale a set distance corresponds to a decade, i.e. from 100 to 10 or from

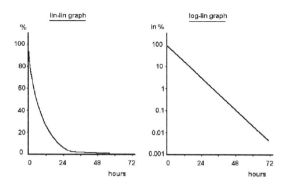

▌ Fig. 1.12 Comparison of linear and log–linear plots of an exponential decay curve. Plotting exponential decay on linear graph paper is seen to be inappropriate. For the decay of activity illustrated in the left figure it becomes too difficult to estimate the activity for times greater than about 24 hours. However, when the log of the activity is plotted, or the activity itself is plotted on the log scale of log–linear graph paper against time, a simple linear graph is obtained. From this linear graph the activity at any time may be estimated quite accurately.

0.1 to 0.01. Thus the five major divisions on the y-axis would correspond to 5 decades and a range of 100% to 0.001%. This, for technetium-99m, would cater accurately for a time scale of 0–100 hours of decay (rather than only 0 to about 24 hours for the conventional plot). The plot of decaying activity (single exponential decay process) against time on semi-logarithmic graph paper is a straight line with a negative slope from which the decay constant k can be calculated easily by identifying how long it takes for the straight line to fall from any activity A to $A/2$. This is the half-life $t_{1/2}$ of decrease. Then

$$k = \frac{\ln 2}{t_{1/2}} \quad \text{or} \quad \frac{0.693}{t_{1/2}}. \tag{1.20}$$

The explanation for equation 1.20 is given above (equations 1.15 to 1.18). Since we are dealing frequently with counting data that is subject to exponential biological or physical decay over time, the use of semi-logarithmic graph paper is important when results have to be plotted manually. Note that the y-axis never reaches zero but simply goes to ever decreasing values .0001%, 0.000001% etc.

Another example of an exponential relationship of importance in nuclear medicine is the equation,

$$y = C(1 - e^{-kx}). \tag{1.21}$$

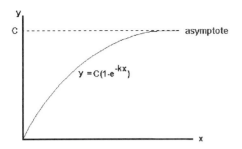

∎ **Fig. 1.13** A plot of the relationship commonly encountered in nuclear medicine, $y = C(1 - e^{-kx})$. As x becomes very large then e^{-kx} (or $1/e^{kx}$) becomes very small so $y \sim C(1 - 0) \sim C$. The curve is said to tend to an asymptote C though the actual value C is never reached.

In this case, as x increases, e^{-kx} decreases exponentially and $(1 - e^{-kx})$ increases in a curve, convex upwards, which approaches a maximum called the *asymptote*, here equal to C (**Fig. 1.13**).

It should be noted that the conventional method, used with linear graph paper, of obtaining the gradient or slope of a line by dividing an increment in the vertical direction by an increment in the horizontal direction does not work with log–lin graph paper because of the non-linear nature of the vertical scale.

1.3.3 Curve stripping

Several processes in nature are the composite or sum of two or more simultaneous exponential processes

which may be described mathematically by a multiexponential curve. When two single exponentials with differing rate constants are added together, a bi-exponential curve results. The reader can perform this task by inventing two mono-exponential curves, adding the two corresponding y-axis values for each x-axis point and plotting the result on semi-logarithmic graph paper as in **Fig. 1.14**.

The reverse of this exercise is curve stripping. Provided the rate constants of the two exponentials are sufficiently different, the composite curve will approach, after a suitably long time, a straight line with a rate constant equal to that of the single exponential with the lower rate constant. This is visually evident when the composite curve has been plotted as a time–activity curve on semi-logarithmic graph paper. 'Backwards' extrapolation of the tail of the bi-exponential curve to $t = 0$ from a t-axis point at which the y-value of the faster exponential has become negligible yields the slower exponential. Subtraction of the slower exponential from the composite curve then yields the faster exponential (**Fig. 1.15**). Theoretically the same manipulation can be performed on multi-exponential curves by again recording the data long enough for the composite curve to reduce to the slowest exponential. Having subtracted the slowest exponential, the composite curve is re-inspected for identification of the next slowest exponential which is subtracted from the composite and so on.

This is a somewhat inexact process to perform by eye unless the composite curve consists of exponentials with widely differing rate constants. The crucial requirement is for the curve to be 'long'

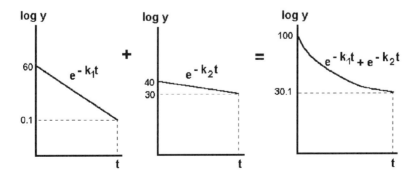

∎ **Fig. 1.14** The addition of two exponentially decaying curves $y = e^{-k_1 t}$ and $e^{-k_2 t}$. This forms a double exponential curve $y = e^{-k_1 t} + e^{-k_2 t}$. Note that while $y = e^{-k_1 t}$ and $y = e^{-k_2 t}$ each form straight lines on the log–lin graph paper, the sum $y = e^{-k_1 t} + e^{-k_2 t}$ forms a curve which when plotted in the same way only tends to straighten at large values of t.

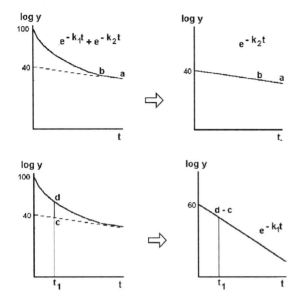

∎ **Fig. 1.15** Demonstration of curve stripping a double exponential curve. Curve stripping is the reverse of the process illustrated in Figure 1.14. Here the curved plot on log–lin graph paper is decomposed into two straight line single exponentials. This is done by assuming that the portion *ab* of the curve is due only to the curve $y = e^{-k_2 t}$ and extrapolating this part of the curve 'backwards' to the y-axis where the intercept has a value, in this example, of 40. The extrapolated line, shown dotted in the lower left figure, is subtracted from the original curve. Thus point *c* is subtracted from point *d*. This forms the 2nd component $y = e^{-k_1 t}$ a straight line with intercept equal to 60.

enough for there to be no doubt that the final exponential has been reached (see equation 2.8). A common error is to perform curve stripping on a multi-exponential curve which has not unequivocally reached the rate constant of its slowest exponential. Because of the errors normally encountered when following decreasing curves over long periods, it is often unrealistic to perform curve stripping for more than two exponential curves. However, there are also dangers in using a computer curve fitting program to fit experimental data to form multi-exponential curves. Unless the data are plentiful and of relatively good quality (i.e. counting errors are small) and unless the computer program is given a reasonable estimate of the values of the expected parameters it may have difficulties in identifying which of several solutions is the best fit. Parameters which have 'unphysiological' values may result

when more than two exponentials are fitted over an inadequate range of sampling times.

1.4 Compartmental analysis

When a tracer is introduced into a complicated system such as the human body it is difficult to describe the behaviour of the tracer and to achieve the aims of distinguishing normal from pathological behaviour of the system unless we simplify the situation. This simplification is often carried out by means of a so-called model.

One simplifying model that is used considers the body as a system consisting only of a number of communicating but quite distinct compartments throughout which the tracer is distributed. The compartments may be real organs (e.g. the liver or the bone marrow) or conceptual and anatomically ill defined (e.g. the extracellular space or the red cell volume). If, after the administration of the tracer into one of the compartments, we can sample how much tracer is in selected compartments at discrete times, we can estimate the general kinetics of tracer distribution throughout the simplified system. Specifically we can derive a set of equations each of which describes the amount or concentration of tracer in each compartment and the fractional rates at which tracer is transferred between adjacent compartments as a function of time. Once a set of equations for 'normal' or expected behaviour of the system is established then the normality of any other findings can be checked.

The basic assumptions underlying conventional compartmental analysis are that:

(1) the kinetics of the system do not change as we perform the experiment;

(2) the mixing of tracer within each compartment is complete and instantaneous;

(3) the flow of tracer out of a compartment is proportional to the concentration of tracer in that compartment.

The simplest situation is that of a compartment containing an amount M of tracer from which tracer is continuously leaving at a rate dM/dt. Then, following the third assumption above

$$dM/dt = -kM. \qquad (1.22)$$

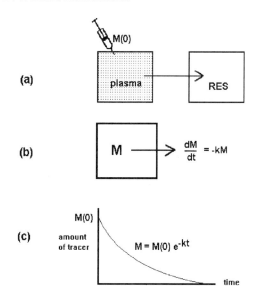

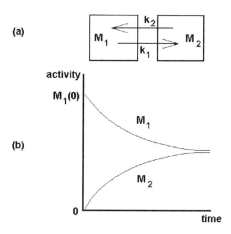

▌ **Fig. 1.16** Compartmental model for a single compartment with exponential loss or decay. The injection of an activity $M(0)$ into plasma (the amount of activity present in plasma at zero time) which is subsequently cleared into the reticulo–endothelial system is illustrated in (a) and shown as a compartmental model representation in (b). A plot of M against time is shown in (c). This is based on the instantaneous injection and a rate of clearance proportional to the plasma activity.

▌ **Fig. 1.17** Compartmental model of two compartments exchanging tracer between themselves. (a) The compartmental model representation of flow of tracer between two compartments after an instantaneous injection of activity, $M(0)$ into the first compartment. Flow from the first compartment (into the second) is proportional to the contents M_1 with rate constant k_1 and flow from the second (into the first) is proportional to the content M_2 with rate constant k_2.

Here k is a constant called the fractional rate constant or the fractional turnover constant since it defines the rate of loss (or gain) to the amount of tracer present in the compartment. An example in nuclear medicine is radiolabelled colloid, which, after intravenous injection, is initially confined to the plasma volume (the first compartment) but is then cleared into the reticulo–endothelial system (the second compartment), see **Fig. 1.16a**.

The solution to equation 1.22 is similar to the exponential decay equation, 1.13, i.e.

$$M = M(0) \cdot e^{-kt}$$

where $M(0)$ is the value of M at $t = 0$. The graph of M against t is the decreasing exponential illustrated in **Fig. 1.16c**.

A more complicated model is illustrated in **Fig. 1.17**, where there is bi-directional movement of tracer between the two compartments. The net change in tracer concentration in compartment 1, given by dM_1/dt, is the difference between

(1) the rate of movement of tracer *out of* compartment 1, which is proportional to the contents of M_1 i.e. equal to $k_1 M_1$. Here k_1 is the fractional rate constant governing the exit from compartment 1

and

(2) the rate of movement of tracer *into* compartment 1, (or out of compartment M_2) which is proportional to the contents of M_2, i.e. equal to $k_2 M_2$, where k_2 is the fractional rate constant governing the exit from compartment 2.

Thus

$$\frac{dM_1}{dt} = k_2 M_2 - k_1 M_1. \qquad (1.23)$$

We can derive the equation expressing the relationship between M_1 and time t as follows. The injected amount of tracer at time $t = 0$ is

$$M(0) = M_1 + M_2$$

so, substituting for M_2 in equation 1.23,

$$\frac{dM_1}{dt} = k_2 M(0) - k_2 M_1 - k_1 M_1. \qquad (1.24)$$

We can simplify the solution to equation 1.24 (which is called a differential equation because one of the variables is a rate of change), by introducing a so-called 'dummy variable' x: let

$$x = \frac{dM_1}{dt} = k_2 M(0) - M_1(k_1 + k_2). \qquad (1.25)$$

Differentiating both sides of equation 1.25 with respect to t and noting that $[k_2 \cdot M(0)]$ is a constant and its derivative therefore zero,

$$\frac{dx}{dt} = -(k_2 + k_1) \cdot \frac{dM_1}{dt} \qquad (1.26)$$
$$= -(k_1 + k_2) \cdot x$$

Therefore $\qquad x = x(0) \cdot e^{-(k_1 + k_2)t}. \qquad (1.27)$

In the same way as if $x = x(0)\, e^{-(k_1+k_2)t}$, $dx/dt = -(k_1 + k_2) \cdot x$.

The role of the dummy variable has been to create an equation, 1.26, of a type similar to equation 1.13, above, in which the rate of change of a variable is proportional to that variable itself; i.e. an exponential relationship.

We can put in some of the initial conditions
At $t = 0$,

$$x = x(0), M_2 = 0 \text{ and } M_1 = M(0).$$

Equation 1.25 can be rewritten for $t = 0$:

$$x(0) = k_2 M(0) - M(0)(k_2 + k_1) \qquad (1.28)$$
$$= -k_1 \cdot M(0).$$

Substituting for $x(0)$ in equation 1.27 and then for x in equation 1.25,

$$-k_1 \cdot M(0)\, e^{-(k_1 + k_2)t} = k_2 M(0) - M_1(k_2 + k_1).$$

Re-arranging

$$M_1(k_2 + k_1) = k_2 \cdot M(0) + k_1 M(0) e^{-(k_1 + k_2)t}$$

from which

$$M_1 = \frac{k_2}{k_1 + k_2} M(0) + \frac{k_1}{k_1 + k_2} \cdot M(0)\, e^{-(k_1 + k_2)t}. \qquad (1.29)$$

Although equation 1.29 looks complicated, it clearly states that the time course of M_1 is the sum of two components, of which the first is a 'lumped' constant. The second represents a single exponential which decreases with rate constant $(k_1 + k_2)$. Furthermore, it is clear that the zero time value of

M_1 is $[M(0) \cdot k_2/(k_1 + k_2)] + [M(0) \cdot k_1/(k_1 + k_2)]$, which reduces to $M(0)$.

If the volume of compartment 1 is V_1 and that of compartment 2 is V_2 then at equilibrium, when the flows between 1 and 2 equalize, then

$$k_1 M_1 = k_2 M_2$$

If the *concentrations* in the two compartments also equalize then

$$\frac{M_1}{V_1} = \frac{M_2}{V_2} \quad \text{and} \quad \frac{k_1}{k_2} = \frac{V_2}{V_1}.$$

An example of this bi-directional flow in nuclear medicine is the equilibration of radiolabelled platelets between blood and splenic pool after injection into the blood. An example in physical chemistry is the distribution of a solute which is both hydrophilic and lipophilic between a layer of chloroform on top and a layer of water below.

In both these examples, concentrations do not equalize at equilibrium and the concentration ratio at equilibrium is called the partition coefficient, λ.

A further model of perhaps more general interest in nuclear medicine and a very important model throughout the biological sciences is illustrated in **Figs 1.18a and 1.18b**. Many seemingly complicated models can, in practice, be reduced to this form. Here, there is bi-directional transfer of tracer between two compartments accompanied by so-called uni-directional 'run-off' or disappearance of tracer from one of them. An example in nuclear medicine is the distribution of DTPA following bolus injection into plasma (compartment 1). DTPA then distributes between plasma and the extracellular fluid volume (compartment 2) whilst at the same time being continuously removed from plasma by glomerular filtration.

The solution of the set of differential equations describing M_1, the activity in the plasma compartment is

$$M_1 = Ae^{-\alpha_1 t} + Be^{-\alpha_2 t}. \qquad (1.30)$$

M_1 is the sum of two exponential terms and the graph of M_1 against t is the double exponential seen before. When $t = 0$, $\alpha_1 t$ and $\alpha_2 t$ are both zero, so $M_1(0) = A + B$. The constants A and B are the zero time intercepts of the two exponentials, with respective rate constants, α_1 and α_2. The bi-exponential curve approaches a slope equal to whichever is the smaller of α_1 and α_2. As t increases, both terms decrease and tend towards zero. If α_1 is substantially larger than α_2, then $Ae^{-\alpha_1 t}$ becomes negligibly small long before $Be^{-\alpha_2 t}$ (providing of course that A and B are comparable). The plot of M_2 against time is more complicated. It starts at zero time with no activity in the compartment. Activity coming from the first compartment causes a rise to a maximum until run-off starts to take effect and the activity falls. The time of maximum *activity* in compartment 2 is also the time of equilibrium, t_{eq}, since, by definition, at the maximum, the rate of change of activity in compartment 2 is zero, a condition that would eventually be achieved in both compartments if tracer was administered as a

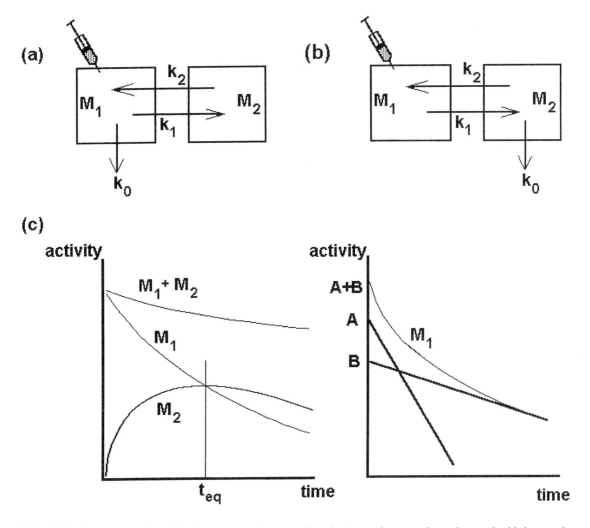

∎ **Fig. 1.18** Compartmental model of two compartments exchanging tracer between themselves and with loss to the outside. (a) Shows a compartmental model representing the situation when, after injection into the first compartment it exchanges tracer with a second and, simultaneously, loses activity, at a rate of k_0, to the outside. The activities of the two compartments are shown as a function of time. M_1 falls as a bi-exponential function since tracer is being continuously lost. (c) M_2 starts at zero value then accumulates activity until a maximum is reached at time t_{eq} then loses activity. The time when the activities cross ("activity equilibrium") and the time when the concentrations cross ("concentration equilibrium") are not necessarily the same as t_{eq}, the time of maximum activity. The overall activity in the system $M_1 + M_2$ falls because of the loss to the outside. (b) Shows a similar compartmental model where activity is lost from the second compartment, at a rate k_0. The time–activity curves in this situation are similar to those in Fig. 1.18a.

continuous infusion at a constant rate (so-called steady state).

At equilibrium, the *rates of flow* between compartments are equal and if the *concentrations* in each compartment are equal then for the model in Fig 18a

$$k_1 M_1(\text{eq}) = k_2 M_2(\text{eq}) \quad \text{and} \quad \frac{M_1(\text{eq})}{V_1} = \frac{M_2(\text{eq})}{V_2}$$

$$\text{and} \quad \frac{k_1}{k_2} = \frac{V_2}{V_1}. \quad (1.31a)$$

So calculation of the fractional rate constants gives the ratio of the volumes of the two compartments. At equilibrium in the model in Fig 18b,

$$k_1 M_1(\text{eq}) = (k_2 + k_0) \cdot M_2(\text{eq})$$

$$\text{so} \quad \frac{V_2}{V_1} = \frac{k_1}{k_2 + k_0} \quad (1.31b)$$

Because of the disappearance of tracer from the system as a whole via compartment 1, the total activity in the two compartments given by $M_1 + M_2$ shows a decrease with time.

The derivation of equation 1.30 is complicated and not shown. However the sense of it can be appreciated. Thus, consider an intravenous injection of technetium-99m DTPA. Initially, the concentration in plasma (the first compartment) will decrease as the combined result of movement into the extravascular extracellular space (the second compartment) and glomerular filtration. As the extravascular concentration builds up, increasingly more DTPA will diffuse back into the intravascular space, and the gradient of the plasma concentration–time curve will progressively decrease (i.e., becomes *less negative*), eventually becoming a function only of glomerular filtration rate.

Because of the symmetrical nature of the compartments, their behaviour following bolus input into compartment 2, rather than into compartment 1 (**Fig. 1.18b**), can be predicted. In this case the activity in compartment 2 will decrease as a double exponential and compartment 1 will show an increase to a maximum followed by a fall off. An example of this might be the injection of an organic anion into the blood compartment which exchanges with and is lost from the liver parenchyma compartment.

Analysis of the bi-exponential time–activity curves obtained by monitoring the activity in the compartment into which the activity has been injected yields four experimental values, the two intercepts, A and B, and the two slopes α_1 and α_2. These can be used to derive values for k_0, k_1 k_2, using the following formulae: For the model in Fig 18a

$$k_0 + k_1 = \frac{A\alpha_1 + B\alpha_2}{A + B} \quad (1.32a)$$

$$k_0 \cdot k_2 = \alpha_1\alpha_2 \quad (1.32b)$$

and

$$k_2 = \frac{A\alpha_2 + B\alpha_1}{A + B} \quad (1.32c)$$

For model in Fig 18b, the equations are different:

$$k_1 = \frac{A\alpha_1 + B\alpha_2}{A + B} \quad (1.33a)$$

$$k_0 \cdot k_1 = \alpha_1 \cdot \alpha_2 \quad (1.33b)$$

$$k_0 + k_2 = \frac{A\alpha_2 + B\alpha_1}{A + B}. \quad (1.33c)$$

(Note the difference between the constants k_0, k_1 and k_2 which are transfer rate constants for the compartments and the constants α_1 and α_2 which are rate constants describing the slopes of the single exponential components of the time–activity curve).

Equation 1.31 for the relative volumes of the compartments can also be expressed in terms of A, B, α_1 and α_2. For the model in Fig 18a

$$\frac{V_2}{V_1} = \frac{k_1}{k_2} \quad (1.34)$$

For the model shown in Fig 18b

$$\frac{V_2}{V_1} = \frac{k_1}{k_0 + k_2} = \frac{A\alpha_1 + B\alpha_2}{A\alpha_2 + B\alpha_1}. \quad (1.35)$$

Again, equations 1.34 and 1.35 assume equalization of concentrations between compartments 1 and 2 as for systems in which λ is unity.

Another situation which often results in the acquisition of a double exponential is when the concentration of a tracer in two separate compartments in parallel is recorded simultaneously (**Fig. 1.19**). The two exponentials are separate mono-exponentials when recorded from each compartment. Provided their rate constants are sufficiently different, one of the exponentials will become negligible while the other continues to be appreciable, at which time the recorded curve becomes mono-exponential;

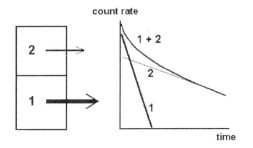

∎ Fig. 1.19 Compartmental model of two compartments both losing activity exponentially at different rates. The concentration of tracer in two separate compartments A and B recorded as one compartment leads to the double exponential curve shown on the right. This curve is, of course, composed of the two single exponential curves from A and B separately.

i.e. identical with the slower of the two curves. By extrapolation to zero time of the tail of the recorded curve, which has a slope equal to the gradient of the slower exponential, the slower exponential can be subtracted from the total (recorded) curve to yield the faster of the two exponentials (curve stripping, see above). Sometimes recorded curves are the sum of three or even four exponentials, and by progressively subtracting the slowest of the remaining exponentials the whole curve can theoretically be resolved into its exponential components by the process of curve stripping. Multi-exponential curves of this sort are encountered in inert gas (e.g. xenon-133) washout studies. Nevertheless, in practice, curve stripping would not be attempted for more than two exponentials for the reasons given above in 1.3. An example of an organ which gives a bi-exponential washout curve following injection of a bolus of xenon-133 into the supplying artery is the brain. The faster exponential is thought to be the result of washout of tracer from grey matter and the slower from white matter. An external scintillation detector obviously cannot distinguish between the two tissues and records their contained radioactivity simultaneously, giving a bi-exponential washout curve.

Equation 1.30 is the sum of two exponentials. A further important compartmental model gives an equation which is the *difference* of two exponentials,

$$M_1 = A\, e^{-\alpha_1 t}$$

while

$$M_2 = B\, e^{-\alpha_2 t} - A\, e^{-\alpha_1 t}.$$

Any biological system in which an agent is cleared exponentially from one compartment into a second compartment in series with it from which it is also cleared exponentially will result in a tracer concentration in the second compartment which is the difference between two exponentials. An example is the clearance from an organ of intra-arterially injected xenon-133 which is then expired from the lungs by ventilation. In this case the organ is the first compartment and the lungs represent the second. The form of the curve recorded with this system (i.e., from the lung in this example) is shown in **Fig. 1.20**. It can be appreciated that the lung builds up in activity, reaches a plateau and then decreases. The decreasing activity approaches a single exponential, either with rate constant α_1 or rate constant α_2, whichever is the smaller.

Rather complex models are routinely used in quantitative positron emission tomography (PET), especially in the measurement of organ perfusion and substrate utilization rates (Section 3.1.3). For a model to be useful, it must adequately describe the biological system being modelled. In theory, an infinite number of models may fit the data obtained about the system although in practice, only a few would be thought reasonable. The one to choose will generally be the one, theoretically generated by the 'parameters' (i.e., the rate constants), which best fits the recorded data and contains relatively few compartments.

A more advanced approach to trying out different arrangements and testing them to see if they are supported by the data is to use a well-established computer software package such as SAAM II. This program, developed by the University of Washington, allows computer models to be constructed using a selection of icons including compartments, inputs, outputs, delays etc.

1.5 Deconvolution analysis

Deconvolution, as the name applies, is a technique of unravelling data that have been made complicated by other factors. An analogy for where it may be applied might be the situation of trying to control a bank account. If a set monthly payment is made into the account and regular withdrawals appear at known times then it is easy to predict the balance. However if the deposits are irregular both in amount and in timing, the money remaining in the bank at a particular time is difficult to predict. Applying the analogy to the kidney so that deposits become activity delivered and withdrawals become activity released then the prediction of the behaviour of the kidney depends on establishing a method of allowing for the irregularity of the delivery system and of simplifying it to correspond to a direct bolus input (the single monthly deposit). Introducing some more physiological terms we can say that the shape of a time–activity curve recorded from a region of interest over the kidney (the recorded function) depends not only on the way the kidney handles the radiopharmaceutical once it has reached the kidney (the retention function), but also on the shape of the curve of activity versus time in arterial blood (the input function), since this determines the delivery rate of the radiopharmaceutical to the kidney.

The shapes of the renogram and the arterial time activity curves are recorded and therefore known (**Fig. 1.21c and Fig. 1.21d**). What we would really like to know, however, is the shape of the curve we would have obtained if we had been able to inject the radiopharmaceutical directly into the renal artery, as

in **Fig. 1.21a** without its having recirculated. This curve, (**Fig. 1.21b**) which we have called the retention curve, is obtainable by deconvolution analysis; i.e. by separating, or deconvolving, the renogram from the arterial input curve (**Fig. 1.21c**).

It is perhaps easier to understand the process of how the complications arise (the process of *convolution*), than how they are unravelled (the reverse process, deconvolution). Figure 1.21 illustrates the process whereby the direct injection curve is convolved on the arterial curve to generate the observed renogram. The response to the theoretical direct sharp bolus input is known as the retention function but it is also called a residue curve because it defines what is retained in the kidney (the residue) or impulse response curve because it is the response to an impulse (or sharp bolus).

The arterial curve is known as the input function because it determines the rate of input of radiopharmaceutical into the kidney. Thus, if $R(t)$ is the observed renogram, $H(t)$ the retention curve and $I(t)$ the arterial curve, then

$$R(t) = H(t) * I(t). \qquad (1.36)$$

The t in brackets indicates that R, H and I are all variables which are functions of time (t). The symbol $*$ signifies the operation of convolution. This

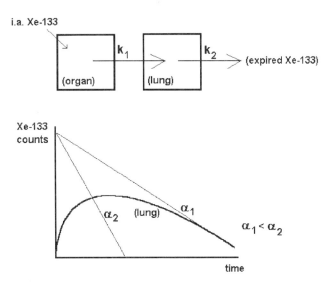

▌ **Fig. 1.20** Compartmental model for a catenary system of two compartments. The curve obtained when activity input into one compartment (organ) is cleared into another from which it too is cleared. Here intravenously injected xenon-133 passes to the lung and is expired. The curve of xenon-133 activity in the lung shows an initial rise to a maximum followed by a fall that tends to the smaller of the rate constants k_1 or k_2. Thus, if $k_2 > k_1$ then k_1 is equal to α_1, otherwise k_1 is equal to α_2.

equation is different from all of those previously encountered in this chapter in that there are no plus, minus or multiplication signs; instead it contains a 'convolution operation' sign. It should also be clear that the terms $R(t)$ and $I(t)$ do not need to be mathematically defined; in other words, the mathematical relationships between R and t, or I and t, are not required and the process of deconvolution or convolution simply disentangles H from I and R or predicts R from H and I, respectively. Any further mathematical treatment of deconvolution analysis and the theoretical conditions such as 'linearity' or 'non-stationary' on which it is founded, is beyond the scope of this text. Simple information that can be obtained from the retention curve is an idea of the transit times of the organ and if they are abnormally long or short or associated with different components of function. For the kidney these may be glomerular and tubular excretion; for the liver and thyroid they may correspond to vascular and parenchymal extraction. The actual procedure itself requires a computer program that is often provided as a part of the suite of nuclear medicine software.

As with any computer program (statistical, compartmental, deconvolution etc.) care should be taken and experience gained with known cases with good data before difficult cases with poor data are explored.

Deconvolution analysis has been applied to many other systems in addition to the kidney. In general, the aim of deconvolution analysis in first pass dynamic studies is to compensate for (i) the spreading of a bolus intravenous injection and (ii) the effects of continuous re-circulation of the tracer. In each case a curve is derived which would be the same as the curve obtained from direct bolus injection of the tracer into an artery supplying the organ of interest.

Deconvolution analysis and compartmental analysis are combined for physiological measurements in position emission tomography (PET). PET is able to quantify the concentration of the tracer in the tissue under study and in the arterial blood, and with the latter as the input, the retention curves of total tracer in the model can be estimated by deconvolution analysis. Using compartmental analysis, equations can then be derived which describe the tracer

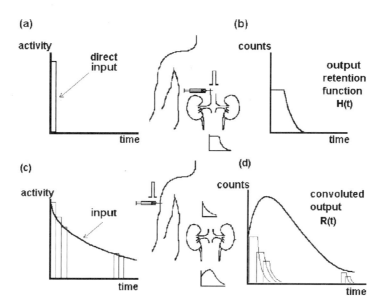

∎ **Fig. 1.21** Illustration of the principle of convolution. A direct bolus, shown in (a) by a narrow bar on the time–activity curve, delivered into the renal artery produces the time–activity curve shown in (b). This idealized curve is called the output retention function and is usually denoted by $H(t)$. It shows a constant activity up to a certain time after which the activity output reduces to zero. In practice the activity is delivered via an intravenous injection that by the time it reaches the renal artery has a shape similar to that shown in (c). This curve can be thought of as being a composite of the narrow bars of (a) but of different heights and appearing at different times. Each of these has the effect shown in (b) which if added together give the convoluted output shown in (d). This is denoted by $R(t)$ (the *renogram*).

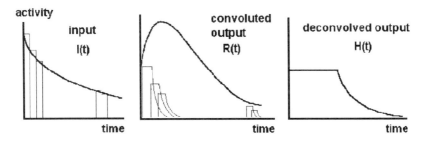

▌ **Fig. 1.22** Illustration of the principle of deconvolution. From the input curve $I(t)$ and the convoluted output curve $R(t)$, the deconvolved output $H(t)$ can be obtained through the mathematical process of deconvolution. The figure shows the reverse process to that illustrated in Fig. 1.21.

disappearance curves from a compartmental model that would result from instantaneous deposition of the tracer into a specific compartment of the model. The description is in terms of the rate constants governing the tracer fluxes between the compartments.

1.6 Statistical techniques relevant to nuclear medicine

At least five different applications of statistical techniques can be found in nuclear medicine:

1. *Estimating the best or most likely result from a set of measurements* This is the traditional use of statistics, often called population statistics, where parameters such as means, standard deviations etc. are used for summarizing data such as measurement of glomerular filtration rate or left ventricular ejection fraction in a number of subjects. Since it is often the case that only a limited number of studies can be performed, usually because of time constraints, then methods of dealing with small populations should be understood. An example might be the measurement, using a particular technique, of cardiac output in, say, 10 patients. Statistical analysis will give the expected range of values of cardiac output for this population against which further subjects can be compared.

2. *Producing reliable estimates of data obtained by detection of radioactivity* Since the emis-

sion of detected gamma rays is a random process, the results of counting are subject to so-called statistical variations. Thus the same activity counted under the same conditions on a number of occasions does not produce exactly the same result each time. Each measurement in fact produces a more or less accurate *estimate* of the activity. Since counting underlies practically all the measurements discussed in this book it is important that the statistics governing the errors involved be taken into account in assessing the accuracy of a measurement.

The statistical analysis is extended from the situation involving counting the same sample many times to considering a single count measurement. Here the probable limits of the result are estimated. Another application is testing the significance of differences in counting results either between repeat measurements or between measurements of 'normal' or 'abnormal' samples or in samples taken with and without a background count. In each case the object is to understand the statistical errors and be able to optimize the accuracy of the measurement.

3. *Comparing the results from one test with those from another or assessing a new method against an old one* Experimental errors in arriving at a clinical measurement may be a combination of counting errors and other experimental errors such as in estimating a sample blood volume. The measurement often has to be compared with other measurements with their own errors. Although traditional tools such as regression and correlation analysis are often applied for these applications

they may not be as useful or appropriate as usually assumed.

4. *Evaluating the usefulness of a test and comparing this with the usefulness of another* Estimates of sensitivity, specificity etc. are involved here.

5. *Using the performance of a number of observers in interpreting and evaluating the results of a test involving images* This includes ROC analysis and κ values.

Only some of the techniques are relevant to this book and will be considered below.

1.6.1 The statistics of conventional experiments — population or descriptive statistics

Population statistics involves measuring a quantity in a number of subjects in order to estimate, for example, the average value of that quantity and the range of values to expect. Consider measurements of cardiac output on 20 subjects. This will produce up to 20 different results. A good way of summarizing the conclusion of the experiment would be to calculate the *average value* (the *population mean*) by summing all values and dividing by the number of values, here 20. For 20 matched subjects (matched using results from a 'gold standard' test) we would expect the individual measurements to be similar. If the results are very different from each other we are faced with the questions: do the subjects really have very different cardiac outputs or is the measurement technique giving erroneous results because of measurement or 'statistical' errors. If we assume that the subjects are well matched then the spread of the results will give an index of how well or how accurately the test itself performs. In order to estimate this spread we could, for each measurements, sum the difference between the measurements and the population mean. This is referred to as summing the deviations from the mean. However, since the deviations are both positive and negative the sum (by definition) would be equal zero. We therefore square the individual deviations to make each of them positive before summing. The average of the squared deviations will be a positive quantity called the *variance*. The variance, derived from squaring numbers, is usually

impracticably large so we use instead its square root, called the *standard deviation* to estimate the spread of measurements in the experiment. The estimation thus quantifies the uncertainty by defining a range over which we can be confident that we have a usefully accurate result.

Another statistical approach often used is called 'hypothesis testing' in which the result obtained is tested in terms of the hypothesis that it could have happened by chance. The question is asked, not how close the results are to a 'true' value but how often the result could have come about by chance and is therefore 'not true'. If many of the results could be 'accidents' or chance results then the measurement or sets of measurements are not very useful. The probability of the result occuring by chance — often denoted by a 'p-value' — is given for different experimental conditions, e.g. population size. Although they are expressed differently the approaches for estimating a range of uncertainties and testing a hypothesis by evaluating p-values are mathematically equivalent.

When large numbers of subjects are involved we often assume that the results obey certain mathematical rules. One rule is that the mean value would be the one we obtain more often than any other value. The further the individual results are from the population mean the less likely we are to obtain that measurement. In fact we assume that the measurements follow a certain theoretical distribution called the *normal distribution*. The distribution results from plotting the value obtained in a measurement (on the *x*-axis) against the probability of actually measuring that particular value in the population (on the *y*-axis) for all the subjects studied. It has the symmetrical shape about the mean value shown in **Fig. 1.23a.** From the properties of the normal distribution it can be stated that if an experiment is carried out a large number of times then the result will lie between the limits of the mean minus the standard deviation (s.d.) and the mean plus the s.d. for about 68% of the measurements. If the mean were 400 and the standard deviation 20 then a result between 380 and 420 would be obtained 68 times out of 100. Also the result will lie between the limits of the mean minus *twice* the s.d. and the mean plus *twice* the s.d. for about 95% of the measurements i.e. in our example we would expect a result between 360 and 440, 95 times out of 100. Thus the result can be used to predict how many of a sampled population would give a result that is within a given range of the mean value. The distribution may also be used to distinguish results from measuring a different population from the original one.

Figure 1.23b shows two overlapped distributions, one from a set of measurements with a mean N_1 and the other from a set of measurements with a mean of N_2. The extent of overlap between the two distributions defines the probability that the set with mean N_1 differs or not from that with mean N_2. In our illustration about half the measurements from the first population could have come from the second population, so there is no significant difference between N_1 and N_2. In practice, an overlap by $< 5\%$ indicates a significant difference.

1.6.2   The statistics of counting

When a radioactive sample is counted a number of times then a range of estimates will be obtained. For example repeat measurements of a sample under the same conditions and with no decay may yield counts of 1, 3, 7, 2, 3 ... However the probability of obtaining a particular results, such as a count of exactly 3, is subject to particular statistical constraints and produces a particular histogram called a *Poisson distribution* represented as in **Fig. 1.24a**. By this is meant that the probability of obtaining each result can be calculated from a unique formula. The formula is different from those used for other sorts of experiments such as tossing a coin or measuring the heights of children in a class which produce other forms of distributions - binomial, normal etc. The figure shows the Poisson distribution representing a set of 100 measurements of a radioactive sample each taken over a time of one second with an average count rate of 3 counts per second. A count of zero in one second is obtained in 5 of the 100 measurements, a count of 1 in 15 of the measurements, of 2 and of 3 in 22 of the measurements and so on. The resulting histogram for this low mean of 3 is asymmetric. However, for any average count greater than about 10 the Poisson distribution

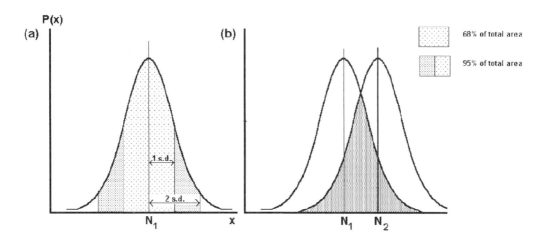

∎ **Fig. 1.23a**   A plot of the normal distribution. The probability of obtaining a result, $P(x)$ is plotted against the result itself x. The distribution is symmetric about the mean value of x equal to N, which is the value corresponding to the maximum of the curve. Two areas are shown. The first is the area under the curve defined by the limits $N \pm 1$ standard deviation. This occupies about 68% of the total area under the curve. The larger area is defined by the limits $N \pm 2$ standard deviations and occupies about 95% of the total area under the curve. The interpretation of these areas is that 68% of the measurements will have a value that lies between the values $N - 1$ s.d. and. $N + 1$ s.d. and that 95% of the measurements will have a value that lies between the values $N - 2$ s.d. and $N + 2$ s.d. The actual value of the standard deviation will depend on the population being studied.
∎ **Fig. 1.23b**   The significance of the difference between two distributions. Two sets of readings, one with mean N_1 and the other with mean N_2, give overlapping distributions. The degree of difference between N_1 and N_2 is given by the relative overlap of the (normalized) distributions. In the example there is about an equal probability that a measurement could have come from either population.

Value of count	Number of times count occurs	Deviation of count from average of 3	Squared deviation	Contribution to variance (No. × Dev^2)
0	5	−3	9	45
1	15	−2	4	60
2	22	−1	1	22
3	22	0	0	0
4	17	+1	1	17
5	10	+2	4	40
6	5	+3	9	45
etc.				etc.
Total Number	100		Total variance	300
			Average Variance	3

∎ **Table 1.1**

approximates closely the more familiar and symmetric normal distribution shown in **Fig. 1.24b**.

The Poisson distribution has a particular property in that the mean or average of the distribution equals the variance of that distribution, using the terms defined above. Consider the results shown in Table 1.1.

In our example of 100 measurements (Fig. 1.24), the average of the measurements is 3. The deviation of a count of zero, the first entry in the table, from

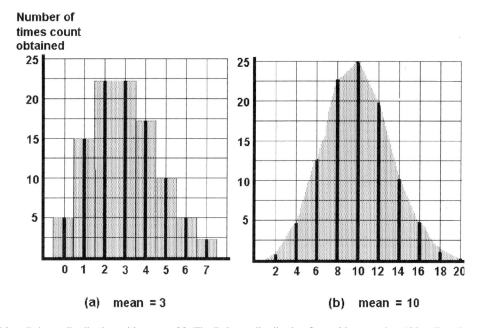

(a)   mean = 3   (b)   mean = 10

∎ **Fig. 1.24a**   Poisson distribution with mean of 3. The Poisson distribution formed by counting 100 radioactive samples with a mean count of 3 is asymmetrical, unlike that of a normal distribution.
∎ **Fig. 1.24b**   Poisson distribution with mean of 10. The Poisson distribution formed by counting 100 radioactive samples with a mean count of 10 has a symmetrical shape approaching that of a normal distribution.

the average is 3 and the square of this is 9. Since from the formula for calculating Poisson probabilities there are 5 counts of zero each with a squared deviation of 9 in our 100 measurements, the contribution to the variance is 45. Repeating this calculation for all the entries in the table gives a total variance of 300 and an average variance of 300/100 or 3, *the same as the average count*. It follows that the standard deviation, the square root of the average variance, is $\sqrt{3}$ or 1.732.

Thus, for example, if a sample were counted 1000 times and the average count was 100 then the variance of the distribution would be the same as 100 and the s.d. would be $\sqrt{100}$ or 10. Following the preceding treatment we can say that twice the s.d. is 20 and a result lying between $100 - 20$ (or 80) and $100 + 20$ (or 120) would occur 95% of the time or in 950 of the 1000 cases. We could thus be fairly definite (i.e. correct in 950 of the 1000 cases) that the result of any one measurement would be between 80 and 120. The standard deviation is often employed to indicate the 'error' in the measurement (though sometimes two standard deviations or even three standard deviations may also be used). The method of defining the error should be stated for all results.

We could not be expected to repeat each count measurement 1000 times on each occasion and usually perform just one measurement. Then the result of that one measurement is taken as the best estimate of the mean we have and the standard deviation of that count is used to estimate the range of possibilities. Thus a single count of 400 will have a standard deviation of $\sqrt{400}$ or 20, and we would be confident that the result would lie between 360 and 440, i.e. ±2 s.d., 95% of the time. The properties of the normal distribution also dictate that 99.8% of the time the count will like between the mean ±3 s.d. Thus we are practically certain that the true count will like between 340 and 460 and that any count outside these limits is very likely to result from a change in the counting conditions.

1.6.3 The statistics of imaging

When a distribution of radioactivity is imaged using a modem digital gamma camera, what is produced is a grid or array or matrix of numbers in the computer memory. The numbers may be translated for the display into gradations along a scale from black to white or along a colour scale to give an analogue display of the distribution. However we are more concerned here with the numbers themselves and the information they yield.

If we consider a single element in the computer matrix called a picture element or *pixel*, the number contained within the pixel represents the activity 'seen' by that part of the detector. Discounting the fact that the number is subject to various distortions due to attenuation, scattering, geometry etc. it is also subject to two forms of statistical variation. One arises from the method of detection used in the gamma camera (Section 5.1). Basically the conversion of scintillations of light into electrons and their subsequent amplification is a statistical process leading to random variations in the positioning signal and thus in variations in the pixel to which a count is allocated or in the numbers of counts appearing in a particular pixel. The other statistical variation is the same as discussed in Section 1.6.2. Each pixel is essentially the result of a counting procedure and therefore subject to Poisson statistics. The statistical error associated with each pixel therefore depends on the total count contained within that pixel so that, for example, a small number of counts in the pixel is associated with a large relative error. In practice the number of counts in a pixel depends on the time of acquisition of the data and the relative size of the pixel. The field of view of the detector is represented by a two-dimensional array of pixels. Even for circular or rectangular crystal detectors the array has the same number of pixels in the y-direction as in the x-direction, for example, 64 pixels height by 64 pixels width. (It follows that not all the pixels correspond to an active detector so that the corners of the matrix for a circular detector are generally blank but this aspect is ignored in the following discussion.) A variety of matrix sizes can be used, ranging from a relatively coarse matrix, consisting of, say, 64×64 elements covering the square matrix to a relatively fine one of 256×256 elements covering the same area. A total of one million counts divided up into the approximately 4000 elements of the coarse 64×64 array will produce an average count per pixel of about 250 while the same total averaged over the fine array consisting of 256×256 or 65 000 pixels will produce a count per pixel of about 16. Each pixel in the 64×64 array will have a error of $\sqrt{250}$ or 16 which, as a proportion of the 250 counts, is a relative error of 4%. Each small pixel in the 256×256 array will have a error of $\sqrt{16}$ or 4 which, as a proportion of the 16 counts, is a much greater relative error of 25%. Thus little confidence can be put in the count from a single pixel of the 256×256 array and only by combining counts from a number of pixels into a 'region of interest' (and therefore losing the resolution of the display) can the total count be increased and the relative error made acceptable. If however the time of acquisition were increased in the above example so that, say, 30 million counts in total were acquired, then the average count in the fine matrix would be 30 million over 65 000 pixels or an average pixel count of 456 with an absolute error of 21 and a relative error of less than 5%.

Count rate data used in the time activity curves discussed elsewhere in this book will be subject to statistical errors due to the activity used, the time interval over which counts were collected and the area in the field of view making up the region of interest. In general, since the total number of gamma photons counted from a patient is limited by the activity allowed to be administered, then the shorter the time interval and the finer the detail of the image seen, the bigger the errors in the resulting data.

1.6.4 Comparing counts

A common calculation in counting activity sampled either physically as in a blood sample or computationally as in a pixel of an image is to estimate the significance of the difference between two counts. Here we could be considering either the difference between two samples or pixels or the difference between a sample count and a background count. If N_1 is one count measurement and N_2 the other, then the difference is $N_1 - N_2$. The error in N_1 itself is equal to the s.d. in N_1 and is $\sqrt{N_1}$. In the same way the error in N_2 is $\sqrt{N_2}$. However the error in the *difference $N_1 - N_2$ is not* $\sqrt{(N_1 - N_2)}$. Since the error has to express the fact that *both N_1 and N_2 are* subject to errors the *error in the difference between N_1 and N_2 is equal to the standard deviation of the sum $(N_1 + N_2)$ or to* $\sqrt{(N_1 + N_2)}$. Thus if one count is 100 and the other 125 the difference is 25 and the error in the difference is $\sqrt{(100 + 125)}$ or 15.

The next question to ask is *whether the difference is significant* or if it could have occurred 'by chance' through the natural variation in counting statistics

discussed previously. Since, as mentioned, the probability of a measurement lying within a range of two deviations from the mean is 95% we can be fairly sure that a difference that is *greater* than two standards deviations is unlikely to have occurred by chance and is due to a *real* difference in counting conditions. In the above example 2 s.d. $= 2 \times 15$ or 30 so, using our criterion, a difference of 25 would *not* be reckoned a *significant* difference. If the two counts were 97 and 128 the difference would be 31, the error in the difference (the s.d.) would be $\sqrt{(97 + 128)}$ or again 15 and 2 s.d. would again be 30. Since the difference of 31 is larger then this value (for two standard deviations) we are fairly certain it is a *real* difference. Just to make sure about differences we could set the criterion as the difference having to exceed 3 s.d. Then all but 0.2% would lie between the range difference ± 3 s.d. In this case 97 and 128 would not constitute very significantly different counts though 90 and 135 would.

1.6.5 Comparing sets of measurements from two different experiments

We often need to compared two sets of measurements made over the same range of subjects. This happens when, for example, we compare one method of obtaining the result with another method. The starting point of analysing the data is to plot one set of measurements on the *x*-axis and the other set on the *y*-axis so that for each subject a point is made with the corresponding *x* and *y* values. For a perfect match of one set with the other the result will be a straight line through the origin at an angle of 45° — the 'line of identity'. More often the results will be ranged about this line and may not tend to go through the origin or even tend to form a straight line. What we would like is a measure of the agreement between the two sets of measurements. Two techniques are often used (and mistakenly so) to help measure this agreement. These are regression and correlation. *Regression* is a method of establishing the liner relationship between two sets of measurements. In its simplest form it establishes the best line of the form $y = mx + c$ to fit the set of points where *m* is the regression coefficient.

However if the original points do not form a straight line (because x is not a linear function of y) then regression will not be appropriate (though the points may be 'transformed' e.g. by taking the log or the square root or the square of the values in one set and replotting in which case a straight line may be indicated). *Correlation* tells us how close to the line the relationship between the two sets makes the points. While regression gives us an equation, correlation gives us r, the correlation coefficient, the measure of how close the points are to a straight line. Sometimes the value of r^2 is given instead of r itself may be positive or negative.

Because what is really required is a measure of agreement, a plot of the *difference* between the values in the two sets against the *average* of the values is to be preferred. Since we do not know the true value of each measurement the average of the two measurements is our best estimate of this. For good agreement the differences will be small. The mean value for the line is calculated and any lack of parallelity with the x-axis shows the bias in the difference between the two sets. Two lines giving the mean ± 2 s.d. can be plotted to show the limits of the agreement. The two methods of analysis are illustrated in **Fig. 1.25**.

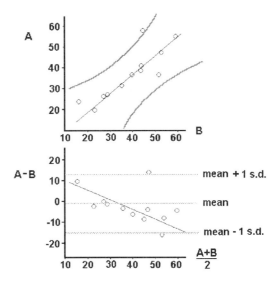

∎ **Fig. 1.25a** Two methods of comparing the results from two experiments or from two techniques. Traditional regression plot of one set of measurements against the other set. A straight line may result, from which a regression equation with an associated regression coefficient r (or r^2) may be obtained.

∎ **Fig. 1.25b** A 'Bland Altman' plot of the same data with perhaps better representation of a trend in the difference between A and B with increase in the value of the mean of A and B and a clearer idea of the confidence limits for the average difference.

2 Transit time, clearance, distribution volume and extraction fraction

Introduction

One of the major attributes of nuclear medicine is its ability to quantify physiological processes, and to do so non-invasively. The most important physiological variables in nuclear medicine are:

- time, usually in terms of a mean transit time T of a tracer or indicator;
- volume, usually in terms of the volume of distribution V of the tracer;
- mass M usually expressed as the mass in mg or activity in MBq of the tracer;
- concentration C of the tracer in mg/ml or MBq/ml;
- Flow Q of tracer in ml/min or ml/sec, or flux, mg/min.

These variables are related to each other by three equations of fundamental importance:

$$T = V/Q \qquad (2.1)$$

$$C = M/V \qquad (2.2)$$

$$dM/dt = Q(C_a - C_v) \qquad (2.3)$$

where the subscripts 'a' and 'v' refer to input (e.g. arterial) and output (e.g. venous).

Equation 2.1 is the transit time equation, equation 2.2 the dilution equation and equation 2.3 the Fick equation. Fick's principle is that when an indicator is introduced into a system it must be conserved within the system, or, in the usual nuclear medicine setting, the rate of change of organ content of a tracer is equal to the difference between the organ tracer input and output rates. The assumption is generally made that the tracer is well mixed in the system.

2.1 Transit and residence time

Many measurements made in nuclear medicine depend on the average time a tracer spends passing through a discrete space (its 'mean transit time') or the average time it spends in a space (its 'mean residence time'). Some physiological variables are expressed as a transit or residence time (for example, perfusion in units of ml/min/ml) or as combinations of time with volume, giving flow rate (ml/min), or time with mass, giving a flux rate (mg/min). Mean transit time is the average time required for tracer molecules to pass from one defined point to another. The proximal point is usually a vascular injection site and the distal point, a vascular sampling site. A space or compartment (such as an organ) may or may not be placed between the two points. Residence time is the average time that tracer molecules remain in a space in which they arrive or are deposited. In both settings, the time is dependent on the rate at which the tracer flows through the space and the volume in which the tracer is dispersed during its transit.

Transit time is usually measured by outflow detection, in which the concentration of the tracer at the distal point is determined by direct sampling (**Fig. 2.1a**). Because of the different paths taken by a tracer through a system, the sampled concentration varies over time and a histogram of transit times is obtained. This is usually recorded as a time–activity or a time–concentration curve, the spread of which is a function of input bolus dispersion and individual transit times. An example of this application is the measurement of cardiac output by the dye dilution technique: the injection site is a central vein while the sampling site is the pulmonary artery or a peripheral artery. Transit time measured by outflow detection is usually combined with simultaneous measurement of

(a) volume (by dilution) to generate flow (as in the measurement of cardiac output — section 3.2), or

(b) flow to generate volume (as in the measurement of lung water with labelled water, flow being cardiac output — Section 8.2.4).

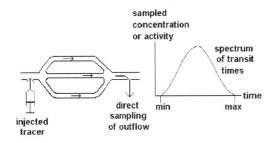

❙ **Fig. 2.1a** Mean transit time. Molecules of the tracer take different times to reach the sampling point. The mean transit time is the average of these. The minimum transit time is that of the molecule that arrives at the sampling point first.

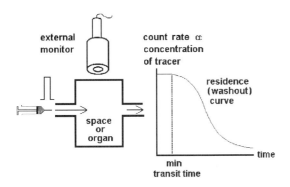

❙ **Fig. 2.1b** Mean residence time. The external monitor records a radioactivity signal from a tracer molecule for as long as that molecule remains in the space. The longer the mean transit time therefore the larger the area under the washout curve. The initial height of the curve is proportional to the number of radioactive molecules instantaneously injected into the space. Mean residence time is the area divided by the initial count, assuming that the molecules remaining within the space are well mixed.

Residence time is determined from residue detection in which the concentration of tracer remaining in the space is measured, usually by external monitoring of radioactivity (**Fig. 2.1b**). It is convenient because it requires no sampling but may be subject to error because the volume measured may not be accurately defined. Examples of residue detection are the measurement of organ perfusion by inert gas washout (Section 3.1.1.1) or pulmonary alveolar epithelial permeability from an inhaled radioactive aerosol (Section 8.4.2).

Transit time and residence time are closely related and in some situations are interchangeable (Swinburne *et al.* 1982). For an instantaneous input, the time–activity curve recorded by outflow detec-tion, which gives mean transit time, can be converted to the corresponding residue time–activity curve, which gives mean residence time, by integrating it backwards from infinite time to zero time (**Fig. 2.2**). Conversely, a residue curve can be converted to an outflow curve by plotting its slope as a function of time (i.e. differentiating it). Mean tracer transit time through, or mean residence time within, an organ, space or compartment is equal to the ratio of the total area under the residue curve divided by its initial height (i.e. the *y* value at zero time). Because the unit of an area is that of the product of the units of *x* and *y*, the ratio area: height has the unit of the *x*-axis (i.e. time), since the unit of of the *y*-axis cancels out (**Fig. 2.3**).

2.1.1 Measurement of transit and residence time

The general equation describing mean transit or residence time T is the summation over time of the individual concentrations of tracer multiplied by their individual transit times divided by the total concentration of tracer (Table 2.1) and is expressed mathematically as

$$T = \frac{\int t \cdot C(t) \cdot dt}{\int C(t) \cdot dt} \qquad (2.4)$$

where C is concentration measured directly at the sampling point (transit) or indirectly within the space (residue) and t is the time of transit or residence of each of the individual tracer molecules. Alterna-tively, in the context of residence time,

$$T = \frac{\int t \cdot M(t) \cdot dt}{\int M(t) \cdot dt}$$

where M is the amount of tracer remaining in the space. Equation 2.4 is sometimes called the first moment of the transit time.

To illustrate equation 2.4, examine Table 2.1 of hypothetical transit times. The total number of molecules is 32 and this is the denominator of equation 2.4. The sum of the products of $N.t$, the numerator in equation 2.4, is the total time spent by all molecules in transit and this is 124 (time units). The average transit time of the 32 molecules is therefore 124/32, or about 4 time units.

When a tracer is deposited instantaneously in a space as a bolus with initial concentration $C(0)$ and proceeds to clear mono-exponentially with rate

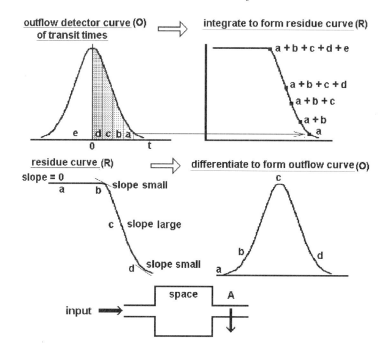

∎ **Fig. 2.2** Relationship between transit time and residence time. When the time–concentration curve recorded by outflow detection O is integrated 'backwards' from time t to 0, the corresponding residue curve R is generated. Conversely, the derivative of R effectively gives O. The average transit time from input to A is equal to the mean residence time in the space, provided that the time of transit of molecules between leaving the space and sampling at point A is

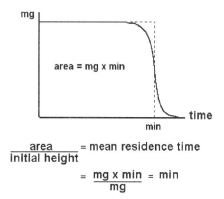

$$\frac{\text{area}}{\text{initial height}} = \text{mean residence time}$$

$$= \frac{\text{mg} \times \text{min}}{\text{mg}} = \text{min}$$

∎ **Fig. 2.3** Measurement of mean residence time expressed as total area under the residence curve (reflecting both the amount of tracer injected *and* the average residence time of tracer molecules) divided by the initial height (reflecting amount of tracer injected).

constant α, the residue concentration at time t, is $C(t) = C(0)e^{-\alpha t}$. The value of T in equation 2.4 is then equal to $1/\alpha$, shown as follows:

$$T = \frac{\int t \cdot C(t) \cdot dt}{\int C(t) \cdot dt} = \frac{\int t \cdot C(0) \cdot e^{-\alpha t} dt}{\int C(0) \cdot e^{-\alpha t} dt}. \tag{2.5}$$

The integral, $\int t \cdot C(0) \cdot e^{-\alpha t} \, dt$ over the time period considered of zero to infinity is represented by

$$\left[\frac{C(0)}{\alpha^2} \cdot e^{-\alpha t}(-\alpha t - 1) \right]_0^\infty .$$

Inserting the values for t of 0 and infinity where $e^{-\alpha 0} = 1$ and $e^{-\alpha \infty} = 0$,

$$\int t \cdot C(0) \cdot e^{-\alpha t} dt = C(0)/\alpha^2. \tag{2.6}$$

Similarly $\quad \int C(0) \cdot e^{-\alpha t} dt = \left[\frac{C(0) \cdot e^{-\alpha t}}{\alpha} \right]_0^\infty ,$

$$= C(0)/\alpha.$$

Therefore

$$T = \frac{C(0)/\alpha^2}{C(0)/\alpha} = \frac{1}{\alpha}. \tag{2.7a}$$

For a bi-exponential function describing tracer concentration over time

$$C(t) = C_1(0)e^{-\alpha_1 t} + C_2(0)e^{-\alpha_2 t}$$

and

$$T = \frac{C_1(0)/\alpha_1^2 + C_2(0)/\alpha_2^2}{C_1(0)/\alpha_1 + C_2(0)/\alpha_2}. \tag{2.7b}$$

A multi-exponential residue curve and the corresponding outflow curve reach terminal exponentials

Number of molecules (*N*) with a particular transit or residence time (equivalent to *C(t)* or *M(t)*)	Transit time or residence time (*t*)	Product (*N · t*) (equivalnt to t·*C(t)* or t·*M(t)*
2	1	2
4	2	8
10	3	30
6	4	24
4	5	20
3	6	18
2	7	14
1	8	8
Sum = 32 = ∫ *C(t)* · d*t*		Sum = 124 = ∫ *t* · *C(t)*.d*t*

▍ Table 2.1

that have the same rate constant. Thus, if t_1 is the time after which the curve has reached its terminal rate constant and t_2 some time later,

$$M(t_2) = M(t_1) \cdot e^{-\alpha(t_2 - t_1)}. \qquad (2.8a)$$

The outflow curve over the same period t_1 to t_2 is the differential dM/dt of the residue curve;

$$Q \cdot C(t_2) = M(t_1) \cdot k \cdot e^{-\alpha(t_2 - t_1)} \qquad (2.8b)$$

(note that blood flow Q is required to maintain consistency of units). The rate constant α is the same for both curves, whereas the intercepts are different by the factor k which has the unit of min^{-1}. So on a semilogarithmic plot the residue and outflow curves eventually become parallel, a state which indicates that the terminal exponential has been reached (Lassen and Sejrsen 1971). It is often important to know for a curve that this is the case, for example when measuring the area under a clearance curve (Section 2.2.1.2).

Several problems are encountered in the measurement of transit and residence times. Transit time following intravascular injection is generally measured from a time–concentration curve which is interrupted by re-circulation of the tracer (e.g. in the measurement of cardiac output). Residence time following bolus injection of the tracer into the compartment of interest, is generally measured from a time–activity curve using the *y*-axis intercept as a measure of the amount of tracer deposited.

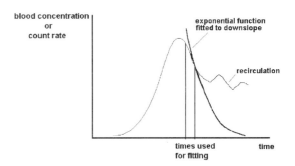

▍ **Fig. 2.4** Correction for tracer recirculation using an exponential fitting function. The downslope of the time–concentration curve (i.e. between the upper part of the downslope and the point of first recirculation) is assumed to be exponential and fitted as such, thereby predicting the time course of the curve had there been no recirculation.

It therefore requires the assumption of instantaneous injection of the tracer (a so-called delta input). In practice the bolus is dispersed in time before reaching the compartment. Like transit time measurement, residue detection also demands no recirculation. These two non-ideal conditions are approached by correction for re-circulation in the case of transit time measurement and correction for bolus dispersion and recirculation by deconvolution analysis in the case of residence time measurement (Section 1.5).

2.1.2 Correction for non-ideal conditions

2.1.2.1 Correction for recirculation

In order to measure transit time from a plasma concentration–time curve, a correction for recirculation of the tracer usually has to be applied. This is achieved by fitting the recorded curve to a 'hypothetical' (mathematically defined) curve which represents an ideal function of the mean transit time and which can be defined mathematically. There are two ideal functions commonly used: an exponential and a gamma function. An exponential function is fitted as the equation

$$C(t) = Ae^{-\alpha t} \qquad (2.9)$$

to the downslope of the curve, prior to the recirculation peak (**Fig. 2.4**). It predicts how the curve would have behaved if there were no recirculation.

On the other hand, the gamma function,

$$C(t) = A \cdot t^{\alpha} \cdot e^{-\beta t} \qquad (2.10)$$

is applied to the major part of the curve enclosed between the upslope and the recirculation point. It predicts the whole of the curve from all the available points before recirculation. A hypothetical first pass curve is shown in **Fig. 2.5** based on hypothetical values of A, α and β in equation 2.10. When the downslope of the gamma fit of the curve is fitted with the exponential function of Fig. 2.5 it can be

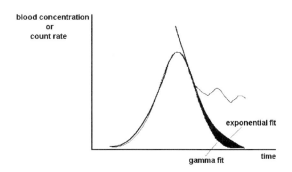

∎ **Fig. 2.6** Relationship between exponential and gamma fits. The total area under a concentration–time curve corrected for recirculation by fitting to a gamma function is about 10% less than that under a curve obtained by correction based on an exponential fit to the downslope.

seen that the area under the curve with the exponential fit is about 10% more than that under the gamma fit (**Fig. 2.6**).

2.1.2.2 Correction for bolus dispersion (instantaneous input)

Since nuclear medicine techniques enable the monitoring of radioactivity in tissues by external detection, measurement of mean transit time T is often carried out by residue detection. Provided the distribution of tracer within its distribution volume in the organ into which it is injected does not change, then T is equal to the area under the residue curve divided by its initial height. If tracer disappears mono-exponentially from the organ (known as first-order kinetics), T is also equal to the reciprocal of the rate constant of disappearance. The requirements of instantaneous injection and no recirculation are adequately met in the two clinical examples of residue detection given above — inert gas washout and alveolar permeability — but in other situations, in which a recirculating tracer is given intravenously, it may be dealt with by deconvolution analysis (Section 1.5). A well-known example of the application of deconvolution analysis for the determination of residence time is to renal transit time (Chapter 11), but many others exist.

Plasma clearance studies are examples of mean residence time measurement in which the tracer is instantaneously deposited into the plasma compartment (Paaske 1980). For tracers that remain in the

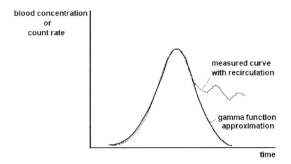

∎ **Fig. 2.5** Correction of tracer recirculation using a gamma fit function. The method of correction for recirculation uses all the points in the recorded curve up to recirculation and fits them to the equation for a gamma function.

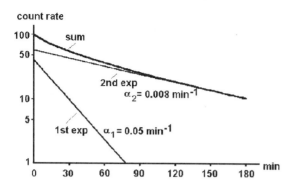

time(min)	1st exp	2nd exp	sum (counts)
0	60	40	100
2	54	39	93
5	47	38	85
10	36	37	73
20	22	34	56
40	8	29	37
60	3	25	28
120	0.15	15	15
180	0.007	10	10

▌ **Fig. 2.7** An example of a typical double exponential time–log concentration curve as it would appear, plotted on log–linear graph paper. The top, curved, line represents the sum of the two straight line components, one a slow exponential with time constant 0.008 min^{-1} and the other a fast exponential with time constant 0.05 min^{-1}. The contribution to the sum curve of the fast exponential becomes negligible from about 100 minutes.

plasma (vascular) compartment, T is equal to V/Q (equation 2.1), where V is plasma volume and the flow Q is the plasma clearance (see Section 2.2). For example, the mean residence time in plasma of technetium-99m labelled colloid is equal to plasma volume divided by plasma colloid clearance, and can be calculated by dividing the area under the time–plasma concentration curve by the zero-time concentration.

In some systems it may be possible to define several different specific residence times. An example of such a situation is the distribution of DTPA or EDTA throughout the extracellular fluid volume (ECF). These 'filtration markers' take about 2 hours to mix throughout the ECF, and this gives rise to a multi-exponential plasma disappearance curve. A typical curve is illustrated in **Fig. 2.7**. Since mixing of the tracer can be assumed to be instantaneous in the plasma, the area under the plasma disappearance curve divided by the total initial height is equal to the mean residence time *in plasma*. This is plasma volume divided by the rate of plasma clearance, i.e. the GFR. The total area under the plasma disappearance curve divided by the total initial height is thus not equal to mean residence time *in the ECF* even though it is distributed throughout the ECF. The mean residence time of DTPA in the ECF is, in fact, ECF volume divided by GFR (assuming this to be the same as plasma DTPA clearance; equation 2.1).

In addition to distinguishing residence times in plasma and ECF it is also useful to make a distinction between 'residence time' itself and the concept of 'sojourn time' (Peters 1993). Imagine a molecule of DTPA passing to and fro between plasma and interstitial fluid. The sojourn time is the random amount of time the molecule spends in either compartment before returning to the other. The residence time in either compartment is the total time (i.e. the sum of the sojourn times) spent in that compartment before the molecule undergoes glomerular filtration. Sojourn time and residence time in plasma are identical in systems in which the tracer is confined to plasma and disappears unidirectionally, as in the case of colloid taken up by the liver. (The concept of sojourn time will be used in Chapter 6 in the discussion of measurement of permeability surface area product.)

2.2 Clearance

Clearance is a very important concept to grasp in nuclear medicine because, except for tracers that label, and remain in, blood itself, the way that radiopharmaceuticals are removed or cleared from the blood into organs allows physiological imaging of those organs. The rate of clearance of a radiopharmaceutical depends on the organ blood flow and the efficiency with which the organ takes up the substance (the extraction efficiency or extraction fraction, discussed below).

In keeping with many physiological variables, the simplest way to understand clearance is to examine its units — ml per min, i.e. units of flow. Clearance is essentially a flow rate; it is the proportion of total blood flow which can be imagined to have been completely cleared of the substance by a tissue. For example, if the incoming arterial concentration is

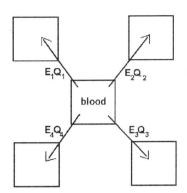

∎ **Fig. 2.8** A model representing clearance from blood of a tracer that leaves the blood by simultaneously entering several organs. Individual organ clearances are E_1Q_1, E_2Q_2 etc. where E denotes extraction fraction and Q organ blood flow. Blood clearance is the same as the sum of the individual organ clearances.

100 mg/ml and the outgoing venous concentration 30 mg/ml, then 70% of the flowing blood can be imagined to have been cleared of the substance (and 30% not cleared at all). If the blood flow through this vascular bed is 100 ml/min, then the clearance is 70 ml/min. Like blood flow, clearance can be expressed in absolute flow units, i.e. as ml/min, or flow per unit volume or mass of tissue (ml/min/ml or ml/min/g), analogously to perfusion. Extraction fraction is the fraction of incoming substance which is removed by a tissue and can also be expressed as efficiency with units of percent. The clearance Z is equal to extraction fraction E multiplied by blood flow Q: i.e.

$$Z = E \cdot Q. \tag{2.11}$$

in the above example $E = 70\%$ and $Q = 100$ ml/min, so $Z = 70$ ml/min.

From equation 2.11 it may be seen that the extraction fraction is equal to clearance divided by blood flow. If the incoming concentration is C_a and the amount removed is $(C_a - C_v)$ the fraction removed E is $(C_a - C_v)/C_a$. So E is unitless with a value between 0 and 1 if expressed as a fraction, or between 0 and 100% if expressed as an efficiency. Extraction fraction can also be thought of as the probability of an individual molecule of the substance being removed by an organ or tissue during one single pass. The probability is the same whether blood or plasma is considered. However if the tracer is confined to plasma, then it is more

appropriate to describe *plasma* clearance or *plasma* flow. For such a tracer, blood clearance will be higher than plasma clearance by a factor equal to the reciprocal of $[1 - H]$, where H is haematocrit.

Clearance may be used in different senses. Most of the time it is used to quantify *removal* from plasma of tracer that does not return to plasma, but it may also be used to quantify the *net movement of tracer* that subsequently does return to plasma (such as technetium-99m–DTPA exchanging across the endothelium). Thus early after injection, DTPA leaves plasma by entering interstitial fluid as well as undergoing glomerular filtration. The net clearance from plasma at this stage is higher than clearance later when DTPA is returning to plasma from the interstitial space. However the clearance of tracer by glomerular filtration and therefore not returning to plasma, remains unchanged and, in the context of measuring renal function using DTPA, is the variable of interest.

So far, we have considered organ clearance. One can also consider whole body clearance which is the sum of the individual clearances of all those organs contributing to the removal of the substance. Although the organs may have different extraction fractions (E) for the substance in question and different blood flows (Q) **(Fig. 2.8)**, the total clearance which is also called whole body clearance, is the sum of the individual clearances; i.e. the sum of the individual values of the product $E \cdot Q$ (which all have units of flow). This may be represented by $\overset{N}{\Sigma}E_iQ_i$.

Para-aminohippurate (PAH) and DTPA are examples of substances which are cleared exclusively by one organ, the kidney. In these cases, the organ (renal) clearances of PAH and DTPA are the same as the whole body clearances. Pertechnetate, di-mercapto succinic acid (DMSA) and meta-iodobenzyl guanidine (MIBG) are examples of agents which are taken up by more than one organ so the whole body clearance is greater than the clearance into each individual organ. It is not necessary to know into which organ(s) the tracer is cleared in order to measure plasma clearance since this is still defined as that volume of plasma (or blood) which is completely cleared in unit time, representing a virtual plasma (or blood) flow.

Apart from plasma clearance, other expressions of clearance are whole body clearance, urinary clearance and organ (e.g. renal) clearance. Plasma (or blood)

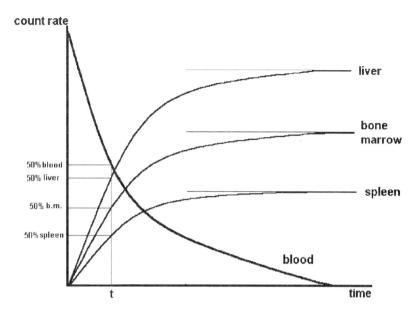

∎ **Fig. 2.9** When a tracer leaves the blood as a result of clearance into several different organs each with a different clearance, such a labelled colloid which is taken up by the liver, spleen and bone marrow, the time courses of organ activity are identical and each a mirror image of the blood clearance curve. Thus for each of the 4 compartments illustrated, the time to 50% uptake or clearance is the same.

clearance is the same as whole body clearance. They can be thought of as the volumes of circulating plasma (or blood) from which the tracer is completely cleared in unit time. It would be appropriate to consider plasma clearance if the tracer, such as DTPA, did not bind to red cells, otherwise clearance can be specified as blood clearance. In the context of blood flow measurement, blood clearance is usually the appropriate variable, whereas in certain other settings, plasma clearance is specifically required, for example measurement of glomerular filtration rate.

Urinary clearance represents that proportion of blood flow (in this case, renal blood flow) that is completely cleared of the radiopharmaceutical ultimately appearing in urine. It is an important concept in renal physiology as it gives quantitative information about the tubular handling of a substance. For example, inulin, which is neither secreted nor reabsorbed by the tubule, has identical urinary and renal clearances. DMSA, on the other hand, is concentrated within the renal parenchyma, although some appears in urine. The sum of parenchymal and urinary activities represents renal clearance, while the urinary activity represents urinary clearance. Thus DMSA has a renal clearance which is greater than its urinary clearance.

In contrast to flowing blood, clearance also applies to the context of a static volume. Thus, if in one minute 10% of tracer leaves a compartment of volume 100 ml in which the tracer is dispersed, then the clearance of tracer from the compartment is 10 ml/min.

2.2.1 Measurement of clearance

Blood or plasma clearance can be measured either under steady state conditions, in which the substance under study is infused at a constant rate, or following bolus injection, in which the rate of disappearance of the substance from blood is recorded. Individual organ clearance can also be measured following bolus injection by quantification of the rate of tracer uptake by the organ.

2.2.1.1 Steady state

Following a continuous intravenous infusion of the agent at a constant rate, the arterial concentration (C_a) eventually becomes constant. From the Fick principle,

$$dC_a/dt = \text{infusion rate} - \text{removal rate from plasma}$$
$$= 0 \text{ (at equilibrium)} \quad (2.12)$$

so, at equilibrium,
removal rate = infusion rate in mg/min.   (2.13)

The removal rate depends on the arterial concentration C_a and on the blood clearance Z; in fact, inspection of the units indicates that the removal rate is the product of the two. Thus C_a is in mg/ml and Z in ml/min, so ml cancels out in their product, leaving mg/min, the same units as the infusion rate. Therefore

removal rate $= Z \cdot C_a$ = infusion rate   (2.14)

and

$$Z = \frac{C_a}{\text{infusion rate}}.$$

If the substance is confined to plasma, with no red-cell binding, then the blood concentration is less than plasma concentration by the factor $(1-H)$ and Z in equation 2.14 is higher by the same factor. If the substance distributes equally between plasma and red cells, then concentration is the same for blood and plasma and equation 2.14 can be based on either blood or plasma. If the substance shows partial binding to red cells then the relationship between blood, C_b, and plasma, C_p, concentration is given by

$$C_b = H \cdot C_{rbc} + (1 - H) \cdot C_p   \quad (2.15)$$

From the partition coefficient, λ, defining the distribution between red cells and plasma we can say

$$C_{rbc} = \lambda \cdot C_p   \quad (2.16)$$

and

$$C_b = C_p[H \cdot \lambda + (1 - H)]   \quad (2.17)$$

The fraction of total blood tracer bound to red cells obviously depends on haematocrit and is

$$\frac{C_{rbc}}{C_b} = \frac{H \cdot \lambda}{H \cdot \lambda + (1 - H)}.   \quad (2.18)$$

Measurement of clearance at steady state is cumbersome but the underlying principle is important, since it is the basis of the gold standard method of measuring glomerular filtration rate (GFR) by urinary inulin clearance. Since it is cleared exclusively by GFR without tubular reabsorption or secretion, the urinary output rate of inulin at equilibrium must be equal to the infusion rate. The input rate of inulin need not be measured since it equals the output rate which can be obtained from measuring urine flow rate (Q_u) and urine inulin concentration (C_u); i.e. urinary clearance. So

$$Z_{inulin} = \frac{Q_u \cdot C_u}{C_a}   \quad (2.19)$$

with units

$$\frac{ml}{min} = \frac{mg}{ml} \times \frac{ml}{min} \times \frac{ml}{mg}.$$

At equilibrium, $C_a = C_v$, so a peripheral venous sample can be used for C_a.

2.2.1.2 Blood clearance following bolus injection

The simplest situation involving clearance is represented by a substance which is (1) confined to plasma (i.e. does not enter the extravascular extracellular space or red cells) and (2) cleared from the plasma into a single organ at a rate which, at any time, is proportional to the concentration of the substance in plasma; i.e. the clearance obeys first-order kinetics (Chapter 1). The disappearance curve from blood will be mono-exponential and the clearance rate equal to the product of the rate constant (α), which has units of a fraction per unit of time, and the volume of distribution (V) of the agent; i.e. plasma volume (Shaldon *et al.* 1962):

$$Z = \alpha V   \quad (2.20)$$

with units

$$\frac{ml}{min} = \frac{1}{min} \times ml.$$

The radiopharmaceuticals which come closest to this simple situation are the radiocolloids, which are taken up by the reticuloendothelial components of the liver, spleen and bone marrow. When, as in the case of a colloid, more than one organ participates in the clearance, the time courses of *uptake* in each organ are identical since each is the mirror image of the time course of blood disappearance. In the case of the mono-exponential removal of a colloid from blood, the time courses of uptake in liver, spleen and bone marrow are also mono-exponential (i.e. approach their final values mono-exponentially) with the same rate constant as the blood disappearance **(Fig. 2.9)**. It should be easy to understand why this is so since at the time when the blood activity concentration has reached, say, 50% of the starting concentration, the rate of input into each organ must be half of what it was at the time of injection (zero time), whilst when all the activity has been cleared

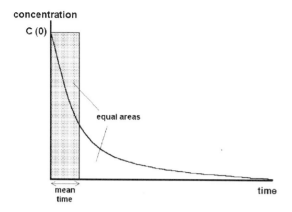

▌ Fig. 2.10 The mean residence time of a tracer in plasma from which the tracer disappears mono-exponentially is the width (on the time axis) of a rectangle of height equal to $C(0)$ and area equal to that under the plasma disappearance curve. This mean time is equal to 1.44 times the half-time of disappearance or to the reciprocal of the rate constant of disappearance.

from the blood there will be none left for each organ to take up, so they will reach their respective final (plateau) uptake values at the same time.

A frequently used way to measure blood clearance by the bolus injection technique is from the area enclosed under the blood disappearance curve. This can be demonstrated from the Fick principle, as for steady state clearance, above. Thus

$$dM_b/dt = Q(C_v - C_a) \qquad (2.21)$$

where M_b refers to the quantity of tracer remaining in blood. Here Q is the volume of blood cleared of tracer in unit time and as such is therefore clearance; C_v is an imaginary venous concentration which represents venous blood from which the tracer has been completely cleared. But by definition, $C_v = 0$, so

$$dM_b/dt = -Z \cdot C_a \qquad (2.22)$$

with units

$$\frac{mg}{min} = \frac{ml}{min} \times \frac{mg}{ml}.$$

Note the minus sign in equation 2.22, which indicates that the blood concentration is decreasing. Integrating equation 2.22 gives

$$M_b = -Z \cdot \int C_a(t) \cdot dt. \qquad (2.23)$$

(The minus sign is accommodated in the integral by reversing the limits, i.e. by subtracting the integral at $t = 0$ from the integral when $t = \infty$.) Also

$$Z = \frac{M_b}{\int C_a(t) \cdot dt}. \qquad (2.24)$$

When the curve is integrated from time infinity to zero, M_b is the total amount of tracer to have left the blood and is equal to the injected activity. Therefore

$$Z = \frac{\text{injected activity}}{\text{total area under plasma curve}}. \qquad (2.25)$$

The units of the area under any graph or curve are the product of the x-axis and y-axis units. In the case of a time–concentration curve, they are (min.mg)/ml; so the units of $Z = mg \times \dfrac{ml}{min \times mg} = ml/min.$

In the case of a mono-exponential disappearance of a tracer confined to the intravascular space, the area under the disappearance curve is equal to the zero-time concentration (mg/ml) divided by the rate constant (units min^{-1}) (Section 1.2.4), i.e.

$$\text{area} = C_a(0)/\alpha. \qquad (2.26)$$

The units are (mg/ml) × min as before.

$$Z = \frac{\text{injected activity} \times \alpha}{C_a(0)}. \qquad (2.27)$$

Note the relationship of equation 2.27 to equation 2.20. For a tracer confined to the intravascular space (when it can be assumed that $C_a = C_v$), the activity/$C_v(0)$ of equation 2.27 is equal to the plasma volume of equation 2.20.

An alternative approach to the derivation of equation 2.26 is to recall that the reciprocal of a rate constant is a mean residence time. The area under the disappearance curve can then be imagined to be that of a rectangle with a height equal to $C_v(0)$ (since $C_v(0) = C_a(0)$) and a width equal to the mean residence time T of tracer in the plasma **(Fig. 2.10)**. Then area $= C_a(0)/\alpha = C_a(0)T.$

If the distribution volume V of the tracer is the intravascular space, such as for a labelled colloid, then, from equation 2.22,

$$\frac{dM_b}{dt} = \frac{-Z \cdot M_b}{V}. \qquad (2.28)$$

According to equation 2.28, dM_b/dt is proportional to M_b, so the blood concentration must decrease

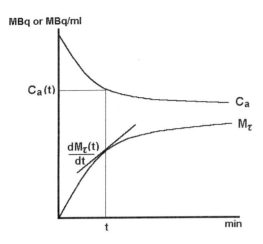

▌ Fig. 2.11 The instantaneous rate of accumulation of tracer at time t, dM/dt, into an organ from which the tracer does not leave, is proportional to the arterial tracer concentration $C_a(t)$ at the same time. The constant of proportionality is the organ clearance rate for the tracer.

exponentially with rate constant Z/V and a tracer residence time in blood of V/Z.

These considerations are important for tracers with distribution volumes greater than the plasma volume and with curves of disappearance from plasma which are more complex than simply mono-exponential. The clearance of DTPA (or EDTA which has very similar pharmacokinetics) is a good example. DTPA diffuses into the extravascular space immediately following injection and then diffuses back into the intravascular space so that by about two hours after injection, the concentrations of tracer in the two compartments decrease with the same rate constant. At the same time, DTPA is cleared into the kidney by glomerular filtration. From compartmental analysis (Section 1.4) it can be shown that, with these pharmacokinetics, the disappearance curve is bi-exponential and resembles that shown in **Fig. 2.7**. The area under a bi-exponential plasma disappearance curve is equal to the sum of the areas under each mono-exponential component of the total curve. Each mono-exponential component has an area equal to its zero-time intercept divided by its rate constant (Section 1.2.4.); i.e. MBq/ml/min^{-1}. The units of area under the time–concentration curve are the same.

From equation 2.25

$$Z_{DTPA} = \frac{\text{injected activity}}{\text{total area}}$$

$$= \frac{\text{injected activity}}{\text{area 1} + \text{area 2}} \qquad (2.29)$$

$$= \frac{\text{injected activity}}{A/\alpha_1 + B/\alpha_2} \qquad (2.30)$$

where A and B are the respective zero time intercepts (i.e. concentrations at zero time) of the two separate exponential components and α_1 and α_2 their corresponding rate constants.

A feature of equation 2.25 (activity/area) for measuring clearance is that the precise mathematical form of the disappearance curve need not be known. The area, at least up to a certain point, can be measured directly, for example, by counting the squares under the curve redrawn on linear graph paper. The area under a time–activity curve recorded by *continuous* monitoring is simply the total number of counts recorded during the entire duration of the measurement; thus the product of counts/min and min has units of counts. If the disappearance curve has become mono-exponential by the end of the measurement period, then the area beyond can be obtained by dividing the last recorded y value by the rate constant of a mono-exponential function fitted to the tail of the curve.

Clearly, if a tracer has a distribution volume larger than the plasma volume (as with chromium-51 EDTA or technetium-99m DTPA), its rate of removal from plasma is slower than it would be if it was confined to plasma; i.e. the rate of removal is inversely proportional to the volume of distribution, or, put another way, its mean residence time within that distribution volume is directly proportional to distribution volume (equation 2.1). However its *clearance* is independent of distribution volume and since clearance is the ratio of volume/time, the mean residence time increases in proportion to the distribution volume.

2.2.1.3 Organ clearance from uptake measurement

Clearance into a single organ can be measured from uptake of tracer into the organ. Separate organ clearance can also be calculated even if several organs are clearing the tracer. The fundamental requirement is that none of the accumulated tracer subsequently leaves the organ, in which case, referring to equation 2.3, the rate of change of organ tracer content M_τ can be stated as follows:

$$\mathrm{d}M_\tau/\mathrm{d}t = Q(C_a - C_v). \tag{2.31}$$

Multiplying top and bottom of the right hand side by C_a,

$$\mathrm{d}M_\tau/\mathrm{d}t = \frac{Q(C_a - C_v) \cdot C_a}{C_a}. \tag{2.32}$$

But $(C_a - C_v)/C_a$ is equal to extraction fraction. Therefore

$$\mathrm{d}M_\tau/\mathrm{d}t = Q \cdot E \cdot C_a \tag{2.33}$$

$$= Z \cdot C_a. \tag{2.34}$$

Note that compared with equation 2.22, there is no minus sign; this indicates that the organ content of the tracer is increasing. Re-arranging equation 2.34 gives,

$$Z = \frac{\mathrm{d}M_\tau}{\mathrm{d}t} \cdot \frac{1}{C_a} \tag{2.35}$$

and integration of which gives

$$Z = \frac{M_\tau}{\int C_a(t) \cdot \mathrm{d}t}. \tag{2.36}$$

Note the similarity of equation 2.36 to equations 2.24 and 2.25. Thus clearance can be measured from the rate of organ uptake at a specified time after injection (equation 2.35, **Fig. 2.11**, Rehling *et al.* 1985), or from the total amount accumulated up to a specified time (equation 2.36, **Fig. 2.12**, Britton and Brown 1971). In either case, it is necessary to determine M_τ in absolute units (MBq) using calibrated (quantitative) imaging (section 5.4.3).

  It should be evident that as the accumulated tracer is not lost from the organ (as would be satisfied, say, for the first 2–3 min of a renogram) then, for either of equations 2.35 and 2.36, the right-hand side remains constant. This provides the basis of a third equation for measuring individual organ clearance, described by several authors for different organs (Rutland 1979, Patlak *et al.* 1983), which is to re-arrange equation 2.36 and divide both sides by C_a: i.e.

$$\frac{M_\tau}{C_a} = Z \cdot \frac{\int C_a(t) \cdot \mathrm{d}t}{C_a}. \tag{2.37}$$

This equation is of the form $y = mx$ which is a straight line of slope m going through the origin. If

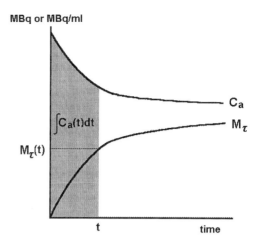

❚ **Fig. 2.12** It may be seen from the same curves as in Fig. 2.11 that the total amount of tracer $M_\tau(t)$ accumulated at time t, in an organ from which the tracer does not leave, is proportional to the area under the arterial concentration curve up to the same time. The constant of proportionality is the organ clearance rate of the tracer.

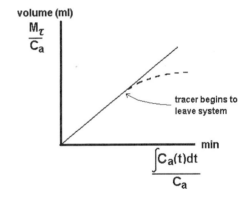

❚ **Fig. 2.13** The Patlak–Rutland plot. The y-axis of the plot is the amount of tracer accumulated up to time t, in an organ from which the tracer does not leave, divided by the instantaneous arterial tracer concentration at the same time (the left hand side of equation 2.37). It has units mg/mg/ml, i.e. ml.. The x-axis is the area under the arterial time–concentration curve up to the same time t divided by the instantaneous arterial concentration at the same time. It has units of [mg/ml × min]/[mg/ml], i.e. min. The slope of the plot, with units of ml/min, is the organ clearance rate of the tracer. If tracer was leaving the organ the slope would not be a straight line. The time axis is sometimes called 'normalized time' to distinguish it from true 'clock' time.

the left-hand side of equation 2.37, M_τ/C_a, is plotted as the y-axis against $\int C_a(t) \cdot \mathrm{d}t/C_a$, a straight line is

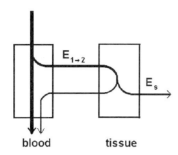

blood   tissue

∎ **Fig. 2.14** Unidirectional extraction fraction and steady state extraction fraction. Unidirectional extraction fraction ($E_{1→2}$) represents the probability of a molecule of tracer entering tissue from blood on arrival in an organ. It does not address the likelihood of that molecule returning to the blood. Steady-state extraction fraction (E_s) does address this probability and determines the uptake rate of tracer by the tissue during continuous infusion at equilibrium defined as constant arterial concentration. It represents the *overall* probability of a tracer molecule being permanently removed from blood.

obtained with slope Z (**Fig. 2.13**). There are several examples in nuclear medicine of the applications of this approach (Peters 1994) and they are discussed more fully in Chapters 3, 6, 8, 11 and 12.

2.2.1.4 Measurement of urinary clearance

Urinary clearance Z_u is a special case of organ clearance. It is defined as the volume of plasma cleared, in unit time, of tracer excreted in the urine. If the amount of tracer M_u appearing in the urine between injection and time t, analogous to M_τ in equation 2.36, is divided by the area under the plasma time–concentration curve up to time t then this gives the urinary clearance

$$Z_u = \frac{M_u}{\int C_a(t) \cdot dt}. \tag{2.38}$$

An error may arise if the urine collection is made too early and the transit time from glomerulus to bladder is a significant proportion of t. Another condition is that the urine collection must be complete, necessitating bladder catheterization. (See also Section 13.2.3 for 'faecal' tracer clearance.)

2.2.1.5 Measurement of organ clearance by positron emission tomography

The basic principles of measurement of clearance by Positron Emission Tomography (PET) and the fundamental assumptions are the same as those described above for single photon tracers. In PET however the quantity of radioactivity in the tissue is usually measured as a concentration C rather than as an absolute amount. Thus, in PET, equation 2.31 is expressed as follows:

$$\frac{dM_\tau}{V \cdot dt} = \frac{Q}{V}(C_a - C_v) = \frac{dC}{dt}. \tag{2.39}$$

Multiplying top and bottom of the right-hand side by C_a,

$$\frac{dC}{dt} = \frac{Q(C_a - C_v) \cdot C_a}{V \cdot C_a} \tag{2.40}$$

Therefore, since $E = (C_a - C_v)/C_a$ and $QE = Z$

$$\frac{dC}{dt} = \frac{Z \cdot C_a}{V}. \tag{2.41}$$

Re-arranging,

$$\frac{Z}{V} = \frac{dC}{dt} \cdot \frac{1}{C_a} \tag{2.42}$$

and integrating over a period from time zero,

$$= \frac{C}{\int C_a(t) \cdot dt}. \tag{2.43}$$

(analogous to equation 2.36)
As an alternative to arterial sampling, C_a can be measured by PET if the tomographic slice includes a cardiac chamber or major vessel.

2.3 Distribution volume

Reference has already been made to distribution volume. For any system, it is most easily grasped from the transit time equation (2.1) as the product of flow and transit time. The flow corresponds to blood flow, as, for example, in the measurement of lung water, where it is equivalent to cardiac output, or it may represent clearance, as, for example, in the relationship between ECF volume, GFR and mean residence time of DTPA in the ECF.

Tracers like DTPA, which rapidly cross the endothelium and enter the extravascular space, have a larger distribution volume compared with tracers such as colloids which are confined to the intravascular space. Tracers which are themselves plasma proteins, such as labelled transferrin, or which are almost completely bound to plasma proteins, such as gallium-67, also have distribution volumes close to plasma volume. However tracers which are able to cross the endothelium, but at the same time undergo partial binding to proteins in plasma, present a more complex situation. Intuitively they should have an effective distribution volume intermediate between the volume they would have if they were not protein bound and the plasma volume itself. Their effective distribution volume is less than the extracellular fluid volume because, upon returning to the intravascular space, their subsequent egress into the extravascular space is hindered by protein binding. This tendency to be held in the intravascular space leads to a greater chance of tracer clearance into those organ(s) responsible for tracer removal than would be the case if the tracer was not protein bound. If an increased removal rate is promoted by protein binding then residence time in the distribution volume must be reduced. Therefore, from the transit time equation $T = V/Q$, the effective distribution volume must also be reduced, since clearance is 'fixed' by extraction fraction and organ blood flow.

Consider two tracers, one 33% protein bound in plasma (and therefore 67% free) and the other 67% protein bound and 33% free. The free portion occupies 13 litres volume (ECF volume) while the portion bound to protein occupies 3 litres (plasma volume). The individual and effective distribution volumes are given in Table 2.2.

Effective distribution volume can be calculated for a tracer occupying the extracellular fluid volume if its degree of protein binding is known. So for tracers with the same clearance rates, removal rates from plasma would be faster for those tracers with the higher levels of protein binding. Examples of tracers with partial protein binding where an understanding of these considerations is important are MAG-3, hippuran and DMSA (see Chapter 11). Quite apart from its higher extraction efficiency by the kidney, MAG-3, for example, gives better renal images than DTPA because of its protein binding in plasma. Furthermore, although renal clearance of MAG-3 is less than that of hippuran, MAG-3 and hippuran have similar residence times in their respective volumes of distribution because MAG-3 is more protein bound.

2.4 Extraction fraction

Extraction fraction is that fraction of incoming tracer that is removed by an organ in one pass through it. It is defined in terms of clearance and blood flow in equation 2.11. It can also be defined in terms of blood concentration as follows

$$E = \frac{C_a - C_v}{C_a} \qquad (2.44)$$

where C_a and C_v are the concentrations of tracer in arterial blood and venous blood draining the organ respectively. Extraction fraction can be thought of as a probability; i.e. the probability of a tracer molecule being retained in the organ during a single pass. When extraction fraction is unity, organ clearance and blood flow are identical. It is important to grasp this since the blood disappearance rates of some tracers are used to measure blood flow, for example, hippuran and para-amino hippurate (PAH) to measure renal blood flow. In recognition of the fact that an extraction efficiency of 100% is not met for this measurement, the term effective renal plasma flow is usually employed. In fact, hippuran has an extraction efficiency of no more than 85%, falling to lower values in the diseased kidney. Another example is the use of colloid clearance as a measure of liver blood flow. An interesting anomaly, until the kinetics were better understood, was the use of heat damaged red blood cells as a measure of splenic reticulo-endothelial function (see Section 10.2.2.2.1). Here splenic blood flow was ignored and the clearance equated with splenic extraction fraction!

Protein bound		Free			
%	Distribution volume (l)	%	Distribution volume (l)	Effective total volume (l)	Transit time
33% (of 3 l)	1	67% (of 13 l)	8.7	9.7	9.7/Q
67% (of 3 l)	2	33% (of 13 l)	4.3	6.3	6.3/Q

▌ Table 2.2

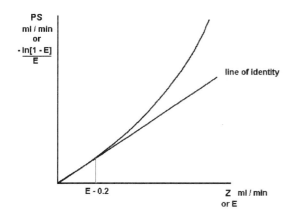

∎ **Fig. 2.15** Relationship between permeability surface area (*PS*) product and clearance. Since $PS = -Q \ln[1-E]$ and $Q = Z/E$, PS is also equal to $-Z \ln[1-E]/E$. Therefore $PS/Z = -\ln[1-E]/E$.

It is important to understand the concept of extraction fraction for a further general reason: that is, the organ uptake of almost all tracers in nuclear medicine is a function of both blood flow and extraction fraction. Thus, in bone scanning, a region of increased uptake of bone tracer (technetium-99m methylene diphosphonate) may be due to increased bone turnover (implying an increased extraction fraction) and/or to increased local blood flow. Another point to remember about extraction fraction is that it is itself dependent (inversely) on blood flow. Thus with high flow rates, the capacity of the vascular bed for transferring a tracer decreases, and extraction fraction consequently falls. This is discussed more fully below and in Sections 3.1.3.2, 6.2.2.1 and 7.1.1.3.

As with clearance, the reader may encounter variants of extraction fraction described in the literature. For example, confusion may be encountered with the use of the terms instantaneous extraction fraction, retention fraction and steady-state extraction fraction. All these terms arise in the situation where a proportion of a tracer that has already passed from blood into a tissue returns to the blood while the remaining proportion is permanently retained in the tissue (**Fig. 2.14**). The instantaneous extraction fraction is the unidirectional extraction fraction in the direction from blood to tissue, while the steady state extraction fraction, which will be equal to or less than the instantaneous extraction fraction, is the *effective* (or net) fraction of incoming tracer permanently removed from blood. These variables have their counterparts in clearance, which may be conceived as an unidirectional clearance of tracer, some of which then returns to blood, or a steady-state clearance of tracer not returning to blood. Sometimes retention fraction is used synonymously with steady-state extraction fraction, and the simultaneous use of extraction fraction in this context is synonymous with instantaneous or uni-directional extraction fraction. Examples which illustrate these concepts and this terminology include (1) the hepatic uptake of organic anions such as IDA, which display bi-directional movement between plasma and hepatocyte but uni-directional movement from hepatocyte to bile canaliculus (Section 9.3); (2) the skeletal uptake of diphosphonate, which, as a small hydrophilic solute displays bi-directional movement between plasma and bone interstitial fluid, but essentially unidirectional movement from bone fluid to bone crystal (Section 13.3); and (3) potassium analogues, such as thallium-201, which display bi-directional movement between plasma and myocardial interstitial fluid but essentially undirectional movement from myocardial intestitial fluid into the myocardial cell (Section 7.1.2). The concept of extraction fraction as a probability helps to explain why, for example in the case of bone uptake of MDP, the steady state extraction fraction is the product of the instantaneous extraction fraction (probability of tracer moving from plasma to bone interstitial fluid) and the extraction fraction of tracer from bone fluid to bone crystal (probability of tracer moving from interstitial fluid to bone crystal rather than back into plasma). Since blood flow, Q, is a single, unambiguous entity, definitions of clearance, corresponding to the variations described above for extraction fraction, must also exist. Similarly, as blood flow can be expressed in absolute units or as 'per unit of tissue volume' (perfusion), the variants of clearance can be described in absolute units or in terms of tissue volume.

2.4.1 Relationships between extraction fraction, clearance and blood flow — PS product

In general, as blood flow to a vascular bed increases, less time is available for uptake of tracer and so extraction fraction falls. The relationship between extraction fraction (*E*) and blood flow (*Q*) for any particular solute in any particular vascular bed can be defined in terms of a constant called the Crone–Renkin constant or, alternatively, the permeability surface area product (*PS* product) (Crone & Levitt 1984). The tracer concentration is assumed to decrease exponentially along the capillary as a result of uptake into the tissue. The rate of this decrease and the length of the capillary determine *E*. Conversely, as *Q* increases, the capillary concentration will decrease at a slower rate, thereby reducing *E*. The Crone–Renkin constant, which is applicable to the transfer of a tracer at any interface, is defined as the tracer flux per unit concentration gradient *C* across the interface. Tracer flux, the amount of material flowing per minute, is referred to as *J*, is proportional to the permeability coefficient and surface area available for transfer and is equal to d*M*/d*t* with units mg/min or MBq/min. That is

$$PS = J/C. \tag{2.45}$$

Because the Crone–Renkin constant was originally applied in the quantification of endothelial permeability to hydrophilic solutes, the derivation of *PS* in terms of *Q* and *E* is covered in detail in Section 6.2.2.1, but the equation is given here

$$PS = -Q \cdot \ln(1 - E) \tag{2.46}$$

or

$$E = 1 - e^{-PS/Q}. \tag{2.47}$$

Substituting *Z*/*E* for *Q* in equation 2.46

$$PS = \frac{-Z \ln(1 - E)}{E}. \tag{2.48}$$

At low values of *E*, $-\ln(1-E)$ is very nearly equal to *E*, so *Z* becomes close to *PS* (**Fig. 2.15**). If *E* falls as *Q* rises, then their product *Z* will tend to be constant. At relatively high values of *Q*, *Z* does indeed approach a constant value, equal to *PS*, because *E* becomes small. The relationship between *E* and *Q* at different *PS* products and their product *Z*, is shown in **Fig. 2.16**. The units of *PS* are the same as those of *Q* and *Z*, yet *PS* may be much higher than *Q*. This is because *PS* defines the clearance of tracer that *could be achieved* if capillary concentration was maintained at the arterial level throughout capillary length. Clearance may refer to plasma or to whole blood, so the same is true of *PS* product, although, as with clearance, plasma is the fluid of reference if the tracer is confined to plasma and *Q* refers to plasma flow rather than blood flow. On the other hand, if the

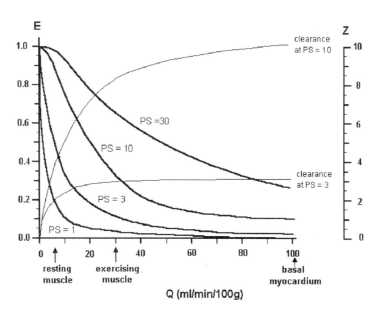

▌ **Fig. 2.16** Non-linear relationship between extraction fraction (*E*) and blood flow (*Q*). For any given *PS* product, *E* decreases as *Q* increases. When *PS* is low, tracer uptake is relatively low, so *E* is low. For any given *PS* product, the clearance (*Z*) increases towards a maximum as *Q* increases. At infinitely high *Q*, *E* becomes very small and the maximum value which *Z* approaches is the *PS* product.

tracer distributes freely between red cells and plasma (i.e. $\lambda = 1$; Section 2.2), then Q is blood flow. If the tracer is partially bound to red cells then more tracer would be transferred from blood to tissue cells (assuming it was available for transfer) for a given extraction fraction, and, to derive the appropriate PS product, Q would need to include an element proportional to the amount of tracer in red cells (see Question 23, Chapter 14). The same applies to partial binding to plasma proteins. Like flow and clearance, PS can be expressed in absolute terms, ml/min, or in relation to tissue volume or mass, ml/min/ml or ml/min/g. As with E and Z, it can also refer to uni-directional transfer (the usual case) or to steady state.

2.5 Expressing variables as quotients

Expressing a physiological variable as a quotient of an appropriate second variable often not only simplifies its measurement but often also makes it more physiologically meaningful. Renal blood flow divided by cardiac output, glomerular infiltration rate divided by extra-cellular fluid volume and mean granulocyte transit time divided by mean red cell transit time are examples. Organ blood flow is not only a function of patient size but in some cases also varies directly with cardiac output. GFR is conventionally expressed in terms of body surface area (the standard of which is 1.73 m^2), but since glomerular filtration regulates the volume and composition of body fluids, it is rational to express it in terms of ECF volume. As explained in Section 11.1.2.1, it is easier, from a technical point of view, to measure GFR/ECF volume than GFR/1.73 m^2. Finally, as explained in Section 10.3.2, granulocytes marginate in vascular beds throughout the body, i.e. are present in excess of the numbers that would be expected from the blood volume of the vascular bed. Such margination can be quantified as total organ granulocyte content or as mean granulocyte transit time. Alternatively, it may be expressed as a quotient of red cell transit time, and since this takes account

of variations in blood volume upon which the margination is not necessarily dependent, it is physiologically rational. Again the two transit times do not have to be measured separately but simply expressed as the ratio of their respective counts rates recorded over the organ, which is technically simpler.

References

Britton KE and Brown NJG. *Clinical renography.* Lloyd Luke, London, 1971.

Crone C and Levitt DG. Capillary permeability to small solutes. In: Renkin EM, Michel CC, eds *Handbook of physiology*, section 2: The cardiovascular system IV. American Physiological Society, Bethesda, Maryland: 1984: 375–409

Lassen NA and Sejrsen P. Monoexponential extrapolation of tracer clearance curves in kinetic analysis. *Circulation Research* 1971, **19**: 76–87.

Paaske W. Microvascular exchange. Kinetic analysis of plasma disappearance curves. *Acta Chirurgica Scandinavica* 1980 supplement **502**: 46–50.

Patlak CS, Blasberg RG and Fenstermacher JD. Graphical evaluation of blood to brain transfer constants from multiple time uptake data. *Journal of Cerebral Blood Flow and Metabolism* 1983; **3**: 1–7.

Peters AM. Graphical analysis of dynamic quantitative data. *Nuclear Medicine Communications* 1994; **15**: 669–72.

Rehling M, Moller ML, Lund JO, Jensen KD, Thamdrup B and Trap-Jensen J. Tc-99m DTPA gamma camera renography: normal values and rapid determination of single kidney glomerular filtration rate. *European Journal of Nuclear Medicine* 1985; **II**: 1–6.

Rutland MD. A single injection technique for subtraction of blood background in ^{131}I-hippuran renograms. *British Journal of Radiology* 1979, **52**: 134–7.

Shaldon S, Chiandussi L, Guevara L, Caesar J and Sherlock SJ. The estimation of hepatic blood flow and intrahepatic shunted blood flow by colloidal heat-denatured human serum albumin labelled with I-131. *Journal of Clinical Investigation* 1961, **40**: 1346–54.

Swinburne AJ, MacArthur CGC, Rhodes CG, Heather JD and Hughes JMB. Measurement of lung water in dog lobes using inhaled $C^{15}O_2$ and $H_2^{15}O$. *Journal of Applied Physiology* 1982; **52**: 1535–44.

3 Measurement of blood flow

Introduction

The relationship between pressure, flow and resistance in the vasculature is the same as that between voltage, current and resistance in Ohm's law, i.e. pressure = flow × resistance. The regulation of blood flow and blood volume is discussed in Section 7.2. The cardiac pump maintains a total resting flow of about 5 litres/min distributed to the major systems of the body as listed in Table 3.1. Blood flow to an organ can be expressed in several different ways; firstly, as blood flow itself, with units of ml/min. Secondly, as perfusion which takes account of the size of the organ, expressed as ml/min/ml of tissue or ml/min/g of tissue, and thirdly, in a unitless form, as a fraction of the cardiac output. There are many descriptions in nuclear medicine of blood flow indices which are often unitless and share the general features of having no physiological definition. No attempt is made to describe these techniques in this chapter. Rather, the several physiological principles upon which blood flow measurement in specific vascular beds may be based will be considered in turn.

3.1 Fick principle

The Fick principle states that when an indicator is introduced into a system it must be subject to the conservation of matter within the system, or, in the usual nuclear medicine setting, the rate of change of organ content of a tracer M_τ is equal to the difference between the organ input and output rates of the tracer. For example, if tracer leaves the organ only through venous outflow, then the arterio–venous concentration difference $(C_a - C_v)$ in the blood flowing through the organ bed multiplied by the blood flow Q is equal to the rate of tracer removal into the organ:

$$\frac{dM_\tau}{dt} = Q(C_a - C_v) \tag{3.1}$$

with units

$$\frac{mg}{min} = \frac{ml}{min} \times \frac{mg}{ml}.$$

If C_a, C_v and dM_τ/dt are known, Q can be calculated in ml/min. If tracer leaves the organ by another route, in addition to venous outflow, at a rate Y, then

$$\frac{dM_\tau}{dt} = Q(C_a - C_v) - Y. \tag{3.2}$$

Organ	Blood flow (ml/min.)	Cardiac output (%)	Weight (kg)	Perfusion (ml/100 g/min.)
Brain	750	14	1.40	55
Heart	300	5	0.33	90
Kidneys	1200	22	0.31	400
Liver	1400	25	1.80	80
(Spleen)	(200)	(5)	0.18	110
(Intestine)	(1200)	(20)	1.00	120
Muscle	1100	20	28.00	4
Skin	200	4	2.60	8
Skeleton	500	9	10.00	5

Table 3.1   Blood flow to the major organs

When equilibrium is reached during continuous infusion of tracer, $dM_\tau/dt = 0$, and

$$Q(C_a - C_v) = Y. \qquad (3.3)$$

If Y is known, then Q is obtainable from the arterio–venous gradient across the organ. If no other organ removes the tracer, then, at equilibrium, the infusion rate can be assumed to be equal to Y. Furthermore C_a can be assumed to be equal to C_v and obtained from a peripheral venous sample.

An example of the Fick principle, applying equation 3.3, for the measurement of blood flow at steady state is the use of an organic anion such as bromo-sulphthalein (BSP) for the measurement of liver blood flow (Section 9.4.1.1). Measurement of the hepatic venous concentration of BSP requires hepatic venous catheterization. Since BSP is removed only by the liver and then excreted in the bile, the infusion rate of BSP at equilibrium can be assumed to be equal to the rate of hepatic BSP uptake (to Y, equation 3.3), and the arterial and peripheral venous BSP concentrations assumed to be equal. The value of C_a can therefore be estimated by measuring the BSP concentration in a peripheral venous sample taken from the arm opposite to the one infused.

The relevance of the Fick principle to nuclear medicine is that it provides the basis of several important general tracer techniques for blood flow measurement, including both steady state and non-steady-state situations.

3.1.1 Inert gas washout

3.1.1.1 Bolus injection

An example of the Fick principle applied to a non-steady state situation is measurement of organ blood flow using radioactive inert gases (Kety 1951), the best known of which is xenon-133. Following injection as a bolus into an artery supplying an organ, the gas rapidly becomes distributed throughout the tissues of the organ, including the intracellular space, because of its high lipophilicity. Mixing is so rapid that equilibrium between intravascular and extravascular spaces is achieved during a single capillary transit; i.e. xenon-133 concentration in blood at the distal end of the capillary is equal to that in the extravascular space of the tissue (**Fig. 3.1**). The gas is subsequently washed out by incoming blood, free of xenon-133, and again equilibrium is established by the time the blood reaches the distal end of the capillary. This free and rapid diffusibility is an important general property of so-called blood flow tracers, the tissue uptake of which is termed 'blood flow' or 'perfusion' dependent.

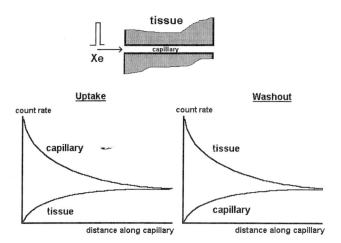

∎ **Fig. 3.1** Perfusion-dependent uptake of a tracer. When the vascular and the extravascular concentrations of a tracer equalize within a tissue at a point proximal to the end of the capillary, the transfer of the tracer between vascular and tissue spaces can be called perfusion dependent. Xenon-133 gives an example of this and as such can be used to measure tissue perfusion. If perfusion is very high however equilibrium may not be reached and, as a result, tracer washout underestimates perfusion.

Using the Fick principle and equation 3.1,

$$\frac{dM_\tau}{dt} = Q(C_a - C_v)$$

where M_τ is the quantity of xenon-133 remaining in the organ following deposition by intra-arterial injection. As it is relatively insoluble in aqueous solution, xenon-133 is almost completely removed in one circulation through the lung where it enters the alveolar air and is ultimately expired. Since there is no recirculation, C_a is essentially zero and

$$\frac{dM_\tau}{dt} = -Q \cdot C_v \qquad (3.4)$$

(note the minus sign, which indicates that the quantity of Xenon-133 in the organ is decreasing). Because equilibrium is established between the blood and tissue, C_v would also be the concentration (C_τ) of xenon-133 throughout the organ if the tracer had the same solubility in tissue and blood (see below), so that

$$C_v = \frac{M_\tau}{V} = C_\tau \qquad (3.5)$$

where V is organ volume. From equations 3.4 and 3.5,

$$\frac{dM_\tau}{dt} = -\frac{Q}{V} \cdot M_\tau. \qquad (3.6)$$

Equation 3.6 states that the rate of decrease in the quantity of xenon-133 is proportional to the quantity present. This is the standard equation seen in Section 1.2.3 in which the rate of change of a quantity is proportional to that quantity itself and represents a mono-exponential decrease with a rate constant equal to Q/V; i.e.

$$M_\tau(t) = M_\tau(0) \cdot e^{-[Q/V]t}. \qquad (3.7)$$

Here Q/V is the organ perfusion, with units of ml/min/ml, or min^{-1}, rather than absolute flow. Xenon-133 washout can therefore be regarded as a technique for measuring mean transit time through the organ. An important factor which affects this transit time is the solubility of xenon-133 in the tissue, which, in turn, largely depends on the lipid content of the tissue (since xenon-133 is so highly lipid soluble). If this is the same as the lipid content of the perfusing blood, then, volume for volume, xenon would partition itself equally between tissue and blood and the partition coefficient would be

unity. However, the partition coefficient λ exceeds unity in tissues with a high lipid content, such as the brain. The xenon therefore tends to be retained and the rate constant of washout is less than expected from tissue perfusion. λ is less than unity in most other tissues, including liver and muscle, because of the greater lipid content of the cell membranes of the erythrocytes of the circulating blood (Conn 1961). For this reason, λ also varies with haematocrit. Equations 3.5 to 3.7 therefore require insertion of the partition coefficient λ defined as:

$$\lambda = \frac{C_\tau}{C_V} \qquad (3.8)$$

where C_τ is the tissue gas concentration and is equal to M_τ/V. Therefore, if α is the rate constant of xenon-133 washout, then for tissues in which $\lambda = 1$, $Q/V = \alpha$. Otherwise,

$$\frac{Q}{V} = \alpha\lambda$$

and

$$\alpha = \frac{Q}{\lambda V}. \qquad (3.9)$$

The quantity λV is sometimes called the *effective volume of distribution* of the gas. Another term often seen in 3.9 is the density ρ of the tissue. This is introduced in order to express perfusion in the conventional units of ml/g/min. As ρ is close to unity for most tissues (except for bone and high lipid-containing tissues such as white matter of the brain), perfusion expressed as ml/min/ml is almost the same. The precise identity of V is not obvious. Is it confined to the extravascular volume of the organ or does it include the blood volume of the organ? It is, in fact, a volume intermediate between them. If equilibrium of xenon-133 between tissue and blood was reached (instantaneously) at the proximal end of the capillary then V would include all of the blood volume, scaled by the partition coefficient. That is

$$V = \frac{Q}{\alpha\lambda} = V_e + \frac{V_i}{\lambda} \qquad (3.10)$$

where e and i refer to extravascular and intravascular respectively. In fact, the capillary concentration of xenon-133 rises with distance along the capillary, equilibrating with the extravascular concentration downstream. Then V becomes less than actual total volume depending on how far down the capillary equilibration is reached (**Fig. 3.2**) and

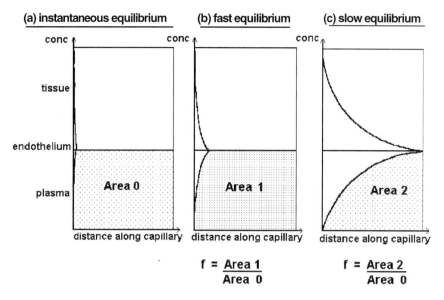

(a) instantaneous equilibrium   **(b) fast equilibrium**   **(c) slow equilibrium**

$$f = \frac{\text{Area 1}}{\text{Area 0}} \qquad f = \frac{\text{Area 2}}{\text{Area 0}}$$

∎ **Fig. 3.2**   The volume included in '*V*' when measuring Q/V with an inert gas (e.g. Xenon-133). If equilibrium was instantaneous between gas-free incoming blood and gas-loaded tissue, as in (a), then V would include tissue blood volume. With equilibrium established at increasing distances along the capillary, as in (b) correspondingly less of the blood volume is included in V. As the gas may have a different solubility in tissue compared with blood, the partition coefficient also influences the precise identity of V. The fraction of the tissue blood volume included in V is proportional to $\text{Area}_1/\text{Area}_0$ in (b) and $\text{Area}_2/\text{Area}_0$ in (c).

$$V = V_e + fV_i/\lambda \qquad (3.11)$$

where f is a scaling factor which depends on the timing of equilibration. (Although separate measurement of organ blood volume is often performed in quantitative PET, it is not attempted with the inert gas technique based on single photon detection.)

Inert gas washout curves are seldom mono-exponential and are more often multi-exponential (**Fig. 3.3**). The number of exponentials into which the washout curve can be confidently resolved varies with the quality of the measurements available for each organ i.e. the adequacy of sampling of each component of the washout curve. For instance, there are usually two in cerebral washout curves recorded after injection of xenon-133 into the internal carotid artery (Section 12.1.1.1), and up to four in renal washout curves (Section 11.1.1.2). The literature is inconsistent for the liver with one, two or three exponentials described by various authors. Each exponential has generally been interpreted to represent washout from a distinct anatomical sub-structure of the organ. The two exponentials for the brain, for example, are considered to represent washout rates from the grey and white matter,

respectively. Analysis of the washout curve into its exponential components by curve peeling (Section 1.3.3), enables separate measurement of perfusion in each sub-compartment, provided the exponentials

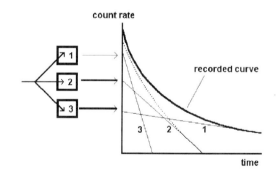

∎ **Fig. 3.3**   The washout curve recorded by an external detector following injection of a radioactive inert gas into an organ that comprises 3 parallel 'compartments' with different perfusions. The curve is the summation of 3 different exponentials. These can be resolved by 'curve stripping'; the relative sizes of the zero-time values (intercepts) are dependent on the relative *absolute* blood flow to each compartment as a result of fractionation of the incoming gas by the blood supply to the compartments.

are very different. The zero time intercepts of the exponentials should reflect the relative fractions of the arterial inflow serving each compartment. This interpretation of a multi-exponential washout curve is almost certainly an over-simplification, and other factors are probably important (Section 9.4.1.5).

Mean perfusion (i.e. total flow/total volume) in organs from which multi-exponential washout curves are recorded can be obtained in a number of ways. One approach is to divide the initial height of the curve by the total area enclosed under it (Zierler 1965). It will be recalled from Chapter 2 that mean transit time is obtained by dividing the area under a residue curve by its initial height. So, if we perform the reciprocal of this and divide the height by the area, we obtain the reciprocal of the mean transit time or the reciprocal of the mean residence time, which is $Q/\lambda V$ (ml/min/ml or min.$^{-1}$). If the compartments representing the separate components of the washout curve have different partition coefficients (for example, the brain), then a 'weighted' mean value should be used (see Question 14.5).

The area under any curve or graph has units which are the product of the x-and y-axis units. So the ratio of area under the curve to its initial height must have the same unit as the x-axis (time, in the case of the xenon washout curve) since the y-axis units cancel out. The height over area technique is essentially a calculation of mean residence or transit time. As shown in Section 1.2.4, the area under an exponential curve is equal to the zero time intercept divided by the rate constant. In principle, it does not matter, therefore, how many exponentials are present in a washout curve as long as the slowest can be identified. At some time t when the washout curve has been reduced to a single exponential with a quantity $Q(t)$ of xenon-133 remaining, the area beyond t is $Q(t)$ divided by α, where α is the rate constant of this slowest exponential. The area up to t, measured directly by summating all the counts recorded up to t, can then be added to the area under the tail (i.e. from t) to give the total area (**Fig. 3.4**). This approach is also used in the measurement of cardiac output by indicator dilution (Section 7.2.1).

Other approaches to mean perfusion include, firstly, measurement of the maximum gradient of the downslope of the washout curve and, secondly, the weighted harmonic mean (whm) of the perfusion of

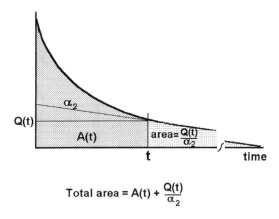

$$\text{Total area} = A(t) + \frac{Q(t)}{\alpha_2}$$

▌ **Fig. 3.4** It is usually not possible to monitor a washout curve until effectively *all* the radioactively has been washed out. If monitoring is continued until time t when the curve has reached its terminal exponential, then the area from t is $Q(t)$ divided by the rate constant of the terminal exponential (α_2).

the separate compartments. The maximum slope is difficult to define but gives a reasonable estimate of mean perfusion and is relatively simple to measure. The whm is defined as follows for an organ with two compartments, giving a bi-exponential washout with respective intercepts $M_1(0)$ and $M_2(0)$, and rate constants α_1 and α_2;

$$\text{whm} = \frac{M_1(0) + M_2(0)}{M_1(0)/\alpha_1 + M_2(0)/\alpha_2}. \tag{3.12}$$

With more components we have to introduce more M terms; i.e. M_3, M_4, and so on. It can be seen from equation 3.12, that the numerator is the sum of the initial heights of each of the individual exponentials, while the denominator is the sum of their enclosed areas. So whm is essentially the same as total height over area, as described above.

A feature of xenon-133 washout curves which results in a difference in mean perfusion measured from height over area on the one hand and from the rate constant of the initial slope or weighted harmonic mean on the other, is the brief plateau seen in the washout curve immediately following xenon-133 injection (**Fig. 3.5**). It is important to be aware of this plateau since it re-emphasizes that perfusion derived from the xenon-133 washout curve is based on xenon-133 transit time. The plateau, which lasts several seconds, represents the *minimum* transit time of the xenon-133 through the organ. This minimum transit time is ignored by

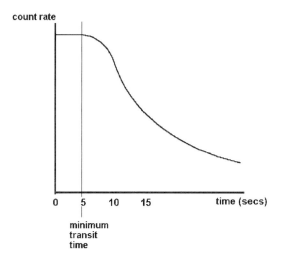

count rate

0   5   10   15   time (secs)

minimum
transit
time

▌ **Fig. 3.5** Since the inert gas washout technique effectively measures transit times, there must be a minimum transit time defined by those molecules which exit the organ first and which is the minimum *intravascular* transit time. This explains why the washout curve has a brief plateau at the beginning. Mean perfusion can be calculated as initial height divided by total area or as the maximum slope of the curve.

the whm and maximum washout slope techniques, which therefore give a higher value for perfusion than height over area. Since, in the height over area approach, V includes the organ's blood volume, the mean transit time through the whole distribution volume is genuinely measured by this technique. In effect, the other two techniques, because they rely on simple compartmental analysis (without a delay compartment), assume instantaneous mixing of the tracer throughout its volume of distribution within the organ as soon as it enters via the afferent vessel. The volume of distribution is effectively underestimated by the limitations imposed by the requirements for equilibration.

One of the major sources of uncertainty associated with the inert gas technique of blood flow measurement is knowledge of the value of the partition coefficient and its variation in disease. It must not be forgotten that the inert gas method primarily measures mean transit time of the tracer. This is heavily influenced by the lipid content of the static (tissue) and moving (blood) phases, and hence by the xenon-133 solubility, so that the washout rate depends not only on perfusion but also on a competition, largely determined by lipid distribution, for xenon-133 between the two phases.

The principal practical drawback of the inert gas washout technique is its requirement for intra-arterial injection, making it an invasive procedure. Nonetheless there is scope for application of the technique in the angiography theatre where, following advances in interventional radiology, the technique has potential value (Kennedy *et al.* 1995).

Most xenon-133 arriving in the lung is extracted into the gaseous phase, although about 5% recirculates and this has been used as the basis of a non-invasive approach to measure blood flow. One technique is to rebreathe the xenon from a closed circuit for a short period and then to measure washout from the organ following 'switchover' to room air. The other is to give the xenon-133 intravenously and to utilize the 5% escaping extraction in the lung to give an adequate signal from the organ for measurement of the rate of washout. A complicating factor in these approaches is that the change in organ count rate will be influenced by the rate of washout from the lung. Thus, since alveolar xenon-133 is in equilibrium with pulmonary venous xenon-133, the arterial input into the organ will be a continuous function of the alveolar xenon-133 concentration. Furthermore, although xenon-133 is rapidly expired, the alveolar concentration is maintained by recirculation to the lungs from all tissues of the body. It is therefore necessary to monitor the time course of radioactivity in the lungs with a separate probe and use deconvolution analysis to correct for the continuing input of tracer into the organ of interest. This approach has been developed particularly for measuring cerebral blood flow, for which it works well because the cranial probes may be placed well away from high radioactivity signal arising from the lungs (Section 12.1.1.1).

3.1.1.2 Steady state

Another inert gas for measuring blood flow is krypton-81m (Turner *et al.* 1976). There are several radioactive isotopes of krypton including the long half-life inert gas, krypton-85. Krypton-81m however has a very short physical half-life of 13 seconds, which requires modification to the theory of the gas washout technique. The rate of change of activity within the tissue is equal to inflow rate minus outflow rate (Fick principle). The outflow rate is the sum of the rate of gas washout by flowing blood *plus* the rate of loss by radionuclide decay (defined by the decay constant δ). That is

$$\frac{dM_\tau}{dt} = QC_a - (QC_v + M_\tau \cdot \delta) \qquad (3.13)$$

(M_τ has units MBq, δ has units min^{-1}, so $M_\tau.\delta$ has units of MBq min^{-1}). The quantity of gas in the tissue M_τ is the product of tissue gas concentration C_τ and tissue volume V. Furthermore, since equilibrium is established between tissue and blood, i.e. $\lambda C_V = C_\tau$,

$$\frac{dM_\tau}{dt} = QC_a - \frac{QC_\tau}{\lambda} - VC_\tau\delta. \qquad (3.14)$$

When the tracer is administered by continuous intra-arterial infusion, a steady state is quickly reached because of the high decay constant, whereupon

$$dM_\tau/dt = 0.$$

Therefore

$$QC_a = Q\frac{C_\tau}{\lambda} + VC_\tau\delta$$
$$= C_\tau(Q/\lambda + V\delta). \qquad (3.15)$$

Re-arranging

$$\frac{C_\tau}{C_a} = \frac{Q}{Q/\lambda + V\delta}$$

and dividing on the right by V

$$\frac{C_\tau}{C_a} = \frac{Q/V}{\dfrac{Q}{\lambda V} + \delta}. \qquad (3.16)$$

Therefore the radioactivity signal at equilibrium, which is represented by C_τ, will be proportional to Q/V and inversely proportional to the sum of perfusion and the decay rate constant, both of which have units, like the numerator, of min^{-1}. The arterial concentration C_a is proportional to the rate of krypton-81m infusion. For tissues with a relatively low perfusion, such as resting muscle and skin, $Q/\lambda V$ (about 0.05 min^{-1}) is negligible compared with δ (3.2 min^{-1}). The term $Q/\lambda V$ in the denominator of equation 3.16 can therefore be ignored, so the count rate is proportional to tissue perfusion. On the other hand, for well-perfused tissues, such as the kidney ($Q/\lambda V = 3$ min^{-1}) and to a lesser extent the liver (1 min^{-1}) and brain (0.5 min^{-1}), perfusion is of the same order of magnitude as the decay rate constant and so the count rate detected can only be said to be 'weighted' by blood flow. Indeed, at very high rates of perfusion, $Q/\lambda V$ becomes larger than δ and C_τ/C_a

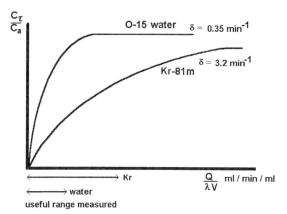

∎ **Fig. 3.6** The relationship between the steady-state tissue signal (expressed in relation to the arterial concentration) and tissue perfusion for two tracers which display perfusion-dependent uptake: oxygen-15 labelled water and krypton-81m (given by continuous infusion; inhalation of CO_2-15 for water and arterial for krypton). Krypton covers a wider range than water because its physical decay rate (δ) is faster.

approaches $(Q/V)/(Q/V\lambda)$ or λ (**Fig. 3.6**). Nevertheless, using the gamma camera, the technique of continuous krypton-81m infusion elegantly demonstrates regional differences in perfusion within a vascular bed. The reader should refer to Section 3.1.3.1 for the use of labelled water for blood flow measurement and also to Section 8.1.1 where a similar set of equations is presented for the theory of imaging regional ventilation from continuous inhalation of krypton-81m.

3.1.2 Measurement of blood flow from clearance

Another important variation of the Fick principle in nuclear medicine is blood flow measurement based on the plasma clearance (as defined in Section 2.2) of a tracer taken up exclusively by a single organ with a high extraction efficiency. An example is para-amino hippurate clearance for measurement of effective renal plasma flow (ERPF; Section 11.1.1.1). Like clearance itself, blood flow based on clearance may be measured at steady state (an example of which, BSP clearance, has already been described) or from blood disappearance following bolus injection. Blood flow may also be measured from organ clearance by quantitative dynamic imaging but the assumption of exclusive uptake does not apply.

3.1.2.1 Blood flow from blood disappearance of tracer following bolus injection

Consider tracer being removed from blood by a single organ, where M is the quantity of tracer in the organ, Q its blood flow and $C_a - C_v$ the arterio–venous concentration gradient across the organ at a specified time after injection: then, from the Fick principle,

$$\frac{\mathrm{d}M_\tau}{\mathrm{d}t} = Q(C_a - C_v)$$

(same as equation 3.1)

If the extraction efficiency is high (greater than 90%), C_v can be assumed to be negligible so

$$\frac{\mathrm{d}M_\tau}{\mathrm{d}t} = Q \cdot C_a \qquad (3.17)$$

Integrating and re-arranging

$$Q = \frac{M_\tau}{\int C_a(t) \cdot \mathrm{d}t}. \qquad (3.18)$$

If the arterial concentration is integrated to infinity, by which time all the tracer will have been taken up, $M_\tau(\infty)$ is the injected dose, and equation 3.18 can be re-stated:

$$Q = \frac{\text{injected dose}}{\text{total area under blood disappearance curve}}. \qquad (3.19)$$

The blood disappearance curve is conveniently based on peripheral venous samples rather than arterial samples, specified in equation 3.18. Therefore, *for tracers that enter the extravascular space,* antecubital venous sampling potentially introduces an error because of an arterio–venous concentration gradient across the forearm vascular bed (Rehling *et al.* 1989). Early on in the blood disappearance curve, C_a is greater than the concentration in antecubital venous blood because of net tracer movement into the forearm interstitial fluid, but this gradient subsequently reverses because of net tracer movement back into forearm plasma. Provided the curve starts from very early samples, the error is minimized as the underestimation of area early in the curve is balanced by a similar overestimation later on (**Fig. 3.7**).

For tracers confined to the intravascular space which mix instantaneously throughout their distribution volume and undergo removal into a single

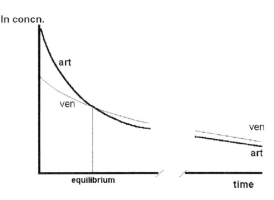

Fig. 3.7 Plasma disappearance curve: difference between arterial and venous sampling. For tracers like technetium-99m DTPA that distribute between the extravascular space and plasma, the antecubital venous curve is not identical to the arterial curve as a result of tracer entering the interstitial fluid of the vascular bed (forearm) drained by the sampled vein. Thus, up to about 15 minutes there is an A–V gradient which reverses after 20 minutes when a net efflux of tracer from the interstitial fluid is established. Nevertheless, because none of the tracer is *actively* retained in the extravascular space, the total areas under the two curves are identical and so provided sampling is started early enough the area under the venous curve can be applied to equation 3.19.

organ, the rate of uptake of tracer *remaining* in the blood M_b is

$$\frac{\mathrm{d}M_b}{\mathrm{d}t} = Q(C_v - C_a) \qquad (3.20)$$

where C_v is the concentration in venous blood draining the organ.

Assuming C_v is zero (i.e., that organ extraction fraction is unity), and substituting $V_b \cdot C_a$ for M_b, where V_b is the volume of distribution (i.e. blood volume),

$$V_b \cdot \frac{\mathrm{d}C_a}{\mathrm{d}t} = -Q \cdot C_a \qquad (3.21)$$

or

$$\frac{\mathrm{d}C_a}{\mathrm{d}t} = -\frac{Q}{V_b} C_a. \qquad (3.22)$$

(Note the minus sign, which indicates that arterial concentration is falling.) So, by analogy with equation 3.6,

$$C_a(t) = C_a(0) \cdot \mathrm{e}^{-[Q/V_b]t}. \qquad (3.23)$$

The blood concentration therefore decreases exponentially with a rate constant Q/V_b. Note here that V_b is *not* the volume of distribution of the tracer within the organ but the volume of distribution of the tracer before removal into the organ; i.e. it is not perfusion that is being measured but the fraction of V_b entering the organ in unit time. The only tracers mixing instantaneously within their volumes of distribution are those confined to the intravascular space. For example, equation 3.23 is applicable to labelled colloids for the measurement of liver blood flow, expressed as the fraction of the total blood volume entering the liver in unit time (Section 9.4.1.4). Since the zero time concentration $C_a(0)$ can be obtained by extrapolation of the disappearance curve, total blood volume can be obtained as [injected activity/$C_a(0)$].

Organ blood flow as a fraction of total blood volume per minute can be measured from more complex models using deconvolution or compartmental analysis. They are best dealt with in their appropriate sections. Examples include splenic blood flow measured with indium-111 labelled platelets (Section 10.1.2.1) and liver blood flow measured with organic anions (Section 9.4.1.1), both of which are based on compartmental analysis of a two compartmental model, and total skeletal blood flow measured with fluorine-18 using deconvolution analysis (Section 13.3.1.3).

3.1.2.2 Blood flow from organ uptake

As for the measurement of clearance, *individual* organ blood flow can be measured from the rate of uptake of a tracer, even if it is not the only organ removing the tracer. The principle is identical to measurement of clearance (Section 2.2.1.3), which is equal to blood flow if the assumption can be made that organ extraction efficiency is 100%. For example, individual kidney ERPF can be measured by quantification of the renal uptake of hippuran. This general approach is frequently used in PET with tracers, such as rubidium-82 (for myocardial blood flow, Section 7.1.1.2) and nitrogen-13 labelled ammonia (for hepatic arterial flow, Section 9.4.2.3 and for myocardial blood flow, Section 7.1.1.2). These agents are regarded as 'chemical microspheres'; i.e. as having extraction fractions of almost unity in several different organs.

Re-stating equation 3.1, $\dfrac{dM_\tau}{dt} = Q(C_a - C_v)$.

If extraction fraction is unity, then $C_v = 0$, and

$$\frac{dM_\tau}{dt} = Q \cdot C_a \qquad (3.24)$$

(note the similarity with equation 3.17).

Integrating

$$M_\tau = Q \int C_a(t) \cdot dt$$

and

$$Q = \frac{M_\tau}{\int C_a(t) \cdot dt}. \qquad (3.25)$$

So again we see the general equation, flow (or clearance) = mass/area, similarly to equation 2.36. Dividing both sides of equation 3.25 by tissue volume V leads to a similar equation for tissue perfusion

$$\frac{Q}{V} = \frac{C_\tau}{\int C_a(t) \cdot dt}. \qquad (3.26)$$

As will be seen later, equation 3.26 is important in measurement of blood flow using PET. Equations 3.25 and 3.26 can be tackled for the measurement of blood flow in the same ways as for measurement of clearance from organ uptake (Section 2.2.1.3), including Patlak–Rutland analysis.

A potential difficulty is that as perfusion (Q) increases, tracer extraction fraction (E) tends to decrease, invalidating equations 3.25 and 3.26 for blood flow. The relationship between Q and E is non-linear and based on an important physiological constant called the Crone–Renkin constant (Crone and Levitt 1984). This was originally applied to the extraction of tracers across the endothelium as the permeability (P)–surface area (S) product (see below, Section 2.4.1 and Section 6.2.2.1), but can be expanded to embrace the relationship between blood flow and the *steady-state* extraction fraction of tracer from plasma to organ parenchyma. We will therefore use the term *PS* product in its wider sense. As will be shown later (Section 6.2.2.1), E and *PS* are related according to the equation

$$E = 1 - e^{-(PS)/Q}. \qquad (3.27)$$

From Table 3.2, showing the relationship between E and Q for various values of *PS*, it may be seen that as the perfusion Q rises, the product $Q \cdot E$ (the clearance Z) fails to rise as fast. Therefore Z is likely to be underestimated by chemical 'microspheres' at high flow rates. If *PS* is known for a given tissue, blood

PS	Q	QE(=Z)
0.1	1	0.095
	100	0.1
1	1	0.63
	100	1
10	1	1
	100	9.5

■ Table 3.2

flow can be measured without having to assume that E approaches a value of 1, since equation 3.25 can be re-stated for clearance (equation 2.36):

$$Q \cdot E = \frac{M_\tau}{\int C_a(t) \cdot dt} \qquad (3.28)$$

and combined with equation 3.27 as simultaneous equations for the separate calculation of Q and E.

3.1.3 Measurement of blood flow by PET

Using compartmental models that are reasonably consistent with physiological systems, PET is a powerful technique for measuring organ blood flow because of its ability to quantify tissue tracer concentrations within tomograhic slices. It depends on the ability to correct for photon attenuation through different amounts of tissue. This correction is not easily available for counting or imaging with single photon emitters. The principles of the kinetic analysis are the same as in single photon work, except that models tend to be more complex and *restricted to the tissue under study*. Thus, in PET modelling, the compartments represent different 'spaces' or volumes within the tissue of interest. In the compartmental models used in single photon imaging for, say, measurement of liver blood flow from plasma colloid clearance, or measurement of glomerular filtration rate from technetium-99m-DTPA plasma clearance, the compartments represent the entire plasma volume, extracellular fluid volume and organ. In fact, because of the way in which PET measures tissue tracer *concentration*, and is seldom concerned with *absolute* amounts of tracer, PET techniques generate blood flow, clearance and substrate utilisation rates in relation to tissue volume or mass, i.e. as ml/min/ml, ml/min/g or mg/min/g. Because of instrumental factors such as resolution in

three dimensions, of the order of 5–10 mm, there is a limit in the accuracy to which volumes and therefore concentrations and masses can be determined.

Analysis of PET data is, in principle, similar to any other tracer kinetic analysis. For example, consider xenon-133 for perfusion measurement. After bolus injection into an artery, xenon-133 is washed out of a tissue at a rate proportional to tissue perfusion. A simple compartmental model is formulated with a differential equation describing the rate of change of tissue concentration in the compartment. With a simple model, the differential equation can be readily solved to produce an equation which describes the moment-to-moment concentration of xenon-133 in each compartment. This is what is also performed in PET modelling. Thus, for whatever model, and into whatever compartment the PET tracer might be directly and instantaneously deposited, the equations expressing the rate of change of tissue concentration can be described. For example, if a PET tracer was injected into an artery supplying an organ which could be modelled as shown in **Fig. 3.8c**, then it would first enter compartment 1. Some would then leave the organ via the venous outflow without entering compartment 2, while some would enter compartment 2. Tracer in compartment 2 might then become trapped in compartment 3, or re-enter compartment 1, and so on. A multi-exponential washout curve from the organ would result, with units of tissue concentration versus time and with an asymptote reflecting the ultimate retention of tracer in compartment 3. Using computerized techniques, several hypothetical curves, all consistent with the model, can be generated. From the one that best 'fits' the recorded curve, best-fit values for the model rate constants (and, secondarily, the volumes of the spaces represented by each compartment) can be generated. Now imagine the tracer being given intravenously. The tissue curve recorded would be influenced by the form of the arterial time–concentration curve, i.e. the shape of the input function. In addition to compartmental analysis, PET techniques, therefore, also use deconvolution analysis in order to derive impulse response curves from which the various parameters of the model can be derived.

The commonest models used in PET are illustrated in **Fig. 3.8** (a–c). The simplest of these is applied to tissue perfusion measurement using

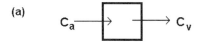

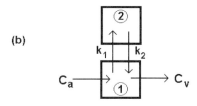

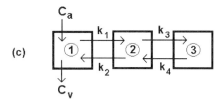

▌ **Fig. 3.8** Models of increasing complexity used in quantitative PET. (a) Simple model used as basis for measurement of tissue perfusion with oxygen-15 labelled water. Because water is highly diffusible between all compartments of the tissues, the latter can be represented by one compartment. (b) More complex model used as basis for measurement of myocardial perfusion with tracers that are freely diffusible between plasma and interstitial fluid (represented by compartment 1) but may be trapped intercellularly (compartment 2). (c) Complex model used as basis for kinetic studies (e.g. fluorine-18 in bone) in which tracer exchanges between plasma and interstitial fluid (compartments 1 and 2) and at the same time enters bone crystal (compartment 3) from which it may or may not return to interstitial fluid.

oxygen-15 labelled water. The tissue can be modelled as a single compartment because water is freely diffusible throughout the spaces — blood, interstitial fluid and intracellular fluid — i.e. it behaves like xenon-133.

3.1.3.1 Positron labelled water

Measurement of perfusion using the positron camera and oxygen-15 labelled water is similar in principle to the inert gas washout technique. Water diffuses across capillary endothelium and cell membranes very rapidly, and, like the inert gases, is almost 100% extracted and equilibrates between tissue and plasma during a single capillary transit. Its uptake into tissue, like the inert gases, is limited by blood

flow rather than by diffusion. As oxygen-15 has a short half-life of 2 min, the similarity with the inert gas technique, in particular with krypton-81m, can be further extended. Thus, using labelled water, blood flow can be measured at steady state because the physical decay rate of the radionuclide, oxygen-15, is sufficiently rapid that radionuclide life span is comparable to the residence time of water in the tissues. Oxygen-15 labelled water can also be given by bolus injection and so used, in essence, like a bolus injection of xenon-133.

3.1.3.1.1 Continuous infusion

The patient receives a continuous intravenous infusion of oxygen-15 labelled water or continuously inhales oxygen-15 labelled carbon dioxide. Under the influence of pulmonary carbonic anhydrase, inhaled carbon dioxide is rapidly converted into labelled water within the lung vascular bed. With either method, the labelled water is delivered continuously at a constant concentration to all the tissues of the body. At equilibrium, when the signal from the organ becomes constant, an equation relating tissue perfusion to tissue concentration of radioactivity can be developed which is identical to that used for krypton-81m (Section 3.1.1.2), i.e.

$$\frac{C_\tau}{C_a} = \frac{Q/V}{\dfrac{Q}{\lambda V} + \delta}$$

which can be rearranged for Q/V:

$$\frac{Q}{V} = \frac{\delta C_\tau}{C_a - C_\tau/\lambda}. \qquad (3.29)$$

So perfusion can be calculated if the arterial and tissue concentrations and the constants λ and δ are known. Since the water content of tissues may vary, it is difficult to estimate λ, which may change in disease. Using PET, the tissue concentration can be quantified in absolute units from three-dimensional images, thereby allowing measurement of regional C_τ. An arterial blood sample is needed for C_a, unless a region of interest can be placed over the cardiac chambers or a large artery when C_a can be measured from the image, in which case a constant γ which relates tracer concentration to recorded count rate N can be introduced into equation 3.29; i.e.

$$\frac{Q}{V} = \frac{\delta \cdot \gamma \cdot N_\tau}{\gamma [N_a - (N_\tau/\lambda)]}. \qquad (3.30)$$

Since γ cancels out, organ perfusion can be obtained from the count rates/pixel respectively recorded from the organ (N_τ) and an arterial region (N_a).

Equation 3.30 reinforces the important concept of expressing variables as ratios in quantitative nuclear medicine (Section 2.5). In this case, Q/V, the reciprocal of mean transit time, can be obtained from count rates without requiring absolute quantification of radioactivity. Nevertheless the value of quantitative PET is that the count rates from different regions of tissue bear the same proportionality constant γ to their respective tracer concentrations. This is because tissue attenuation effects can be corrected. In planar scintigraphy and in SPECT, however, attenuation effects are only partially corrected and γ does not necessarily cancel out, as in equation 3.30. So, for quantification of tissue blood flow, whereas PET is almost always based on quantification of tissue tracer concentration, planar scintigraphy is based on a diversity of approaches, including blood and organ clearance rates, organ uptake rates, quantification of absolute *total* organ tracer content, dilution measurements and direct transit time measurements. This also explains why physiological variables determined by PET are almost always expressed in relation to organ volume; e.g. in the case of blood flow, as perfusion rather than total, or absolute, flow.

As with krypton-81m, the relationship between C_τ and $Q/\lambda V$ for oxygen-15 labelled water is almost linear for values of $Q/\lambda V$ that are small compared with δ, since, under these circumstances, the denominator of equation 3.29 reduces to δ and

$$\frac{C_\tau}{C_a} = \frac{Q}{V} \times \frac{1}{\delta}. \qquad (3.31)$$

For higher values of $Q/\lambda V$ on the other hand, δ becomes small compared with Q/V, which ultimately cancels out in equation 3.29, leaving:

$$C_\tau / C_a = \lambda. \qquad (3.32)$$

For krypton-81m, with a half-life of 13 seconds, δ has a value of 3.2 min^{-1}, about 9 times that of Oxygen-15, 0.35 min^{-1}. Figure 3.6 compares the respective relationships between C_τ/C_a and $Q/\lambda V$ for these two agents and shows that for tissues with high perfusion rates (such as the kidney in which $Q/\lambda V$ is approximately 3.0 min^{-1}) C_τ/C_a is rather insensitive to changes in $Q/\lambda V$, particularly for labelled water, and ultimately approaches the value of the partition coefficient λ. For xenon-133, δ is essentially zero, so

at steady state C_τ/C_a is equal to λ for all values of perfusion. Thus the xenon-133 signal at equilibrium depends on the tissue solubility of xenon-133.

By multiplying both sides of equation 3.29 by V, we obtain an expression for M_τ, the total quantity of radioactivity in the organ.

$$\frac{M_\tau}{C_a} = \frac{Q}{\frac{Q}{\lambda V} + \delta}. \qquad (3.33)$$

Nevertheless, the denominator on the right still includes perfusion, Q/V, so perfusion still determines the shape of the relationship between total radioactivity in the organ and absolute blood flow (ml/min). Although, on account of its longer half life, oxygen-15 is apparently at a disadvantage compared with krypton-81m, it has the advantage, as a positron emitter, of being amenable to quantification by PET, i.e. C_τ can measured. Krypton-81m, on the other hand, gives information only on *relative* distribution of blood flow. Because it is a steady-state situation, it is possible to perform SPECT with krypton-81m, but quantification of blood flow is not possible because of unknown attenuation effects.

3.1.3.1.2 Bolus injection

Positron-emitting labelled water can be given intravenously for measurement of perfusion because, unlike the inert gases, it is not trapped in the lung (**Fig. 3.8a**). The theory, following bolus injection, has to be modified in comparison with xenon-133 washout since the labelled water recirculates, and also decays rapidly (Bergmann *et al.* 1989). However it is easier to understand the mathematics of the technique if the fast decay constant is, for the time being, ignored. This is acceptable because unlike the continuous infusion approach, the fast physical decay rate is not fundamental to the theory of the bolus injection technique. Obviously the raw data would have to be corrected for physical decay, but this can be treated as a separate operation.

In the simplest analysis, oxygen-15 labelled water can be treated theoretically like xenon-133 since its washout rate is proportional to tissue perfusion. Thus after administration by intra-arterial injection into an extremity, for example, recirculation can be accounted for by subtracting the time–activity curve recorded from the opposite limb, and limb perfusion calculated in exactly the same way as for xenon. For most tissues, it is not possible to adopt this simple approach to recirculation, which instead has to be approached with more complex mathematical techniques, such as deconvolution analysis. If the water was completely extracted in a tissue, then the concentration C_τ in the tissue would be given by re-arrangement of equation 3.26

$$C_\tau = \frac{Q}{V} \int C_a(t) \cdot dt. \qquad (3.34)$$

However the tissue signal is modified by continuous washout of labelled water from the tissue, at a rate governed by the rate constant $Q/\lambda V$ (**Fig. 3.8a**), and then by recirculation of radioactivity. The time course of C_τ is therefore a function of the arterial input *convolved* (Section 1.5) on the washout rate, and is given by

$$C_\tau = \frac{Q}{V} \int C_a(t)^* e^{-[Q/\lambda V]t} \cdot dt. \qquad (3.35)$$

The symbol * denotes the operation of convolution, which is the reverse of deconvolution. Deconvolution analysis generates a tissue time–activity curve which represents the tissue washout curve that would be obtained following bolus injection of tracer into an artery supplying the tissue and from which Q/V can be calculated, analogously to a xenon-133 washout curve. Remember that for water, λ is determined by relative water content between tissue and blood, while for xenon, λ is determined by relative lipid content.

Instead of taking an 'instantaneous' image of C_τ at time t, an image is acquired continuously over a period of time t from injection in order to improve statistical accuracy. Acquisition of an image itself represents integration (i.e. integration of the counts recorded over time t) and this leads to the formulation of equation 3.36, a double integral which, when re-arranged, can be written for Q/V;

$$\frac{Q}{V} = \frac{\int C_\tau(t) \cdot dt}{\int [\int C_a(t)^* e^{-[Q/\lambda V]t} \cdot dt] dt} \qquad (3.36)$$

The principle of double integration is illustrated in Fig. 12.4. Although at first sight a complicated process, double integrations are performed quite routinely in nuclear medicine, for example, in quantification of differential renal function from renography, in which the function of the kidney is based on an image acquired up to 3 min after injection (Section 11.1.2.2). Thus the amount of tracer $M(t)$ accumulated in the kidney up to time t is

a function of the integrated arterial activity; the image acquired of the kidney is then an integral of all the values $M(t)$. In other words, the image itself is a function of a double integral of the arterial activity, just as in equation 3.36.

The concentrations C_a and C_τ can be measured by PET (either in absolute units of concentration or, if the slice includes an arterial blood region, as a count rate per pixel as in equation 3.30), from which Q/V can be obtained. An advantage of the bolus technique, compared with the continuous infusion technique, is that it is applicable to tissues with high perfusion (**Fig. 3.6**).

3.1.3.2 Non-linear regression analysis

Another approach for measuring blood flow using PET, which in principle is the same as the deconvolution approach above, is to use a technique called, rather inappropriately, non-linear regression analysis. Equation 3.14 gives

$$\frac{dM_\tau}{dt} = Q(C_a - \frac{C_\tau}{\lambda}) - V\delta C_\tau$$

and dividing by V

$$\frac{dC_\tau}{dt} = \frac{Q}{V}(C_a - \frac{C_\tau}{\lambda}) - \delta C_\tau. \qquad (3.37)$$

Non-linear regression analysis is then be used to generate Q/V from continuous measurements (i.e. curves) of C_a and C_τ. The principle of the technique is to first make a realistic guess of Q/V and then to convolve it on the recorded arterial concentration time curve, C_a vs. t. The tissue curve resulting from this convolution is then compared with the recorded tissue curve, C_τ vs. t. If the fit is acceptable using a least-squares criterion, Q/V is accepted; if not, another value of Q/V is tried and so on until the best fit, defined as that which gives the lowest sum of squared deviations (see Section 1.3.1.1), is obtained. The technique is therefore perhaps more appropriately termed non-linear least-squares iteration.

Non-linear regression analysis or non-linear least-squares iteration can be applied to more complex models, as shown in Fig. 3.8b, and tracers other than water. The model shown in Fig. 3.8b is used to represent the kinetics of tracers which rapidly and freely diffuse between plasma and interstitial fluid but which, at the same time, have a certain probability of being metabolically trapped in the tissue, for example nitrogen-13 ammonia (Schelbert *et al.* 1981). The trapped tracer is represented by the second compartment in the model. In the case of ammonia, aminated derivatives may diffuse out of the trapped compartment, hence the inclusion of rate constant, k_2 (**Fig. 3.8b**). The model also applies to tracers like rubidium-82 (Goldstein *et al.* 1983) which can be regarded as diffusible tracers with respect to exchange between plasma and interstitial fluid, while the second compartment represents intracellular rubidium maintained by the sodium/potassium pump. Rubidium-82 slowly diffuses out of the intracellular compartment and so k_2 also applies, although for short-duration dynamic studies, this diffusion can be ignored and k_2 assumed to be zero.

A set of differential equations defining this model can be described as in Section 1.4. Each equation defines the individual fluxes into and out of the compartment. Assuming that k_2 is zero and ignoring radionuclide physical decay, the rate of change of tissue tracer concentration in compartment 1, where the tracer is 'free', is given by the difference between (i) input rate and (ii) the sum of output rates with respect to the compartment:

$$\frac{dM_f}{dt} = Q \cdot C_a - (k_1 \cdot C_f + Q \cdot C_v) \qquad (3.38)$$

where k_1 is a proportionality constant, with the same units as Q, relating the concentration C_f of free-tracer in compartment 1 to the flux into compartment 2, and is equivalent to the *PS* product at the interface between the compartments per unit of tissue volume.[†]

A further assumption that can be made is that, since the tracer behaves as a freely diffusible tracer, the venous outflow concentration C_v is equal to the concentration C_f in the free compartment (λ is usually assumed to be unity.) This is analogous to the assumption of equilibration of xenon-133. So

$$\frac{dM_f}{dt} = Q \cdot C_a - (k_1 \cdot C_f + Q \cdot C_f). \qquad (3.39)$$

Dividing by the tissue volume V and replacing M_f by $V_1 C_f$, where V_1 is the volume of compartment 1, gives

$$\frac{V_1}{V}\frac{dC_f}{dt} = \frac{Q}{V} \cdot C_a - C_f\Big(\frac{Q}{V} + \frac{k_1}{V}\Big). \qquad (3.40)$$

The term V_1/V scales concentration in compartment 1 to concentration with respect to total tissue volume.

The differential equation for compartment 2, where the tracer is bound or 'trapped' is

$$\frac{V_2}{V} \cdot \frac{dC_\chi}{dt} = \frac{k_1}{V} \cdot C_f \qquad (3.41)$$

where V_2 is the volume of compartment 2. The tissue concentration C_τ recorded by PET is the sum of the bound and free concentrations C_χ and C_f. However C_χ and C_f are concentrations with respect to the volumes of their respective compartments. Since PET records the tracer concentration with respect to *total* tissue volume C_χ and C_f must be scaled down according to the proportion that these volumes occupy of total tissue volume, i.e.

$$C_\tau = (V_1/V) \cdot C_f + (1 - V_1/V) \cdot C_\chi. \qquad (3.42)$$

There are five unknown variables in these three equations (3.39–3.41), namely C_χ, C_f, V_1/V, k_1/V and Q/V — and so it is not possible to solve the equations for all five. It is therefore necessary to assume values for V_1/V and k_1 in order to derive Q/V.

3.1.3.3 Significance of *PS* product

The term k_1/V is the *PS* product per unit of tissue volume for tracer exchange from compartment 1 to compartment 2. From Sections 2.4.1 and 6.2.2.1, it can be seen that the *PS* product for transcapillary exchange is the constant of proportionality that relates the unidirectional flux J of a tracer across the capillary to the mean capillary blood concentration C_p; i.e. at steady state

$$J = PS \cdot C_p = E \cdot Q \cdot C_a \qquad (3.43)$$

where E is the extraction fraction (of tracer into compartment 2. (Note that, in the present context, $[E.Q.C_a]$ is the steady-state tracer clearance into the 'trapped' compartment.) Since C_p is considered to be equal to C_f the flux of tracer per unit tissue volume from compartment 1 to compartment 2 is $(k_1 C_f)/V$, and

$$\frac{k_1}{V}C_f = E \cdot \frac{Q}{V} \cdot C_a. \qquad (3.44)$$

[†]As will become apparent later, the *PS* product is the flux rate per unit concentration gradient; i.e. $J/C = PS$ and $J = PSC$, which is why k_1 is a *PS* product.

In the compartmental modelling of PET, since the tracer present in a compartment is expressed as a concentration, the rate constant determining the flux from one compartment to another must be the equivalent of a *PS* product (acting at that compartmental interface). The steady-state extraction fraction of tracer by the tissue represented by the model in Fig. 3.10b must therefore be the flux of tracer from compartment 1 to compartment 2 divided by the incoming arterial flux $Q \cdot C_a / V$ (mg/min/ml of tissue). Assuming that $C_v = C_f$ (as in equation 3.39), then the outflux from the tissue is the product $(Q/V) \cdot (C_f)$. Therefore, the arterial influx rate

$$\frac{Q}{V} \cdot C_a = \frac{k_1}{V} \cdot C_f + \frac{Q}{V} \cdot C_f. \qquad (3.45)$$

This is the same as equation 3.40 for the condition $dC_f/dt = 0$ (i.e. steady state). So

$$E = \frac{(k_1/V) \cdot C_f}{(k_1/V) \cdot C_f + (Q/V) \cdot C_f}, \text{ i.e } \frac{(\text{flux } 1 \to 2)}{(\text{arterial influx})}, \qquad (3.46)$$

$$= \frac{k_1/V}{k_1/V + Q/V}. \qquad (3.47)$$

Equation 3.47 is frequently seen in the PET literature and, if E is known, it can be combined with equations 3.39–3.42 to derive both k_1/V and Q/V, and then it is necessary to assume only V_1/V.

The reader will note from Chapters 2 and 6 that the relationship between *PS, E* and *Q* was shown to be

$$PS = -Q \cdot \ln (1 - E) \qquad (3.48)$$

which can be re-arranged to the form of equation 3.27

$$E = 1 - e^{-PS/Q}.$$

Recalling that $PS = k_1$,

$$E = 1 - e^{-(k_1/V)/(Q/V)}. \qquad (3.49)$$

Why are the right-hand sides of equations 3.47 and 3.49 different? The answer is the assumption that C_f is equal to C_v (equation 3.39). At low levels of k_1, E from equation 3.47 agrees with E from equation 3.49, but at higher values, E from equation 3.47 progressively underestimates E from equation 3.49 (**Fig. 3.9**). The concentration C_v must in fact be less than C_f, because although they may equalize at the distal end of the capillary, the *average* concentration of tracer in compartment 1 is higher than the concentration in the venous outflow. The effect is

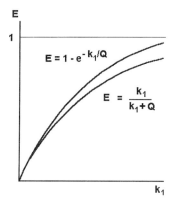

❙ **Fig 3.9** Relationship between extraction fraction E and PS product k_1 with respect to transfer of tracer from compartment 1 to 2 in Fig. 3.8b. The derivation of equation 3.47 assumes that the mean tracer concentration C_f in compartment 1 is equal to the venous outflow concentration C_v. As E rises, C_f increasingly exceeds C_v and $k_1/(k_1 + Q)$ becomes progressively less than $1 - e^{-k_1/Q}$

for Q/V in equation 3.47 to be overestimated since in reality Q/V should be multiplied by C_v. E is consequently underestimated. At increasingly lower values of E, C_f will equalize with C_v more proximally in the capillary, and the assumption that $C_v = C_f$ will become increasingly valid.

3.1.3.4 Blood flow measurement by PET based on a three-compartmental model

The third model frequently used in quantitative PET is a three-compartmental model (**Fig. 3.8c**), different from the two-compartmental model of Fig. 3.10b in that the vascular and interstitial fluid compartments are not considered to be a single compartment. The differential equations defining the various tracer fluxes are as follows, although, in this model, the concentrations, except for C_p, are those of the tracer in the compartment expressed in relation to *total tissue volume* rather than compartmental volume. As will be seen below, the inclusion of C_p is a crucial difference compared with the two compartmental model.

For the first compartment

$$dC_p/dt = k_2 \cdot C_i - k_1 \cdot C_p \qquad (3.50)$$

for the second

$$dC_i/dt = k_1 \cdot C_p + k_4 \cdot C_x - k_2 \cdot C_i - k_3 \cdot C_i \qquad (3.51)$$

and for the third

$$dC_\chi/dt = k_3 \cdot C_i - k_4 \cdot C_\chi. \tag{3.52}$$

Here C_p is the mean capillary plasma concentration *relative to plasma volume, not tissue volume*, so k_1 is the *PS* product per unit of tissue volume for the tracer moving across the capillary into the interstitial fluid. The other constants are fractional rate constants (see a few lines below), and are therefore conventionally given a small k, while K_1, a physiological parameter in its own right, is sometimes written with a capital K. Whilst the flux of tracer from compartment 1 to compartment 2 is equal to $k_1 \cdot C_p$, it is also equal to unidirectional clearance, Z/V (from 1 to 2), multiplied by the arterial, as opposed to capillary, tracer concentration[†]: i.e. $Z/V \cdot C_a = k_1 \cdot C_p$. Therefore, as non-linear regression analysis is based on the recorded *arterial* time–concentration curve and not capillary concentration, instead of generating k_1, it generates unidirectional *clearance* per unit volume of tissue. It would only generate k_1 if E was low, such that $C_p = C_a$ and therefore $Z/V = k_1$. The model therefore effectively measures clearance (from compartments 1 to 2) which can only be equated with blood flow if E is close to unity (in which case $C_a \gg C_p$ and $k_1 \gg Q/V$). The technique is therefore analogous to other techniques for measuring blood flow from organ uptake of a substance with a high extraction fraction. Again however if *PS* product for the tracer with respect to transfer from compartment 1 to compartment 2 is known, it is not necessary to assume that E is unity.

In many systems to which this model is applied, k_4 is essentially zero, for example, fluorine-18

uptake from bone interstitial fluid (compartment 2) to bone crystal (compartment 3). Steady state extraction fraction E_s from plasma (compartment 1) to bone crystal (compartment 3) is the product of unidirectional extraction fraction from plasma to interstitial fluid and the extraction fraction from interstitial fluid to bone crystal:[‡]

$$E_s = E_{1,2}. \frac{k_3}{k_3 + k_2} \tag{3.53}$$

But from (3.44) $\quad E_{1,2} = \dfrac{k_1 \cdot C_p}{C_a \cdot Q/V} \tag{3.54}$

Substituting for $E_{1,2}$ in equation 3.54

$$E_s = \frac{k_1 C_p}{C_a \cdot Q/V} \cdot \frac{k_3}{k_3 + k_2} \tag{3.55}$$

and multiplying both sides by Q/V

$$\frac{Q}{V} \cdot E_s = \frac{Q}{V} \cdot \frac{k_1 C_p}{C_a \cdot Q/V} \cdot \frac{k_3}{k_3 + k_2}. \tag{3.56}$$

But

$$Q \cdot E_s = Z_s$$

so

$$\frac{Z_s}{V} = k_1 \cdot \frac{C_p}{C_a} \cdot \frac{k_3}{k_3 + k_2}. \tag{3.57}$$

Steady state clearance (Z_s/V) is equal to the gradient of a Patlak–Rutland plot (Section 2.2.1.3) in which the recorded tissue concentration (from all compartments), C_τ is plotted as C_τ/C_a (ordinate) against $\int C_a(t) \cdot dt/C_a$ (abscissa). If $C_p = C_a$, the gradient of the plot is $(k_1 \cdot k_3)/(k_3 + k_2)$, the steady state *PS* product; if $C_p < C_a$, the gradient of the plot is $(Z_{1,2}/V \cdot k_3)/$

[†] *Since*

$$k_1 \cdot C_p = [Z/V] \cdot C_a$$

$$\frac{k_1}{Z/V} = \frac{C_a}{C_p}$$

When extraction fraction is low, $C_p = C_a$, and $k_1 = Z/V$. This is also the case for endothelial solute transfer (Section 6.2.2.1) for low E, under which circumstances *PS* product and clearance from plasma to interstitial fluid space become identical.

[‡] The reader may have difficulty grasping the concept of an extraction fraction from a compartment through which no blood is flowing. Extraction fraction can be regarded as a probability (of a molecule moving across a boundary). At steady state, under conditions of continuous infusion, the tracer concentration in compartment 2 is constant whereas in compartment 3 it is rising at a rate equal to the infusion rate. Steady-state extraction fraction is the probability of a molecule, arriving in the arterial inflow of the organ, entering compartment 3 and is the product of the respective probabilities of (a) the molecule first entering compartment 2 from compartment 1 and then (b) the relative likelihood of the molecule entering compartment 3 rather than returning to compartment 1. So if 50% of incoming tracer enters compartment 2 and the steady-state extraction efficiency is 25%, extraction efficiency from compartment 2 to compartment 3 must be 50% (i.e. $0.5 \times 0.5 = 0.25$).

$(k_3 + k_2)$, the steady-state clearance. The question of whether C_p is equal to or less than C_a determining whether the model generates *PS* product or clearance, has its counterpart in relation to *PS* product generally, in that for any system $Z = PS$ if E is low.

It is interesting to compare steady-state clearance from the Patlak plot with steady-state clearance obtained from use of non-linear regression analysis (equation 3.57), as it provides mutual validation of the two approaches. Such a comparison has been made for cerebral and myocardial glucose utilization rates using fluorine-18–fluorodeoxyglucose and skeletal fluorine-18 uptake in bone, and agreement has been close.

A final note of caution is offered to those who venture into the PET literature and that is the difference between a fractional rate constant and a *PS* product. In many cases they are identical, as can be appreciated from their respective units — min^{-1} for a rate constant — and, when expressed in terms of tissue volume (analogously to perfusion), ml/min/ml for a *PS* product. They become different when the two 'ml's in the PS product units do not refer to the same volume. *PS* product is a special case of clearance. Clearance is a volume of fluid cleared in unit time; *PS* product has the same units and is the volume of fluid that would be cleared in unit time if the 'driving' concentration was not allowed to decrease, as does the capillary concentration of a tracer as the tracer diffuses into the tissue. Consider the transfer of a small hydrophilic solute from capillary plasma to interstitial fluid in the forearm. Here *PS* product is usually expressed as ml of plasma cleared of solute per min per ml of forearm tissue. If it was expressed as ml of plasma cleared of solute per min per ml of forearm *plasma*, then it would be a fractional rate constant. The relevance of this is that a fractional rate constant will vary with the volume of the space containing the tracer, whereas a *PS* product relates specifically to the properties of the interface across which transfer occurs and, as such, is a physiological constant. Fractional rate constants are usually abbreviated with a small case k and *PS* products (or clearances) with an upper case K. If the reader returns to equation 3.51, which has for example been applied to the skeletal handling of fluorine-18 (Hawkins *et al.* 1992), it will be seen that, with the exception of k_1, the terms describing the individual fluxes contain concentrations which are not expressed in relation to the volumes of the individual compartments themselves. The concentrations are, in contrast, expressed in relation to total tissue volume, and the rate constants are therefore fractional rate constants which describe the fraction of tracer in each compartment transferred in unit time. The plasma fluorine-18 concentration is not related to bone volume, but to the measured plasma concentration, so the transfer rate is expressed as ml of plasma cleared per min per *ml of bone*, and k_1 is therefore a *PS* product.

Now look at equation 3.39, where C_f, is the concentration of tracer with respect to the volume of compartment 1. This means that k_1 in this model is a *PS* product rather than a fractional rate constant. Why vary the way in which concentration is expressed? The reason is that these techniques aim to measure blood flow and clearance, and so require the derivation of *PS* products. In contrast, because of the added uncertainty of the relative compartmental volumes, there would be little physiological advantage in expressing k_2, k_3 and k_4 as anything other than fractional rate constants. In general, when a proportionality constant precedes a concentration it is a *PS* product denoted by K and when it precedes a mass, it is a fractional rate constant denoted by k.

3.1.3.5 Correction of organ blood volume in PET

When organ perfusion is measured by PET, it is the usual practice to express it in terms of organ tissue volume rather than total volume; i.e. to correct it for organ blood volume, unlike perfusion measured with the single photon-emitting inert gases, in which blood flow is usually expressed in terms of the entire volume of distribution. The latter is valid provided equilibration of tracer between capillary blood and tissue is achieved rapidly (i.e. proximally in the capillary — see section 3.1.1.1). For the measurement of organ blood volume V_b as a fraction of total organ volume V_τ the patient inhales oxygen-15 labelled carbon monoxide, which labels red cells by forming carboxyhaemoglobin. The recorded tissue concentration C_τ is then compared with that in an arterial region of interest or in an arterial blood sample C_a: since, within a region, wih respect to blood,

$$C_\tau \cdot V_\tau = C_a \cdot V_b$$

$$\frac{V_b}{V_\tau} = \frac{C_\tau}{C_a}. \qquad (3.58)$$

If Q' is perfusion per unit of extravascular volume and Q perfusion per unit of total volume then

$$\frac{Q}{Q'} = \frac{V_\tau - V_b}{V_\tau}$$

and

$$Q' = Q/1 - (V_b/V_\tau). \tag{3.59}$$

So, for instance, if V_b/V_τ were 0.1, and $Q/(V_b + V_\tau)$ were 100 ml/min/100ml, then Q/V_τ would be 100/ 0.9 = 111 ml/min/100ml.

3.2 Indicator dilution

A static volume can be measured by observing the extent to which an added tracer is diluted. A moving volume (i.e. blood flow Q) can be measured using the same principle, called indicator dilution. Imagine a flowing river (**Fig 3.10**), and imagine sprinkling an amount M of dye into the river while a colleague downstream repeatedly took samples of water from the river and measured the dye concentration C in each sample until all the dye had washed away. From a curve constructed of dye concentration versus time, it can be seen intuitively from the units that

$$\text{flow} = \frac{\text{amount of dye added}}{\text{area under dye concentration} - \text{time curve}}, \tag{3.60}$$

$$\text{with units mg} \times \frac{\text{ml}}{\text{mg} \times \text{min}} = \text{ml/min},$$

or

$$Q = \frac{M}{\int C(t) \cdot dt}. \tag{3.61}$$

The assumption is made that the dye has completely mixed with the water by the time it reaches the point of sampling. If the river was joined by a tributary between the site at which the dye was sprinkled into the river and the sampling site, then the inflow of the tributary would further dilute the dye, the area in the denominator of equation 3.61 would be less and the flow measured would include that of the tributary. If the river divided into two branches between the place where the dye was added and the sampling site, then the concentration of dye in the water would be the same irrespective of which branch of the river the water was sampled from, assuming that

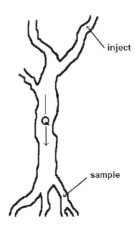

∎ **Fig. 3.10** Principle of indicator dilution for measuring blood flow. After complete mixing the injected tracer is diluted by the entire flow, irrespective of the tributary into which it is injected, down to a concentration which will be identical in all branches, irrespective of which are sampled. The sampled concentration will then depend only on (a) how much tracer was injected and (b) the flow. Q is the total flow.

the dye completely mixed in the water before the branching point. In other words, flow measured in this situation would be that of the river before the branching point, or equal to the sum of the two branch flows. Imagine that several tributaries joined to form one river which, downstream, divided again into several branches. If dye was sprinkled into any one of these tributaries upstream, and sampled from any one of the branches downstream, the flow measured would be that of the whole system, i.e. the total of the tributaries or the single main river or the total of the branches, to whichever tributary the dye was added and from whichever branch the water was sampled.

Moving from the example of a river to a vascular bed, the derivation of equation 3.61 can be formally proved. Thus we can say that a small amount of indicator or tracer dM_r, passing a sampling point, distal to the vascular bed, at time t during a small interval dt is equal to the product of tracer concentration at the sampling point and the flow Q_r in the sampled vessel (**Fig. 3.11**) i.e.

$$dM_r = Q_r C_a(t) \cdot dt. \tag{3.62}$$

Integrating between $t = 0$ and $t = \infty$, in which case M_r is the total amount of tracer passing along the

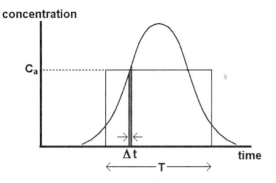

T = average transit time

▌ **Fig. 3.11** A treatment of the indicator dilution principle for measuring blood flow, more formal than that shown in Fig. 3.10. The area under the bell shaped time–concentration (or indicator dilution) curve is the summation of all the infinitesimally small areas, $C_a(t) \cdot \Delta t$ $C_a(t)$. $\Delta t \cdot C_a(t)$ has units of [mg/ml] × min and is equal to amount of tracer injected (mg or MBq) divided by flow (ml/min), i.e. [mg or MBq/ml] × min.

vessel,

$$M_r = Q_r \cdot \int C_a(t) \cdot \mathrm{d}t$$

and

$$Q_r = \frac{M_r}{\int C_a(t) \cdot \mathrm{d}t}. \qquad (3.63)$$

If mixing is complete prior to sampling then the tracer will fractionate between branching vessels in proportion to the fractionation of the total blood flow, So

$$\frac{Q_r}{M_r} = \frac{Q}{M}. \qquad (3.64)$$

So, if M is the amount of tracer administered, then Q is the flow in the vascular bed, provided mixing is completed before the sampling point and if there are no losses of indicator between the points of administration and sampling. If the indicator is given into a vein, pulmonary vessel or a cardiac chamber and the sampling point is an artery, then Q will be cardiac output. If, on the other hand, indicator is injected into the renal artery, and sampled from the renal vein, then renal blood flow would be measured. Similarly, tracer injected into the hepatic artery with sampling from the hepatic vein would yield *total* liver blood flow (not hepatic arterial flow), since the indicator would be diluted

by both hepatic arterial and portal venous blood before reaching the sampling site. An important problem encountered in the human circulation, not encountered in the example of the river, is recirculation of the indicator before the 'tail' of the initial injection has passed the sampling site for the first time. This is solved by applying a correction which essentially extrapolates the curve of activity versus time forwards from the point of recirculation to the x-(time) axis (see Sections 2.1.2.1 and 7.2.1).

Measurement of blood flow by indicator dilution is invasive but non-invasive modifications are possible such as detection of the radioactivity residue signal in the lungs following intravenous injection of a known dose of an intravascular tracer. The recorded time activity curve represents the dilution curve and can be calibrated in units of ml/min using a single blood sample taken at a time when the tracer has mixed in the blood and the time activity curve has become stable (see measurement of cardiac output — Section 7.2.1). Measurement of blood flow by dye dilution also underlies one method for measuring the permeability surface area product as an index of capillary permeability (see Section 6.2.2.4.1, Fig. 6.6)

3.3 Fractionation of cardiac output

When particles of a size greater than the diameter of a capillary are injected into an artery, they are retained in the distal vascular bed. When such particles are injected into the left ventricle, they become distributed throughout the vascular beds of the body. If the particles are completely mixed within the left ventricle and are not streamlined as they travel in arterial blood, they become distributed throughout the capillary beds of the body in proportion to the fraction of cardiac output delivered to each capillary bed. Microspheres of denatured human serum albumin can be labelled with technetium-99m or radio-iodine and, after an injection into the left ventricle, can be used to measure the fraction of cardiac output supplying an organ by external counting. If M_τ is the total amount of radioactivity deposited in the organ (MBq) and Q is organ blood flow (ml/min).

$$\frac{Q}{\text{cardiac output}} = \frac{M_\tau}{\text{injected dose}} \quad (3.65)$$

and M_τ can be measured by quantitative scanning as described in Section 5.4.3 (Crean *et al.* 1986).

The main practical difficulties of this technique are (1) it is invasive; (2) quantification is difficult because of the widespread deposition of activity; and (3) injected dose is difficult to measure because the microspheres stick to the injection syringe, catheter and anything else they come into contact with, all of which require counting after the injection in order to determine the residual, non-injected, radioactivity. However it exemplifies an important principle of blood flow measurement — fractionation of cardiac output — and is the basis of a number of non-invasive modifications for measuring blood flow, including renal blood flow (Section 11.1.1.3), splenic blood flow (Section 10.1.2.1.3), the regional distribution of blood flow (as in lung perfusion imaging, Section 8.2.2) and right to left shunt measurement (Section 8.2.5). It is also a principle used in PET measurement of blood flow using so-called 'chemical microspheres'.

Local arterial or intra-ventricular injection of radio-labelled microspheres is widely used in the experimental animal for measurement of absolute organ blood flow and has been extensively used in the PET literature as a 'gold standard' for blood flow. Particles of a range of sizes and materials, labelled with long-lived radionuclides of distinct emissions, are commercially available, but not suitable for human use. If arterial blood down-stream to the injection site is withdrawn at a constant, known rate during the injection, then the radio-labelled microspheres fractionate between the withdrawn blood and the distal capillary bed (**Fig. 3.12**). Say the withdrawal rate is 1 ml/min and the withdrawn blood contains a total of 10 units of radioactivity, while the organ itself ultimately receives 400 units of radioactivity, then the organ blood flow must be 40 ml/min. The assumptions are that the microspheres mix completely between injection and sampling sites, that the withdrawal itself does not affect organ blood flow and that the period of withdrawal completely encompasses the width of the bolus (i.e. it starts before injection and finishes only after all the

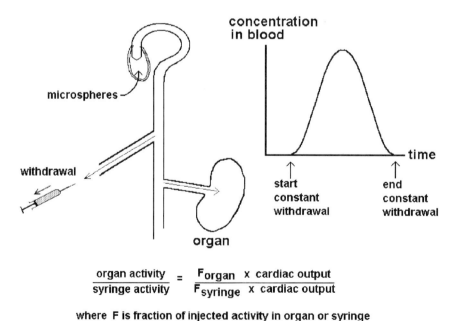

$$\frac{\text{organ activity}}{\text{syringe activity}} = \frac{F_{\text{organ}} \times \text{cardiac output}}{F_{\text{syringe}} \times \text{cardiac output}}$$

where F is fraction of injected activity in organ or syringe

∎ **Fig. 3.12** Principle of blood flow measurement based on fractionation of cardiac output. Provided arterial blood is withdrawn (from an artery) over a period which completely encloses the whole of the arterial time–concentration curve recorded following intraventricular injection of labelled microspheres, then the amount of radioactivity in the syringe (expressed either as the total or per ml of blood) will bear the same relation to the radioactivity trapped in the organ (total or per ml of tissue) as their respective blood flows (ml per min) or 'perfusions' (ml per min per g).

microspheres have passed the sampling site). Microspheres labelled with different radionuclides can be injected in sequence so that it is possible to study the effects of interventions on blood flow before sacrificing the animal, isolating the tissues of interest and performing multiple isotope analysis. Counts are usually expressed per gram of tissue so flow is expressed as tissue perfusion and only a representative sample of tissue needs to be counted and weighed.

Although invasive, the technique has been applied to man using radiolabelled albumin microspheres and PET (Weisenberg *et al.* 1981), which is able to quantify the absolute tissue concentration of radioactivity. In addition to microspheres, several other agents behave similarly to microspheres in that they undergo almost complete extraction in tissue beds on a single pass despite being in solution. They are consequently known as 'chemical microspheres' and include analogues of potassium, such as rubidium-82 and thallium-201, nitrogen-13 labelled ammonia, and technetium-99m HMPAO. In order to be used for absolute quantification of blood flow, these compounds must approach complete extraction on one pass, although for the purpose of simply providing images of regional blood flow distribution, they need only have an extraction fraction which is relatively constant from tissue to tissue, or from region to region within a tissue (Sapirstein 1958). For example, this is how technetium-99m HMPAO is used to provide images of regional cerebral blood flow. Since many of these chemical microspheres have found widespread use in cardiology, the technique of tissue quantification combined with arterial sampling has most often been applied to the measurement of myocardial blood flow (see Section 7.1).

Tracers that freely recirculate, without trapping, can also be used to measure blood flow using the cardiac output fractionation principle. This is based on the premise that any organ has a *minimum* (in contrast to *mean*) intravascular transit time, during which any tracer behaves as though it was trapped (Mullani and Gould 1983). The increase in tissue concentration within this period can then be compared with the arterial concentration, obtainable from a region of interest over a large artery or cardiac chamber. Approaching this from the fractionation principle, as though the tracer was a labelled microsphere,

$$\frac{Q/V}{CO} = \frac{M_\tau/V}{\text{injected activity}} = \frac{C_\tau(\infty)}{\text{injected activity}}. \tag{3.66}$$

Now, similar to equation 3.19,

$$CO = \frac{\text{injected activity}}{\int C_a(t) \cdot dt}, \tag{3.67}$$

So combining equations 3.66 and 3.67,

$$\frac{Q}{V} \int C_a(t) \cdot dt = C_\tau(\infty).$$

Therefore

$$\frac{Q}{V} = \frac{C_\tau(\infty)}{\int C_a(t) \cdot dt}. \tag{3.68}$$

For a recirculating tracer, the integrated arterial curve has the same shape as the tissue curve recorded within the minimum intravascular transit time of the tissue, during which the tracer behaves as a microsphere (which has a minimum transit time of infinity).
Therefore

$$\frac{C_\tau(t)}{\int\limits_0^t C_a(t) \cdot dt} = \frac{C_\tau(\infty)}{\int\limits_0^\infty C_a(t) \cdot dt} \tag{3.69}$$

Where t is less than the minimum intravascular transit time. Combining equations 3.68 and 3.69,

$$\frac{Q}{V} = \frac{C_\tau(t)}{\int\limits_0^t C_a(t) \cdot dt}. \tag{3.70}$$

A difficulty with equation 3.70 is that there is a time interval of a few seconds between the take-off points of the arterial and tissue curves so that the values of t in the numerator and denominator are different. It is necessary therefore to 'shift' one of the curves so that their take-off points are identical.

Note however that the maximum slope of the tissue curve, $dC_\tau/dt(max)$, is directly proportional to the maximum slope of the integrated arterial curve (the denominator in equation 3.70), which itself is equal to the peak height of the arterial curve (**Fig. 3.13**), so we can also say

$$\frac{Q}{V} = \frac{dC_\tau/dt(max)}{C_a(max)} \tag{3.71}$$

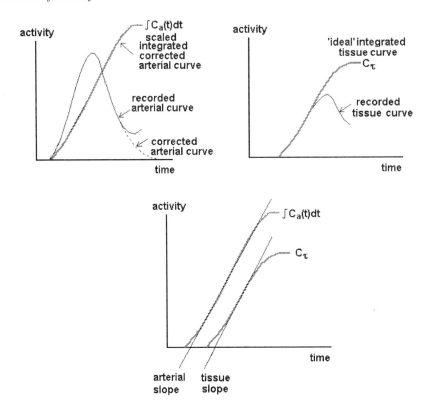

∎ **Fig. 3.13** Principle of blood flow measurement by 'non-invasive' fractionation of cardiac output. If microspheres were injected into the left side of the heart, the arterial and organ curves shown top left would be obtained. The organ curve is the integral of the arterial curve. The curves shown top right would be obtained following intravenous injection of a recirculating tracer. Correction for recirculation in the arterial curve followed by integration of the corrected curve would generate an organ curve reproducing the situation with microscopes. Scaling this hypothetical curve so that its upslope is parallel to the upslope of the real organ curve effectively predicts the plateau height that the real curve would have reached if all the tracer arriving in the organ on first pass were retained like microspheres (bottom). This plateau activity, expressed as a fraction of the injected activity, represents the blood flow to the organ as a fraction of cardiac output.

Equation 3.71 is independent of the time difference between arterial and tissue curves.

In equation 3.70, the numerator and denominator have been differentiated to produce 3.71.

Equation 3.71 has been used for the measurement of tissue perfusion by dynamic computed tomography (CT) and the construction of CT colour flow images (Miles 1991, Miles *et al.* 1991) because the attenuation by radiological contrast medium is directly proportional to tissue concentration, and the theory is essentially identical to that of PET.

Multiplying both sides of equation 3.69 by organ volume V followed by re-arrangement, gives

$$M_\tau(\infty) = M_\tau(t) \cdot \frac{\int\limits_0^\infty C_a(\infty) \cdot dt}{\int\limits_0^t C_a(t) \cdot dt}. \qquad (3.72)$$

This is the approach adopted for single photon imaging since M_τ can be measured by quantitative scanning and $\int C_a(\infty) \cdot dt$ obtained by correcting the input curve for recirculation of tracer using a gamma function or exponential fit to the downslope (see Section 2.1.2.1) (Peters *et al.* 1987). Remember that t is less than the minimum intravascular transit time. Note that $M_\tau(\infty)$ as a fraction of the injected dose is organ blood flow as a fraction of cardiac output.

Multiplying both sides of equation 3.71 by organ blood volume V

$$Q = \frac{dM_\tau/dt(\max)}{C_a(\max)}. \qquad (3.73)$$

Administering an intravascular tracer and calibrating the time–activity curve over a blood pool region using a timed blood sample, absolute blood flow can be obtained (see Section 11.1.1.3).

3.4 Plethysmography

Venous occlusion or impedance plethysmography is a classical non-invasive method of measuring limb blood flow in man. If a cuff is applied to a limb and rapidly inflated to a pressure just above venous pressure, venous return is briefly occluded. For a short period immediately after inflation, the arterial inflow continues unimpeded, and the rate of blood inflow can be measured as the rate at which the volume of the limb increases. Isotope plethysmography is a modification of this technique. Two approaches are possible. In the first, instead of measuring the rate of volume increase (after application of the cuff), the rate at which the radioactivity signal increases after having first injected an intravascular tracer (and allowed it to mix in the circulation) can be measured. By measuring the concentration of activity in a blood sample, it is possible to calibrate the rate of increase of activity in units of volume increase (or flow).

In the second approach, the cuff is placed on the proximal part of the limb and inflated to above systolic arterial pressure. An intravascular tracer is then injected in another limb and allowed to mix in the blood volume over a period of 2–3 minutes, before the cuff is rapidly deflated. The rate of increase in count rate in the limb distal to the cuff, which, before deflation, contained no radioactivity, is proportional to the rate of blood flow into the limb at the time of deflation. A blood sample, taken after complete mixing of the tracer in the blood volume, is required for calibration. A correction for photon attenuation in the limb is required for both approaches. The volume of the limb, which can be measured by simple water displacement, is also required in order to express the flow rate as perfusion. These techniques have been applied to measurement of limb blood flow in patients with peripheral arterial disease (Section 6.1.3.1).

3.5 Blood flow measurement based on transit time

Blood flow can be measured using the transit time equation defined in equation 2.1. Thus, if mean tracer transit time (T) and the volume (V) of distribution of the tracer within the organ are measured, blood flow to the organ can be calculated as the quotient V/T. Measuring perfusion as flow per unit volume with xenon-133 is an example of this approach in which V is the entire tissue volume and is left unmeasured so that flow is expressed as perfusion. This section, however, concentrates on flow measurement using an intravascular tracer which can also be used to measure the distribution volume (i.e. organ blood volume), hence allowing calculation of Q as an absolute flow. It lends itself well to measurement of cerebral blood flow (Section 12.1.5). Labelled red cells or human serum albumin is injected as an intravenous bolus and the time–activity curve is recorded over the brain and also over the arch of the aorta. Applying deconvolution analysis to the aortic and cerebral curves, the residue curve over the brain is obtained from which T is calculated as height over area. Cerebral blood volume V is then measured from the count rate recorded over the brain and the simultaneous activity in a blood sample taken after the tracer has mixed within the total blood volume and the count rate over the brain has stabilized.

Then

$$V = \frac{\text{brain count rate}}{\text{blood sample count rate}} \times \frac{\gamma}{\Gamma} \qquad (3.74)$$

where γ and Γ are constants relating gamma camera count rate to quantity of radioactivity and well-counter count rate to blood radioactivity concentration, respectively. The units are

$$\frac{\text{MBq}}{\text{MBq/ml}} = \text{ml}.$$

V is then inserted into the transit time equation; i.e. $Q = V/T$. Assumptions have to be made about the shape of the brain in comparison with a phantom, filled with radioactivity and taken to be the same shape as the brain, and corrections made for non-cerebral counts recorded from the scalp.

An alternative approach in which volume of distribution is not measured has also been applied to the brain. It involves measurement of regional intravascular transit time from a first-pass curve over the vertex following an intravenous bolus injection of pertechnetate (Merrick *et al.* 1991). The technique generates an image in which the grey or colour scale reflects Q/V (i.e. tracer transit time) in each pixel. This is an example of a parametric image; i.e. an image in which the colour in a pixel is scaled for a physiological variable rather than a count rate. These techniques are further discussed in Section 12.1.4.

References

Bergmann S, Herrero P, Markham J, Weinheimer CJ and Walsh MN. Non-invasive quantitation of myocardial blood flow in human subjects with oxygen-15 labeled water and PET. *Journal of the American College of Cardiology* 1989; **14**: 639–52.

Conn HL. Equilibrium distribution of radioxenon in tissue: xenon–hemoglobin association curve. *Journal of Applied Physiology* 1961, **16**: 1065–70.

Crean PA, Pratt T, Davies GJ, Myers MJ, Lavender JP and Maseri A. The fractional distribution of the cardiac output in man using microspheres labelled with technetium-99m. *British Journal of Radiology* 1986, **59**: 209–15.

Crone C and Levitt DG. Capillary permeability to small solutes. In: Renkin EM and Michel CC (eds) *Handbook of physiology*; section 2: The cardiovascular system IV. American Physiological Society, Bethesda, Maryland: 1984: 375–409.

Goldstein RA, Gould KL, Marani SK, Fisher DJ, O'Brien HA and Loberg MD. Myocardial perfusion imaging with rubidium-82. 1. Measurement of extraction and flow with external detectors. *Journal of Nuclear Medicine* 1983, **24**: 898–906.

Hawkins RA, Young C, Huang S-C, Hoh CK, Dahlbom M, Schiepers C, Satymurthy N, Barrio N and Phelps ME. Evaluation of the skeletal kinetics of fluorine-18-fluoride ion with PET. *Journal of Nuclear Medicine* 1992; **33**: 633–42.

Kennedy AM, Banks LM, MacSweeney JE, Myers MJ, Peters AM and Allison DJ. The use of xenon-133 for measurement of blood flow through systemic arteriovenous malformations before and after therapeutic embolization. *British Journal of Radiology* 1995, **68**: 844–9.

Kety SS. The theory and applications of the exchange of inert gas at the lungs and tissue. *Pharmacological Reviews* 1951, **3**: 1–41.

Merrick MV, Ferrington CM and Cowen SJ. Parametric imaging of cerebral vascular reserves. 1. Theory, validation and normal values. *European Journal of Nuclear Medicine* 1991, **18**: 171–7.

Miles KA. Measurement of tissue perfusion by dynamic computed tomography. *British Journal of Radiology* 1991, **64**: 409–12.

Miles KA, Hayball M and Dixon AK. Colour perfusion imaging: a new application of computed tomography. *Lancet* 1991, **337**: 643–45.

Mullani NA and Gould KL. First-pass measurement of regional blood flow with external detectors. *Journal of Nuclear Medicine* 1983, **24**: 577–81.

Peters AM, Gunasekera RD, Henderson BL, Brown J, Lavender JP, de Souza M, Ash JM and Gilday DL. Non-invasive measurement of blood flow and extraction fraction. *Nuclear Medicine Communications* 1987, **8**: 823–37.

Rehling M, Hyldstrup L and Henriksen JH. Arterio venous concentration difference of [51$_{Cr}$] EDTA after a single injection in a man. Significance of renal function and local blood flow. *Clinical Physiology* 1989, **9**: 279–89

Sapirstein LA. Regional blood flow by fractional distribution of indicators. *American Journal of Physiology*, 1958, **193**: 161–8.

Schelbert HR, Phelps ME, Huang S-C, MacDonald NS, Hansen H, Selin C and Kuhl DE. N-13 ammonia as an indicator of myocardial blood flow. *Circulation* 1981, **63**: 1259–72.

Turner JH, Selwyn A, Jones T, Evans TR, Raphael MJ and Lavender JP. Continuous imaging of regional myocardial blood flow in dogs using krypton-81m. *Cardiovascular Research* 1976, **10**: 398–404.

Weisenberg G, Schelbert HR, Hoffman EJ, Phelps ME, Robinson GD, Selin CE, Child J, Skorton D and Kuhl DE. *In vivo* quantitation of regional myocardial blood flow by positron-emission computed tomography. *Circulation* 1981, **b3**: 1248–58.

Zierler KL. Equations for measuring blood flow by external monitoring of radioisotopes. *Circulation Research* 1965, **16**: 309–21.

4 Pharmacokinetics of agents routinely used in nuclear medicine

Introduction

The appropriate use of radiopharmaceuticals demands a clear understanding of their physiological handling, in particular the kinetics of bio-distribution and the physiological data they generate. The kinetics of most radiopharmaceuticals are well understood. However there are examples of agents, which, although having specific clinical applications, are not fully understood in terms of kinetics. Radioiodine and DTPA are agents with kinetics that are well understood, while those of DMSA and IDA analogues, for example, remain controversial.

4.1 Renal agents

Renal agents, all those of which listed in Table 4.1 are small molecules (<1000 Da), provide good examples of the interplay of several physiological factors determining the pharmacokinetics of a radiopharmaceutical (**Fig. 4.1**).

4.1.1 DTPA

DTPA is a hydrophilic chelating agent which, following intravenous injection, diffuses between the intravascular and extracellular extravascular spaces. At the same time it is filtered at the glomerulus and excreted in the urine without tubular secretion or reabsorption. It does not enter the intracellular space or red cells. Soon after injection, more enters the extravascular space from plasma than returns to plasma, but as the extravascular concentration rises, the *rates of tracer movement* in the two opposite directions become, for an instant, equal. After this time, the extravascular concentration exceeds the intravascular and the rate of tracer movement back into plasma is the greater. If this were not the case, the tracer could never be cleared from the body. By two hours after injection, the *fractional disappearance rates* from extravascular and intravascular spaces become equal, at which time the tracer is said to have equilibrated throughout its distribution volume, i.e. throughout the total extracellular fluid volume (**Fig. 4.2**). Although this

Label	Renal agent	Protein binding (%)	Uptake mechanism	Extraction efficiency (%)	Effective distribution volume (V) (litres)	Residence time in blood (V/Z) (min)
Tc-99m	DTPA	< 5	Filtration	20	13	110
Cr-51	EDTA	0	Filtration	20	13	110
I-123/131/125	Iothalamate	0	Filtration	20	13	110
(I)	(X-ray contrast)		Filtration	20	13	110
I-123/131/125	OIH	≈ 50	Tubular secretion	80	8	18
	(PAH)	≈ 50	Tubular secretion	90	8	16
Tc-99m	MAG3	≈ 80	Tubular secretion	50	5	18
Tc-99m	DACH	≈ 20	Tubular secretion	≈ 20	11	90
Tc-99m	Glucoheptonate	< 5	Tubular secretion	≈ 20	≈ 13	
Tc-99m	DMSA	≈ 80	Tubular Uptake	6	5	100

Table 4.1

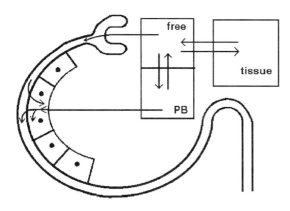

❚ **Fig. 4.1** Scheme for renal handling of radiopharmaceuticals. Most renal agents are small molecules and if circulating 'free' in plasma such as DTPA, EDTA or radiological contrast medium, will undergo diffusional exchange between plasma and interstitial fluid and simultaneous glomerular filtration. Protein binding in plasma limits both of these processes. Agents which are almost entirely protein bound in plasma such as DMSA and MAG-3 are handled largely at a tubular level with (for MAG-3) or without (for DMSA) tubular secretion. Some tracers such as glucoheptonate are re-absorbed by the tubules following glomerular filtration.

definition of equilibrium is frequently used in nuclear medicine, equilibration is more strictly the instant at which the rates of tracer movement in the two directions are equal (see Section 13.1.1.2), i.e. when the concentrations are the same. For DTPA in skeletal muscle this is at about 20 minutes after injection.

These kinetics are common to almost any hydrophilic solute (e.g. iothalamate, EDTA) with a molecular weight of less than about 6000 daltons. Above this size, diffusion across the endothelium becomes increasingly restricted (see Section 6.2.2.2). The rates of movement and partition between the intravascular and extravascular spaces are dependent on molecular size, ionic charge, degree of protein binding and renal clearance. Technetium-99m DTPA has a molecular weight of 492 daltons and less than 5% in plasma is protein bound. The DTPA filtered at the glomerulus is not reabsorbed by the tubule and since there is no significant tubular secretion or extra-renal uptake, DTPA is a good marker for glomerular filtration. The plasma clearance rate of DTPA almost equals the glomerular filtration rate (GFR), its distribution volume almost equals the extracellular fluid volume and its renal extraction fraction almost equals the

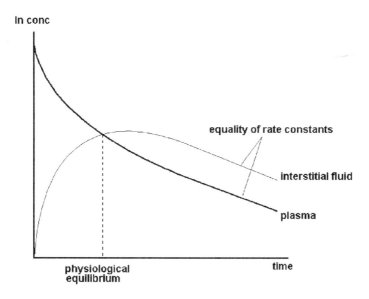

❚ **Fig. 4.2** When a small molecule such as DTPA exchanges between plasma and interstitial fluid, a concentration gradient becomes established across the endothelium. Equilibrium according to the traditional physiological definition is the point at which the interstitial and plasma concentrations are identical. The loose definition of equilibrium used in nuclear medicine is the state in which the extracellular fluid space is completely 'mixed' and the rate constants with which the plasma and the interstitial concentrations are falling are identical. It should be appreciated that the interstitial fluid concentration must eventually exceed the plasma concentration otherwise the interstitial space would never be cleared of tracer.

filtration fraction. In spite of its slight imperfections, DTPA is a good surrogate for the ideal filtration marker, inulin. Chromium-51 EDTA and iodine-125 iothalamate have molecular weights similar to DTPA and are handled almost identically. All three agents are adequate for the routine clinical measurement of GFR.

4.1.2 DMSA

Technetium-99m DMSA is at the opposite end of the spectrum to DTPA in terms of kinetics. To begin with, it is predominantly protein bound in plasma. Secondly, it binds to metalloproteins in the renal cortex, probably via sulphydryl group interactions with protein resulting in the formation of disulphide bonds. If it were completely protein bound in plasma, it could only get into the renal cortex by direct extraction from peri-tubular capillaries. In fact, it is not completely protein bound, with estimates varying between 75% and 90%. Since technetium-99m DMSA is a small molecule, about the same size as DTPA, any non-protein-bound fraction would be filtered at the glomerulus (and would also enter the extravascular space). Some DMSA could therefore gain access to the tubular epithelium by reabsorption following glomerular filtration. This can be estimated from the renal extraction fraction of DMSA and the extent of protein binding. Thus the sum of the two extraction fractions (one by glomerular filtration E_{glom} and the other by direct removal from peri-tubular blood E_{direct}) will be equal to the total renal extraction fraction (E) (**Fig. 4.3**), i.e.

$$E = E_{glom} + E_{direct}. \qquad (4.1)$$

The term E_{glom} should be equal to the filtration fraction, which is normally 0.2, multiplied by [1–protein-bound fraction]. Thus for protein binding of 75% and 90%, the corresponding values of E_{glom} are given by

$$E_{glom} = [1 - 0.75] \times 0.2 = 0.05$$

and

$$E_{glom} = [1 - 0.9] \times 0.2 = 0.02. \qquad (4.2)$$

Total extraction fraction, measured by renal venous sampling and by other indirect methods is 0.05–0.08. This means that the ratio $E_{glom} : E$ will be critically dependent on protein binding and, for the examples of protein binding and extraction fraction given above, will be somewhere between unity (0.05 : 0.05) and 0.25 (0.02 : 0.08). On the other hand, micropuncture

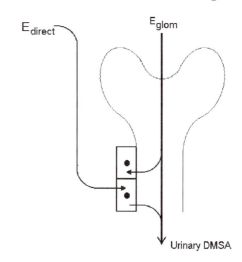

∎ **Fig. 4.3** Probable mechanism of renal uptake of technetium-99m DMSA. Although DMSA is 80–90% protein bound plasma, a significant fraction of renal uptake is likely to be through glomerular filtration followed by tubular re-absorption. Thus overall DMSA renal extraction fraction is only about 0.06. With a filtration fraction of 0.2, the extraction fraction of DMSA as a result of glomerular filtration would be [0.2 × 0.2] if protein binding was 80%; i.e. 0.04 which is a significant contribution to the total of 0.06.

experiments in the rat kidney suggest that, although some DMSA is filtered, it is not reabsorbed from the tubular lumen. If this applies in the human clinical situation, most of the urinary activity, which amounts to about 15% of the injected dose, would arise from filtered DMSA. Because of protein binding, technetium-99m DMSA tends to be held within the intravascular space and its effective volume of distribution is therefore considerably less than the extracellular fluid volume. Based on quantitative estimates of renal uptake and the rate constant of uptake by the kidney, the effective volume of distribution of technetium-99m DMSA can be estimated and shown to be more in keeping with protein binding in plasma of 75% rather than 90%.

Approximately half of the injected dose of technetium-99m DMSA is ultimately cleared by the kidneys, and, of this total renal handling, about one fifth to one quarter appears in the urine. In adult humans, extra-renal clearance is predominantly into the liver and spleen. In young infants, on the other hand, there is significant extra-renal uptake in the skeleton (probably bone marrow). From the distribution of whole body activity into renal and extra-renal compartments at the completion of blood clearance, renal and extra-renal DMSA clearance rates can be estimated from the total blood clearance. Thus plasma clearance is normally about 50 ml/min, of which about two-thirds is renal because about two-thirds of a dose is cleared by the kidney (including the tracer which ends up in the urine).

4.1.3 Hippuran and mercaptoacetyl-triglycine (MAG-3)

Both these agents are partially protein bound in plasma and are excreted unchanged in the urine as a result of tubular secretion and glomerular filtration, without retention in the tubular epithelium. The extraction fraction of hippuran is normally about 80%, greater than that of MAG-3, which is about 50%. Thus their renal clearances (with respect to whole blood) are normally about 800 and 500 ml/min, respectively. Nevertheless the urinary excretion rate of MAG-3, i.e. its rate of removal from the body, is similar to that of hippuran because its effective volume of distribution is smaller. In other words, mean transit times in their respective volumes of distribution are similar. The lower distribution volume of MAG-3 results from its greater protein binding in plasma which is about 80% compared with about 50% for hippuran. Some MAG-3 is also taken up by the liver, and so its plasma clearance slightly exceeds renal clearance. Taking a level of protein binding of 80%, at plasma clearance of 300 ml/min, the mean residence time of MAG-3 in its distribution volume is about 18 minutes; it is almost the same value for hippuran.

4.1.4 Glucoheptonate

Glucoheptonate combines the properties of the above mentioned compounds in that it is minimally protein bound, undergoes glomerular filtration and is partially reabsorbed by the tubules. Although the majority is excreted in the urine, about 6% is retained by each kidney, enough to allow reasonable delayed static imaging and to yield information similar to technetium-99m DMSA. Glucoheptonate is used in North America but very little in the UK.

4.2 Hepatic agents

Imaging the liver with radionuclides has become less important over the last few years as a result of developments in ultrasonography, computerized tomography and magnetic resonance imaging. Nevertheless dynamic imaging of the liver with biliary agents (IDA analogues) remains important.

4.2.1 IDA analogues

The renal imaging agents described above have corresponding analogous agents in liver imaging. For example the IDA agents (IminoDiAcetic acid analogues) are, in principle, handled in the same way as the kidney handles hippuran and MAG-3. They circulate in plasma, partially bound to plasma protein, are actively removed from plasma by the hepatocytes (equivalent to the tubular epithelium) and are ultimately transported into the biliary tree (equivalent to tubular secretion into the urinary collecting system). Not so much is known about the effective distribution volumes of IDA agents but protein binding is probably quite extensive, although variable from analogue to analogue. The IDA agents are more lipid soluble than the renal agents. Protein binding varies directly with lipid solubility. The protein binding and rapid selective clearance by the liver prevents much IDA from appearing in the urine, although there is some spill-over into the kidneys. This increases with decreasing liver function and increasing analogue hydrophilicity.

The IDA analogues are organic anions (i.e. weak acids) and use the same carrier system into the hepatocyte as substances such as rose bengal, indocyanine green and bromosulphthalein (BSP), which are also organic anions. Bilirubin also uses this carrier system, which explains why urinary IDA excretion increases in jaundiced patients. Bilirubin also displaces IDA from its protein binding sites in plasma, and this adds to the urinary excretion of IDA in jaundice. The IDA analogues, such as butyl IDA, which have been developed specifically for use in patients with jaundice owe their success, in this respect, to their higher lipophilicity, and therefore protein binding in plasma. However, their clearance rates from blood and intrahepatic parenchymal transit times are also slower. So, although useful in jaundiced patients, they offer no advantage in the absence of jaundice. Here they may be inferior to the analogues, like diethyl-IDA, which give good images of the biliary system because of the rapidity of their arrival there. These considerations underline the care that should be exercised when comparing

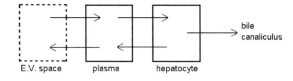

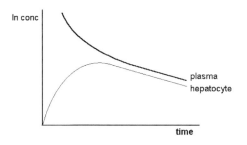

▌**Fig. 4.4** Model illustrating the hepatic handling of IDA analogues. There is bidirectional movement of IDA between plasma and hepatocyte which, with simultaneous uni-directional 'run-off' into bile canaliculus, would be predicted to give a bi-exponential plasma clearance curve which is, in fact, observed. The effective size of the extrahepatic extravascular space with respect to IDA is probably small as a result of extensive protein binding in plasma.

sequential IDA scans, such as in the follow-up of patients who have undergone drainage procedures, when different analogues may have been used.

It is well recognized that organic anions, such as BSP, rose bengal and indocyanine green, undergo reversible uptake in the hepatocyte, as does bilirubin; in other words, transfer of these agents across the hepatocyte membrane is bi-directional. Their transfer from hepatocyte to bile canaliculus however is uni-directional. A closed two-compartmental model with run-off would therefore be appropriate for these agents. Although not widely recognized, the model is applicable to IDA analogues (**Fig. 4.4**). This has important implications for the interpretation of IDA imaging and for liver blood flow measurement, as discussed in Section 9.4.1.1.

4.2.2 Colloids

Colloids are removed from the circulation as a result of uptake into the reticuloendothelial elements of the liver, spleen and bone marrow. Removal is rapid, because liver blood flow is substantial and hepatic extraction fraction high, about 0.8. The distribution volume of a colloid is the plasma volume, so with an extraction efficiency of 80% and a liver blood flow

of about 30% of total blood volume per min, a colloid would be cleared from blood into liver with a plasma disappearance rate constant of 0.8×0.3, or 0.24 min^{-1} (i.e. 24% cleared from plasma per min). The actual rate constant is a little higher than this because, although splenic blood flow enters the portal vein and is therefore included in liver blood flow, there is additional clearance into the bone marrow. At completion of uptake about 85% of an injected dose of technetium-99m labelled sulphur colloid is present in the liver, about 10% in the spleen and about 5% in the bone marrow.

4.3 Bone agents

The bone agents comprise polyphosphates and phosphonates. Several are commercially available, of which technetium-99m methylene diphosphonate is the most popular. They are taken up by bone in proportion to bone turnover. Increased uptake is also seen if regional bone blood flow is increased, either as the result of primary bone pathology such as Paget's disease or a result of a surrounding inflammatory process such as a neighbouring soft tissue infection. Bone agents are deposited at the interface between new osteoid and mineralized bone; i.e. at the advancing edge of osteoid calcification. Although bone agents are not taken up by the osteoblasts themselves, increased osteoblastic activity is associated with increased bone turnover. Bone agents also localize in areas of soft tissue calcification and other pathological processes, not necessarily associated with calcification, such as infarction and neuroblastoma.

The bone agents are small hydrophilic solutes and consequently have an extra-skeletal bio-distribution similar to DTPA. The diffusion kinetics of MDP across bone capillaries are similar to the kinetics of DTPA diffusion across capillaries with continuous endothelium, such as in muscle and skin. Having diffused into bone interstitial fluid, MDP may be deposited in bone, as described above, or re-enter the bone capillary, as shown in the model in **Fig. 4.5**. From inspection of this model, it can be appreciated that there is a complex relationship between the respective roles of bone blood flow, bone capillary permeability and bone metabolic activity in steady state skeletal MDP clearance (Section 13.3.1).

As a hydrophilic solute, MDP is cleared through the kidneys by glomerular filtration. Early images

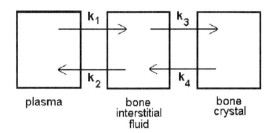

∎ **Fig. 4.5** Model illustrating the handling of diphosphonates and fluorine-18 in bone. Bone interstitial fluid is a significant space, into which small hydrophilic solutes diffuse from plasma with similar kinetics to those in muscle and skin. Very little tracer returns to bone interstitial fluid from bone crystal.

taken over the kidneys following injection of technetium-99m MDP are almost indistinguishable from images taken at the corresponding time after technetium-99m DTPA and indeed MDP gives the same information concerning urinary tract drainage as DTPA. In the normal subject, slightly more than half of an injected dose of MDP is cleared by the kidneys. Of this renal handling, almost all is excreted in the urine. However a small amount is taken up into the parenchyma and so MDP is handled by the kidney more like glucoheptonate than DTPA. Parenchymal uptake is increased in some conditions, including sickle cell disease and after chemotherapy.

The level of renal function has an important bearing on the quality of technetium-99m MDP bone images. One might imagine that in renal failure bone uptake would be increased since the kidneys offer less competition for uptake than normal. This is indeed the case in the tertiary hyperparathyroidism of renal osteodystrophy, but not in renal failure without osteodystrophy in which the target (bone) to background ratio is poor, at least at the conventional imaging time, 3 hours, after injection. This is because the skeleton and the kidney between them clear the MDP from the entire extravascular space. If the contribution of either is reduced, then the extravascular space is not adequately cleared of radioactivity by 3 hours; consequently background is elevated and lesion detectability reduced. For this reason, imaging should be delayed beyond 3 hours in patients with renal failure. High target-to-background ratios can be achieved at 12 hours, and indeed this applies to normal subjects as well.

Because of its access to the extravascular space, technetium-99m MDP enters extravascular fluid collections such as pleural effusions and ascites and this represents an important mechanism for non-osseous localization. Turnover of fluid in these collections is slow and consequently they may remain 'hot' for hours.

4.4 Lung agents

Lung agents can be divided into perfusion and ventilation agents, and agents which assess the integrity of the blood-gas barrier (alveolar/endothelial permeability).

4.4.1 Perfusion agents

Radioactive agents that are trapped in the lung following intravenous injection can be used to image the regional distribution of pulmonary blood flow. They can be divided into inert gases which enter the alveolar spaces from blood, and the microparticles, which embolize in the lung.

4.4.1.1 Microparticles

Macroaggregates of denatured human serum albumin of diameter 10–60 μm are routinely used to image pulmonary blood flow. These particles are too large to pass through pulmonary capillaries and therefore microembolise in the lung immediately following intravenous injection. Provided the particles completely mix in the blood between the injection site and the lung, their regional distribution in the lung is proportional to the distribution of pulmonary blood flow. A major factor which may prevent mixing is streamlining, which means that, according to local hydrodynamic and rheological factors, particles and plasma may partially separate from each other. Streamlining is related to particle size, decreasing with decreasing particle size.

Microspheres of denatured human serum albumin have a narrower range of sizes than macroaggregates, a preparation of which may contain some particles of relatively large size. Although more expensive and of limited availability, they may therefore be preferable to macroaggregates in patients with right to left shunts. Other patients in whom there is at least a theoretical objection to microembolization in the lung are those with pulmonary hypertension, although the fraction of the pulmonary vessels actually occluded is very small, and there is no convincing evidence that lung scanning compromises the right side of the circulation in pulmonary hypertension.

It should also be realized that the distribution of particles in the lung is a statistical event governed by the laws of probability. The greater the number of injected particles therefore the closer their distribution reflects the distribution of blood flow. Since relatively more activity is carried on larger particles and since the number of large particles is relatively small, microspheres are also preferable to macroaggregates on statistical grounds.

4.4.1.2 Inert gases

Other agents with which to assess perfusion include radioactive inert gases, such as xenon-133, xenon-127, nitrogen-13 and krypton-81m, which because of their relative insolubility in water, rapidly diffuse from pulmonary capillary blood into alveolar gas. Thus, following intravenous injection, the distribution of xenon in the lung during a brief period of breath holding (which prevents the gas from being expired from the lung) is proportional to the distribution of blood flow to aerated alveoli. Since the tracer is dissolved in plasma water, the problems relating to mixing do not significantly apply to this technique. On the other hand, the approach is much less convenient than that based on microembolization of particles and is consequently limited to physiological studies. Krypton-81m is an interesting perfusion agent. It has a physical half-life of only 13 seconds and so can be infused continuously to monitor the 'real-time' distribution of lung blood flow (notwithstanding the rather prominent radio-activity signal from the right side of the heart). See Section 8.4.1 for the quantitative kinetics of this approach.

4.4.2 Ventilation agents

Agents used for ventilation imaging include inert gases which may either be ultra-short-lived or long-lived, and aerosols.

4.4.2.1 Inert gases

4.4.2.1.1 Xenon

Two isotopes of xenon, xenon-133 with a half-life of 5.2 days and xenon-127, with a half life of 36 days are useful for ventilation imaging. Xenon is an inert gas with a low aqueous solubility and high lipid solubility. Following a period of continuous inhala-

tion from a closed circuit (so that expired xenon is re-inhaled) the concentration of gas in the alveoli becomes equal to that in the re-breathing circuit. At this point the regional count rates over the lung are proportional to the regional lung gas volumes (see Section 8.1.1). Following the first few breaths, well before equilibration, the count rates are weighted by regional ventilation — the so called wash in phase. If, following equilibration, the xenon circuit is removed so that the patient breathes room air, the xenon is washed out of the lungs at a rate determined by the ratio of ventilation to lung volume (the ventilatory turnover rate — see Section 8.1.2). This is the so called wash out phase.

An asthmatic patient with regional broncho-constriction may have areas of lung with air trapping and a reduced wash in rate, reflecting reduced ventilation, and other areas perhaps with normal wash in rate. At equilibrium, broncho-constricted regions have a higher count rate than normally ventilated regions because of the expanded volume associated with air trapping. In addition, the time to equilibrium will be delayed. During the wash out phase, air trapping shows as a delay in the washout rate with a persisting signal. Bullae in the lung have very little ventilation, and re-breathing has to be prolonged in order for them to reach equilibrium when, again, their count rate reflects volume. During washout, the signal persists much longer than in normal regions, not so much because of air trapping but because of the very low ventilatory turnover rate. In circumstances in which there is absent ventilation, such as in lobar consolidation, no signal is seen at any stage.

4.4.2.1.2 Krypton-81m

Because of its very short half-life of 13 seconds, krypton-81m rapidly reaches equilibrium although the kinetics are different. Thus instead of reaching an equilibrium in which the inspiration rate of gas equals the expiration rate, krypton-81m equilibrates as a result of the inspiration rate becoming equal to the sum of the physical decay rate and the expiration rate. Since the ventilatory turnover in the adult human breathing at rest is small compared with the rapid physical decay rate of krypton-81m, expiration has only a small effect on the count rate recorded over the lung. Because the decay rate is constant, the regional distribution of radioactivity predominantly reflects regional inspiration rate (i.e. ventilation).

The following general equation derived in Section 8.1.1, summarizes the kinetics of both xenon and krypton-81m:

$$C_{alv} \cdot V_{alv} = M_{alv} = \frac{\dot{V} \cdot C_i}{\frac{\dot{V}}{V_{alv}} + \delta} \qquad (4.3)$$

and we see that comparing units:

$$MBq = \frac{\frac{ml}{min} \cdot \frac{MBq}{ml}}{\frac{ml}{min \cdot ml} + \frac{1}{min}}$$

$$= MBq$$

where $\dot{V}$ is ventilation, C_i inspired concentration, C_{alv} alveolar concentration of radioactive gas, V_{alv} regional alveolar volume and δ radionuclide physical decay constant. The product $C_{alv} \cdot V_{alv}$ is the amount M_{alv} of activity in a lung region and therefore proportional to the recorded regional count rate. In the case of xenon-133 and xenon-127, δ (with units of min^{-1}) is negligible compared with $\dot{V}/V_{alv}$ (also min^{-1}) so M_{alv} becomes closely proportional to V_{alv}. In the case of krypton-81 m however $\dot{V}/V_{alv}$ is generally small compared with δ, so M_{alv} becomes approximately proportional to $\dot{V}$. In small children, $\dot{V}/V_{alv}$ may not be small compared with δ for krypton-81m, and the count rate over the lung may be 'weighted' by volume as well as ventilation.

For the purpose of imaging the lung in pulmonary embolism, xenon-133, xenon-127 or krypton-81m may be used. There is no need to re-breath xenon-133 to equilibrium in order to determine whether or not a perfusion defect is matched on the ventilation image and, if prolonged re-breathing is avoided, more projections can be obtained, since, after a limited period of inhalation, xenon-133 can be more quickly expired. Krypton-81m is ideal for imaging ventilation defects and, because of its very short half-life, views from multiple projections can be obtained. Furthermore, since its energy of 190 keV is higher than that of technetium-99m (140 keV), ventilation images can be obtained after, or simultaneously with perfusion images, in contrast to xenon-133, which, because of its lower energy of 80 keV, has to be administered before technetium-99m, i.e. at a time when the distribution of any perfusion defects that may be present is not known. Xenon-127 has higher energy gamma emissions (177, 203 and 375 keV) than technetium-99m and can therefore be administered after imaging perfusion.

For imaging lung disease other than pulmonary embolism, both agents have their advantages.

Xenon-133 is suitable for studying air trapping whilst krypton-81m is useful for studying clinical pulmonary physiology, such as the effects of gravity on the distribution of ventilation (Section 8.2).

4.4.2.2 Aerosols

The principle underlying the use of labelled aerosols for imaging the distribution of ventilation is self-evident. The particles are re-breathed for a limited period. Most are exhaled again but a minority are deposited in the airways where they remain. A major problem with this approach is the deposition of particles in the larger airways rather than in the terminal bronchi and alveoli. Main airway deposition increases with increasing particle size and with increasing airways turbulence, as occurs in chronic obstructive pulmonary disease (COPD) and asthma. This is unfortunate as COPD is the very clinical setting in which high-quality ventilation images are desirable for the diagnosis of pulmonary embolism. The newer ventilation agents are the so-called pseudo-gases of which technegas and pertechnegas are examples. The former is a labelled hydrophobic particulate material and the latter is hydrophilic. Technegas particles are very small and hexagonal in shape with sides about 3×13 nm (1000 nm = 1 μm). It is produced by heating pertechnetate in a carbon crucible to a temperature of 2500 °C. Following rapid cooling and inhalation, the labelled carbon particles are deposited in the periphery of the lung. They have a relatively long clearance half-time through the alveolar epithelium which may necessitate computer subtraction of the ventilation images from the subsequent perfusion images for the evaluation of pulmonary vascular disease. Following inhalation, pertechnegas behaves essentially like pertechnetate and is cleared through the alveolar epithelium much more rapidly.

4.5 Blood cells

4.5.1 Erythrocytes

Intravenously injected radiolabelled erythrocytes label the circulating blood. Their main use is for cardiovascular imaging, particularly multiple-gated (MUGA) cardiac studies, and for the detection and localization of gastrointestinal bleeding. Apart from some degree of splenic pooling and variations in organ haematocrit, the distribution of labelled red cells needs little further discussion. The other main applications of labelled red cells are haematological, when the label employed is usually chromium-51. This long-lived radionuclide is the best available for labelling red cells for the measurement of red cell life span, which normally is 120 days, falling to values of a few days in certain haemolytic anaemias. The detection of gastrointestinal bleeding by counting radioactivity in the faeces (in contrast to locating the site of bleeding in a patient known to have GI bleeding) is another application of chromium-51 labelled red cells.

4.5.2   Platelets

Like red cells, platelets can be labelled with chromium-51, technetium-99m or indium-111. Chromium-51 labelled platelets were, for many years, used in haematological studies of platelet distribution and mean platelet life span. With the availability of other gamma emitters, the applications of labelled platelets now also includes the imaging of platelet deposition, as in deep venous thrombosis and arterial disease. The most striking feature of the distribution of platelets is their pooling within the spleen. Pooling in this context describes a situation where blood cells are present in a vascular bed in a higher concentration relative to plasma compared with their concentration in central blood but, at the same time, are in free dynamic exchange with the circulating population. About one third of the total platelet population is at any time pooled in the normal spleen which, in consequence, shows up very prominently after injection of indium-111 or technetium-99m labelled platelets. The concentration of platelets, relative to plasma, is about 50 times higher than that in central blood. A small pool also exists in the liver with a concentration of about 1.5 times that of central blood. The time course of platelet uptake in the splenic pool, immediately following injection, approaches an asymptote mono-exponentially with a half-time of about 5 minutes; i.e. it takes 20–30 minutes for equilibration to take place between blood and the spleen. The fraction of the injected platelets recoverable in the circulation at equilibrium, which is normally somewhat less than two thirds, is sometimes known as the recovery. The recovery is reduced in splenomegaly because of expansion of the splenic platelet pool. Recovery may also be reduced as a result of cell damage sustained from *in vitro* manipulation during the labelling procedure.

In normal subjects, the disappearance of labelled platelets from the blood is almost linear; i.e. platelet removal or destruction is largely the result of platelet senescence, rather than a random process. The normal platelet life span is 9 days, after which the platelet is removed by the reticulo–endothelial system. Estimates of the numbers of platelets finally taken up by the liver, spleen and bone marrow vary, but are of the order of 20, 40 and 30% respectively.

4.5.3   Granulocytes

Like platelets, the kinetics of granulocytes have been studied for many decades with inefficient or non-gamma-emitting agents such as chromium-51 and phosphorus-32 labelled di-isopropylfluoro-phosphonate (DFP-32). The most important feature of granulocyte kinetics is the distribution of the cells between the so-called circulating and marginating pools. This distribution was quantified largely on the basis of the earlier work with DFP-32. Following their injection, only about 40% of labelled granulocytes can be accounted for in circulating blood because the remainder enters the marginating granulocyte pool. Although the marginating granulocyte pool has, until recently, been considered to be widely distributed throughout the body, kinetic studies with indium-111 labelled granulocytes have shown it to be largely present in the spleen and bone marrow, with smaller fractions in the lung and liver. The gamma-emitting radionuclide indium-111 has, in other words, allowed us to map the distribution of the marginating granulocyte pool. The kinetics of granulocytes in the spleen are almost identical to those of platelets, which have a very similar mean intrasplenic residence time. The lower recovery in blood of granulocytes (about 40%), compared with platelets, is the result of additional sites of granulocyte margination. Since granulocytes are more sensitive to *in vitro* manipulation than platelets, some of the difference in recoveries is also the result of artefactual granulocyte sequestration resulting from granulocyte activation and/or damage. Activated granulocytes are retained in the lung for variable periods (up to about one and a half hours), following which they are taken up by the liver. Early lung and subsequent liver activity are both, therefore, sensitive *in vivo* criteria of cell integrity following *in vitro* labelling.

Although granulocytes have a life span of about 15 days (most of which is spent in the bone marrow prior to release), they disappear from the circulation exponentially, with a half-time of only about 6 hr, corresponding to a mean residence time in blood of 10 hr. If they migrate into the tissues they may remain viable for up to a further 4 days. Granulocytes are removed from the circulation at random by the reticulo–endothelial system, and do not undergo migration into the tissues in the absence of inflammatory disease. Thus, although they differ from red cells and platelets insofar as their removal for destruction is not based on senescence, they are similar to red cells and platelets with respect to their destruction in the reticulo–endothelial system.

4.6 Myocardial agents

For many years thallium-201 was essentially the only agent for imaging regional myocardial blood flow, but more recently, technetium-99m labelled agents have become established. The mechanisms of uptake of these agents remains unclear and, following early development, it is being appreciated that, whilst they are excellent for evaluating coronary artery disease following injection into the stressed patient, thallium-201 is probably superior for the assessment of viability of ischaemic myocardium.

4.6.1 Potassium analogues

Thallium-201, which is used for myocardial perfusion imaging, is a potassium analogue and therefore taken up by tissues in general. Following intravenous injection, potassium analogues rapidly enter the intracellular space with extraction efficiencies ranging from 30 to 80%, depending on the analogue and myocardial blood flow. For a given analogue, the extraction fraction varies little between different tissues. The high extraction efficiency of radioactive potassium was exploited many years ago to quantify the fractional distribution of the cardiac output, an approach made possible by the low extraction of potassium analogues by the lung and by the fact that many tissues have an extraction fraction which is very similar to whole body extraction fraction for any given analogue. Thus, for a potassium analogue to be used for measuring the fraction of cardiac output supplying an organ, it need only have an

extraction efficiency in the organ similar to whole body extraction efficiency and not necessarily 100%. Thus the distribution of thallium-201 soon after injection reflects blood flow distribution, and this property has been exploited for imaging the regional distribution of myocardial blood flow.

Potassium and its analogues redistribute with time, such that about 4 hours after injection the distribution reflects the distribution of the potassium pool, or potassium 'volume'. This is analogous to xenon-133 inhalation, which initially reflects the distribution of ventilation but at equilibrium, after rebreathing, reflects the distribution of lung volume. Redistribution of thallium-201 forms the basis of distinguishing between myocardial ischaemia and myocardial infraction or, more precisely, identifying ischaemic but otherwise viable myocardium. A two compartmental model has been developed for measurement of myocardial blood flow using potassium analogues or nitrogen-13 labelled ammonia (**Fig. 4.6**). The transfer rate from the second to the first compartment represented by the PS product k_2 is assumed to be zero for the duration of blood flow measurement. Thallium-201 moves along this pathway when it slowly re distributes after injection. Although viable ischaemic myocardium usually takes up thallium-201 within 4 hours as a result of redistribution, it is now well recognized that, under some circumstances, it may fail to do so, even 24 hours after injection, and therefore be falsely interpreted as infarcted. This failure to redistribute can be explained on the basis of the two compart-

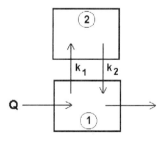

▌ **Fig. 4.6** Model illustrating the myocardial handling of myocardial perfusion agents, such as potassium analogues and nitrogen-13 ammonia. Compartment 1 represents plasma and interstitial fluid, regarded as one compartment because of the freedom of diffusion across the vascular endothelium. Compartment 2 represents the myocyte into which thallium-201, technetium-99m-MIBI and nitrogen-13 ammonia are essentially trapped, at least over the short term.

mental model and the fundamental observation that the ratio of the PS products k_1 to k_2 (**Fig. 4.6**) is similar for both normal and ischaemic viable myocardium. At equilibrium

$$k_1/k_2 = C_\tau/C_p \qquad (4.4)$$

so

$$C_\tau = \frac{k_1}{k_2} \cdot C_p \qquad (4.5)$$

where C is tracer concentration and subscripts p and τ refer to tracer in plasma and 'trapped' in tissue, respectively.

If k_1/k_2 is similar for ischaemic and normal myocardium, then C_τ is dependent on the circulating plasma thallium-201 concentration to the same extent in ischaemic as in normal myocardium, and at equilibrium their tissue concentrations will be similar. Since the whole body represents a large thallium 'sump', C_p is very low, and equilibrium may be delayed, explaining the failure of the tracer to redistribute. An injection of thallium-201 at rest ('re-injection'), which maximizes the availability of isotope to ischaemic myocardium, may be required to demonstrate the viability of a myocardial segment shown to be ischaemic following injection at stress. Furthermore it is important to appreciate that a zone of myocardium may be sufficiently ischaemic at rest to appear as a defect on the immediate reinjection images, and a period of redistribution may still be required after a rest injection in order to assess viability.

In addition to myocardial imaging, thallium-201 has been used to image skeletal muscle, the parathyroid glands and tumours. The basis for all these applications is the same, namely rapid generalized intracellular uptake. Thallium's counterpart in PET is the positron-emitter rubidium-82, which has a similar first-pass extraction fraction and similar redistribution kinetics to thallium-201.

4.6.2 Isonitriles

The isonitriles, of which MIBI is an example, are, like thallium-201, cations but are complex organic molecules. The first-pass extraction efficiency by myocardium of MIBI is slightly less than that of thallium-201. Unlike thallium-201 however it does not significantly redistribute from normal to ischaemic myocardium because it remains relatively firmly bound following uptake, clearing from the myocardium at a rate of only about 5% per hour. If the agent is injected during stress, the distribution of radio-activity — which represents the distribution of myocardial blood flow during stress — remains the same after recovery, in spite of a return of myocardial blood flow to resting levels. In this respect, it behaves more like microspheres and indeed, like technetium-99m HMPAO, it is a 'truer' chemical microsphere than, for example, thallium-201. In cardiac nuclear medicine therefore the MIBI has to be given separately (preferably on separate days) for comparison of rest and stress perfusion patterns. The lack of redistribution can be perceived as an advantage for comparison of rest and stress perfusion patterns since the patient can be injected under stress (at the time, for example, of stress electrocardiography) or at rest (for example in a patient in the accident and emergency department suspected of a myocardial infarction) and then imaged several hours later. On the other hand, lack of redistribution is a disadvantage compared with thallium-201 for the identification of hibernating myocardium, since a zone of severe ischaemia may appear as a defect even after injection at rest and therefore be misjudged as an infarct.

Technetium-99m-MIBI is being used increasingly for tumour imaging, especially of the parathyroid and breast. In common with several other compounds, many of which are anti-cancer chemotherapeutic agents, MIBI is a substrate for an intracellular mechanism which actively eliminates such compounds. The gene which regulates this 'multi-drug resistance' is over-expressed in many forms of cancer and may be responsible for rapid elimination of MIBI from cancer cells and consequent false-negative studies. Pharmacologic suppression of the mechanism may enhance the uptake.

4.6.3 Teboroxime

Technetium-99m teboroxime is a neutral lipophilic organic molecule which is taken up by the myocardium in proportion to blood flow. Its main difference compared to MIBI is a much faster rate of washout from myocardium. Its blood clearance is also faster, such that 90% is cleared into the tissues by 3 min after injection, compared with about 60 min for MIBI. Its washout from the myocardium is so fast that it has been compared to xenon-133 as a blood flow tracer. In keeping with this, its washout rate is proportional to myocardial perfusion. Like thallium-201, images have to be acquired very soon after injection, and, in this respect, it is again unlike MIBI, for which imaging is not conventionally started until about an hour after injection. Although teboroxime washes out rapidly from the myocardium, it does not redistribute like thallium-201 and there is no re-uptake in previously ischaemic myocardium. Like MIBI, therefore, it has to be given in two separate injections for the comparison of rest and stress perfusion. Whereas with MIBI, the rest and stress injections are best given on separate days, they can be done on the same day with teboroxime owing to its rapid washout.

4.6.4 Ammonia

Ammonia can be synthesized to incorporate nitrogen-13, a positron-emitting radionuclide with a half-life of 10 min. It is used for myocardial imaging and blood flow studies using PET. Following injection it exists almost exclusively as the ammonium ion, which, like the potassium analogues, is a univalent cation. Although, like potassium analogues, it has a high first-pass extraction fraction and redistributes slowly, its uptake is not mediated by the sodium/potassium pump mechanism. Instead, it probably penetrates cell membranes as non-ionic ammonia, which is highly diffusible. As the small amount of non-polar (i.e. neutral) ammonia present in capillary blood diffuses into cells, it is rapidly replenished in the blood by dissociation of the circulating ammonium cation. Once inside the cell, ammonia is rapidly utilized for amination and trapped intracellularly, maintaining dissociation of the ammonium ion in blood. All this happens so rapidly in the capillary that about 60% of the incoming ammonium ion is extracted. Ammonia can only be used for short-term studies, since arterial blood soon becomes contaminated by aminated metabolic derivatives exported (via pathway k_2, **Fig. 4.6**) from the tissue.

4.6.5 Fatty acids and glucose

The myocardium can be imaged with the radiolabelled substrates from which it generates energy, namely fatty acids (and their analogues) and glucose. Under normal circumstances the myocardium uses fatty acids for 80% of its energy requirements. Under conditions of ischaemia, the myocardium relies increasingly on glucose for its energy requirements since glucose can be catabolized to lactate anaerobically. The energy from fatty acids, in contrast, is derived from metabolism in the citric acid cycle, which requires oxygen for energy production. Palmitic acid can be synthesized with carbon-11 incorporated into the molecule. A less satisfactory agent for tracing myocardial fatty acid metabolism are the fatty acid analogues labelled with iodine-123. Nevertheless both agents reflect fatty acid kinetics and their alterations in ischaemic heart disease. The glucose analogue frequently used to image glucose utilization is fluorine-18 labelled 2-deoxyglucose (FDG). Although this analogue is taken up by myocardial cells by the same process of facilitated diffusion which results in glucose uptake, and is phosporylated to deoxyglucose-6-phosphate, the analogue (a) cannot be utilized in any forward metabolic pathway and (b) cannot be exported back to plasma since the myocardium contains no glucose-6-phosphatase. The tracer therefore becomes metabolically trapped. The rate of native glucose clearance from plasma by the myocardium exceeds that of FDG by a factor that appears to be similar for normal and ischaemic myocardium. This factor, called the lumped constant, is about 1.5. Unlike native glucose, FDG is excreted in the urine, possibly as a result of different rates of tubular reabsorption, reflecting a lumped constant similar to that of the myocardium.

The relative uptake of glucose is increased in viable ischaemic myocardium whilst fatty acid uptake is decreased. The value of FDG in this setting is that it can distinguish between viable and infarcted myocardium. Thus, when combined with a flow tracer such as nitrogen-13 labelled ammonia, viable ischaemic myocardium shows decreased ammonia uptake and increased glucose uptake, whereas infarcted myocardium shows a decrease in the uptake of both. Agents labelled with technetium-99m are now appearing which also show selectivity for hypoxic myocardium and, like the impact technetium-99m HMPAO has made on brain imaging, may give similar scintigraphic information as the positron-emitting agents.

4.7 Brain agents

As with the liver, the emphasis in radionuclide brain imaging has changed over the last few years as a result of developments in other imaging modalities. Whereas diffusible hydrophilic solutes image regional breakdown in the blood–brain barrier, the newer agents are lipophilic and image the regional distribution of cerebral blood flow.

4.7.1   Diffusible solutes

Technetium-99m DTPA, glucoheptonate and pertechnetate have all been used to image focal brain disease on the basis that, whilst unable to cross the intact blood brain barrier, they freely diffuse across abnormal endothelium of pathological tissue. Pertechnetate was used many years ago but is inferior to the other two because of partial protein binding in plasma, which limits its transfer into abnormal tissue. X-ray contrast materials, although having a slightly larger molecular size than DTPA and glucoheptonate, are also small diffusible solutes with similar biokinetics. Scintigraphy cannot compete with computerized tomography in terms of image resolution and consequently radionuclide brain imaging of this type has almost disappeared.

4.7.2   Technetium-99m HMPAO and iodine-123 iodoamphetamine

HMPAO and amphetamine are lipophilic agents and therefore readily cross the blood brain barrier. Because of their high first-pass extraction by the brain, they have been developed for imaging the distribution of cerebral perfusion. Technetium-99m HMPAO becomes metabolically trapped, intracelluarly, as result of conversion to secondary hydrophilic species by mechanisms which involve glutathione. The whole body distribution of HMPAO remains stable for several hours after injection and this conveniently allows imaging to be performed some time after injection and also by SPECT. It behaves, in other words, like a chemical microsphere. The lipophilicity of HMPAO confers certain other useful applications in nuclear medicine. Firstly, it is a successful cell-labelling agent, with good stability resulting, again, from intra-cellular conversion to hydrophilic species, which, because they are polar (i.e. ionic) cannot cross the cell membrane. Secondly, it rapidly enters pulmonary blood following inhalation as an aerosol. Thus its transfer across the pulmonary blood gas barrier is blood flow rather than diffusion dependent and it could therefore be used to image pulmonary vascular disease. Thirdly it is taken up by tumours and has been used to image them.

Important PET agents for imaging the brain are oxygen-15, oxygen-15-labelled water, oxygen-15-labelled carbon monoxide and fluorine-18 labelled-2-deoxyglucose (FDG). Labelled water, which is generated in the lung enzymatically by carbonic anhydrase following inhalation of oxygen-15-labelled carbon dioxide, is a tracer for cerebral perfusion. The kinetics of this approach are described in Section 3.1.3.1 and Section 12.1.2. Oxygen-15 and FDG are used respectively to image cerebral oxygen and glucose utilization. By combining these tracers with labelled water, images of oxygen and glucose extraction efficiency can be generated. Labelled carbon monoxide binds rapidly and stably to red cells, and, when given by inhalation, provides a positron-emitting red cell and therefore blood pool label.

4.8   Gallium-67 and indium-111

4.8.1   Gallium-67

Gallium-67 is used for imaging inflammation (infective or non-infective) and tumours. With respect to pyogenic inflammation, it has to a large extent been replaced by labelled white cells. However it retains an important role in the investigation of pyrexia of unknown origin, in which its non-specific uptake into inflammatory and neoplastic lesions is exploited as a means of localizing pathology. The normal distribution of gallium-67 includes the reticulo–endothelial system (particularly liver and bone marrow), breasts, testes, gut, nasal mucosa, and, to a smaller extent, lacrimal glands, salivary glands and female perineum. It enters gut directly and via the hepato-biliary tree. Slight symmetrical renal activity is normal up to 24 hours after injection. The skeletal uptake that is seen reflects both bone turnover (analogous to MDP bone scanning) and reticulo–endothelial (i.e. marrow) uptake. Intravascular gallium-67 is bound predominantly to plasma protein and circulates in blood with a half-time of about 20 hours. A number of mechanisms explain its localisation in inflammatory foci. Firstly, protein-bound gallium-67 enters the extravascular space as a result of protein 'leakage' through abnormal endothelium. Secondly, because of its structural similarity to ferric ion, gallium-67 binds to lactoferrin, which is a product of degranulating neutrophils. The lactoferrin–gallium complex is then taken up by local macrophages. Thirdly ferric iron and gallium-67 bind to siderophores, which are low molecular weight products of bacteria concerned with bacterial ferric iron utilization. Its relatively long residence time in the circulation (at least compared with indium-111-labelled white cells) and its uptake into macrophages may explain why gallium-67 localises in chronic inflammation, while its affinity for bacterial siderophores may explain why it localizes in sites of infection, even in neutropenic patients. Its mechanism of uptake into tumours is less well understood but includes increased endothelial permeability.

4.8.2 Indium-111

Indium-111 has many similarities with gallium-67. It is protein bound in plasma, mainly to transferrin, and circulates with a half-time similar to that of gallium-67. Its normal distribution is confined to the reticulo-endothelial system, mainly liver and bone marrow. The bone marrow uptake is into both erythroid and reticulo–endothelial compartments. Indium-111 has been used as a substitute for iron in ferro-kinetic studies but suffers in this respect from a number of dissimilarities with iron. It has also been used for imaging inflammation both as the chloride and complexed with lipophilic chelating agents like oxine and tropolone, but with limited success.

4.9 Agents localizing in endocrine glands

Localization of endocrine agents is generally based on the targeting of specific biochemical pathways.

4.9.1 Adrenal gland

4.9.1.1 Adrenal medulla

Meta-iodo-benzyl guanidine (MIBG) is an analogue of noradrenaline and as such is taken up into the sympathomimetic storage vesicles of sympathetic nerve endings. Its affinity for chromaffin tissue results in localization in the adrenal medulla. The normal distribution of MIBG therefore includes the salivary glands, myocardium, and adrenal medullae. In addition, it shows some uptake into the lungs, mainly the lower zones, the gut (into which it is secreted directly) and into the urinary tract. Less commonly, physiological activity may be seen in the gall bladder and uterus. Some gut activity may reflect free iodine uptake by the stomach. Since the urinary activity is largely filtered unchanged MIBG, and the agent is not significantly protein bound in plasma, its half-time in blood is short. Dynamic imaging over the kidneys immediately following injection gives data very similar to DTPA renography and may be useful for subsequent anatomical localization of a suspected abnormality. The finding that neuroblastoma may be seen with iodine-131 MIBG some days after injection, but not with iodine-123 MIBG, which has a relatively short physical half-life, has concentrated attention on the kinetics of MIBG redistribution.

MIBG uptake into pheochromocytoma and neuroblastoma can be reduced by some drugs, such as cocaine, dimethylimipramine, insulin, and reserpine, and can be increased by others, such as catecholamines and 6-hydroxydopamine. It has also been suggested that myocardial uptake, which is quite prominent in normal individuals, is minimal in the presence of neuroblastoma (as a result of competition) and this been used diagnostically. Myocardial uptake is also reduced in heart failure as a result of a decrease in sympathetic innervation.

4.9.1.2 Adrenal cortex

Radiolabelled analogues of cholesterol are used for imaging the adrenal cortex. In order to image the zone glomerulosa, such as in patients with Conn's syndrome, the rest of the cortex has to be suppressed with dexamethasone administration for a period of several days before administration of the radiopharmaceutical. Unilateral adenoma is visualized as a unilateral focus of uptake within 5 days of injection, while, with bilateral hyperplasia, uptake is bilateral (although not necessarily symmetrical). Imaging beyond 5 days after injection gives images which are difficult to interpret because the normal gland becomes refractory to dexamethasone suppression (i.e. 'escapes').

Cushing's syndrome may be ACTH dependent, as a result of a pituitary tumour or ectopic source, or ACTH independent, as a result of bilateral cortical hyperplasia, unilateral adenoma or carcinoma. ACTH dependence is seen as symmetrical bilateral adrenal visualization. This can be suppressed with dexamethasone treatment when the ACTH originates from a pituitary tumour but is usually not suppressible with an ectopic source. In Cushing's syndrome, which is ACTH independent, bilateral hyperplasia is seen as bilateral (usually asymmetrical) uptake, adenoma as unilateral visualization and carcinoma as bilateral non-visualization as a result of bulky, biochemically differentiated but poorly functioning tissue on the abnormal side with suppression of the contralateral side.

4.9.2 Parathyroid glands

Abnormal parathyroid glands may be difficult to visualize, depending on their size. They are usually demonstrated by subtraction imaging, in which the thyroid gland is imaged with pertechnetate and the thyroid gland plus parathyroid glands with thallium-201. Subtraction of the pertechnetate image from the thallium-201 image leaves, in theory, uptake to be seen only in the parathyroid glands. There are three possible approaches. Firstly, to give the thallium-201, image immediately, give pertechnetate and then repeat the image 20 minutes later. This has the advantage that there is no interference in the thallium-201 window from the higher energy of the pertechnetate, but has the disadvantage of movement artefacts. Secondly, to give pertechnetate, wait 20 minutes and then commence imaging. After acquiring the technetium-99m image, the patient is given thallium-201 and imaging repeated immediately. This reverses the advantages and disadvantages for the first procedure although the cross over of pertechnetate into the thallium-201 window can be corrected for. The third approach is to give the agents simultaneously and image by dual photon acquisition. If dual energy acquisition is available with the camera/computer system and the detector can adequately differentiate the energies of the two isotopes, then this is the ideal approach.

The new myocardial perfusion agent, MIBI (sestamibi), is being increasingly used for parathyroid imaging in place of thallium-201. Since it is labelled with technetium-99m, it has to be used with iodine-123 (in place of pertechnetate). Initial results with this approach are encouraging. The feasibility of dual photon imaging (including SPECT) is improved with iodine-123 (169 keV) and technetium-99m (140 keV). It has also been claimed that the parathyroid retains MIBI for longer than normal thyroid tissue and can therefore be distinguished from the thyroid in single tracer studies by sequential imaging over several hours. A focus of persisting activity favours abnormal parathyroid tissue. The influence of multi-drug resistance on this approach is discussed above.

4.9.3 Thyroid gland

The thyroid can be imaged with either technetium-99m pertechnetate or radio-iodine. Pertechnetate is concentrated (i.e. trapped) within the gland but, in contrast to radioiodine, is not organified. Nodules which retain the capacity for concentration but not organification can therefore be positive with pertechnetate but cold with iodine. Quantification of uptake is important during thyroid imaging for several reasons and is performed by comparison with a neck phantom. Technetium-99m uptake is usually quantified 20 minutes after intravenous injection and iodine-131 at 24 hours after oral administration. Typical normal ranges are 0.4–3% for technetium-99m and 20–50% for iodine-131. The procedures with iodine-123, which is less often used, are variable; uptake values at 24 hours are the same as for iodine-131 (after correction for the 13 hour half-life of 1-123).

4.9.4 Somatostatin receptor imaging

Somatostatin receptors are widely distributed throughout the body. The physiological actions of somatostatin, a polypeptide hormone, are in general opposite to those of growth hormone, hence its name. Secreted from the hypothalamus into the local portal circulation, it inhibits the release of growth hormone and thyroid stimulating hormone from the pituitary. It is also secreted widely in the gastro-intestinal tract, where it inhibits the release of insulin and glucagon, and in the nervous system where it functions as a neurotransmitter. Somatostatin receptors can be imaged with indium-111-labelled somatostatin analogues such as octreotide. The physiological distribution of this agent includes the liver, kidneys and especially the spleen. The thyroid and pituitary glands may also be seen. Much of the renal uptake is due to tubular reabsorption of filtered tracer and this can be competitively blocked by the intravenous administration of large doses of native amino acids. Although somatostatin receptors are present on lymphocytes they are insufficient to result in physiological uptake of the agent in lymph nodes. Somatostatin receptors are up-regulated in several neoplastic and neoplastic-like conditions, especially tumours of the alimentary tract, and this forms the basis for the wide range of clinical applications of indium-111 octreotide.

4.10 Pertechnetate

The biochemistry of pertechnetate is complex. Its normal distribution includes the salivary glands, gastric mucosa and thyroid gland. There is minimal uptake in the choroid plexus and breast. Pertechnetate gains access to breast milk. In plasma, it is partly bound to albumin and pre-albumin. The unbound fraction is excreted unchanged in the urine, although there is some retention in the renal parenchyma. Pertechnetate uptake at its three main sites is reversible. As result of luminal transport, activity may be seen in the mouth and gut lumen. Uptake into the thyroid gland is reversible with perchlorate.

Free pertechnetate is used to image the thyroid gland, salivary glands and ectopic gastric mucosa as in Meckel's diverticulum. Since the fraction in plasma that is not protein bound readily enters the extravascular space, pertechnetate has also been used to image soft tissue inflammation, particularly in joints. The mechanism underlying the rationale of this approach accounts for one of the causes of false positive results in Meckel's diverticulum, namely uptake into inflammatory bowel disease. Because of convenience, pertechnetate is often used for first-pass flow studies, for which, in effect, any gamma photon-emitting radionuclide would be suitable. One particular application in this respect is testicular torsion, in which total testicular ischaemia is present and can be distinguished, on radionuclide angiography, from inflammatory causes of a swollen painful testis. Bilateral non-visualization indicates bilateral torsion, a eunuch or a female.

Technetium-99m that dissociates from a radiopharmaceutical *in vivo* is taken up by the thyroid and stomach. Uptake in these organs indicates the existence of free pertechnetate and reflects radiopharmaceutical impurity and/or instability *in vivo*. Pertechnetate that fails to become incorporated into the radiopharmaceutical at the time of *in vitro* preparation may form a colloid which is subse-

quently seen on imaging as hepatic uptake. Occasionally dissociated technetium-99m may form a colloid *in vivo* with resulting liver uptake but this only occurs if the patient is receiving drugs such as those containing aluminium.

4.11 Proteins

The plasma proteins are classified according to eletrophoretic mobility (i.e. electrical charge) into albumin and globulins. The latter are further divided into α, β and γ globulins, the last being the immunoglobulins. Radiolabelled proteins imaged in nuclear medicine include albumin, pre-albumin, transferrin, proteins of the coagulation system, particularly fibrinogen and plasmin, the immunoglobulins, both monoclonal and polyclonal, and the acute phase proteins, particularly serum amyloid P component.

4.11.1 Albumin

Albumin, labelled with technetium-99m or iodine-123, is widely used as a blood pool imaging agent. Labelled with iodine-125, it is also used for measuring plasma volume. For albumin turnover studies it is generally labelled with iodine-131. Native albumin has a long survival time in the body, with a half-time of about 18 days. Since it is the smallest of the plasma proteins (molecular weight, 66 000 daltons), about half of it is extravascular. During the first hour following bolus intravenous injection, two exponentials are present in the radio-iodinated albumin plasma clearance curve. The first exponential is 'buried' in the dispersion (or mixing) phase. The rate constant of the second exponential is generally taken to represent the transcapillary escape rate of labelled albumin and has been used as a measure of capillary permeability but may instead represent penetration into the 'gel meshwork' of the interstitial fluid from the surrounding fluid phase of the interstitial space (Section 6.2.2). Over a period of days, a third exponential, which represents the degradation of the protein-label complex, can be identified with a half-time of about 10 days. Albumin can be labelled with chromium-51 for detection and quantification of gastrointestinal protein loss. Technetium-99m labelling of albumin is only suitable for relatively short-term studies, such as blood pool imaging, because the elution rate is rather rapid. Pre-albumin, which is actually a globulin, is only of importance because it loosely binds pertechnetate given intravenously.

4.11.2 Transferrin

Transferrin is labelled in several settings in nuclear medicine, either intentionally or unintentionally. It is in the globulin fraction and is relatively small (molecular weight, 76–81 kDa). It is intentionally labelled with iron-59 for ferrokinetic studies, including plasma iron clearance, red cell iron utilization and plasma iron turnover. Although the normal half-time of plasma iron-59 clearance is 60–140 min, this reflects the rate of transfer of iron from transferrin to the erythron rather than the survival of transferrin. Indeed, transferrin, like albumin, has a long half-life in the body. Transferrin is also intentionally labelled with indium-111 for detecting and quantifying (by whole body counting) gastro-intestinal protein loss (Section 9.5.1) and for capillary permeability studies, particularly involving the lung, where it has been used in conjunction with technetium-99m labelled red cells (Section 8.4.3). Successful gallium-67 imaging probably relies on transferrin labelling *in vivo*. When gallium-67 citrate is given to patients whose transferrin binding sites are saturated, such as following multiple transfusions, more of it is taken up by the skeleton in proportion to bone turnover and less is available for uptake in target pathological tissues. It may, under these circumstances, undergo glomerular filtration and partial tubular reabsorption resulting in renal parenchymal and urinary activity. Transferrin is unintentionally labelled during indium-111 white cell scanning as a result of the injection of non-cell-bound radionuclide and also as a result of a small amount of elution *in vivo*. Binding of non-cell-bound indium-111 by transferrin explains why the urinary tract is not normally seen in an indium-111 white cell scan.

4.11.3 Proteins of the coagulation pathways

Coagulation proteins include fibrinogen and plasmin. Radioiodinated fibrinogen is famous for the detection of post-operative deep venous thrombosis by surface probe counting but is now essentially obsolete for this application. This is partly because proximal vein thrombosis, which, in contrast to calf thrombosis, is thought to be the principal source of pulmonary emboli (although see below), is obscured by counts from urinary iodine. Technetium-99m labelled plasmin was briefly investigated in the early eighties as a clot localizing radiopharmaceutical.

Fragment E_1 is a fragment of fibrinogen which binds to cross-linked fibrin but not fibrinogen and labelled with iodine-123, has shown promise as a thrombus-localizing agent. More recently technetium-99m labelled tissue plasminogen activator has been proposed for thrombus localization. A recombinant version, with reduced or absent biological activity, should be used, since localization of the native thrombolytic molecule may result in localized clot lysis with subsequent loss of tracer from the thrombotic site. Peptide sequences are now being developed. Recently a small peptide derived from fibrinogen has been explored for thrombus imaging. This agent, known as RGD, binds to the fibrinogen receptor of platelets following their activation. It has the theoretical advantage of being selective for platelets that have already accumulated in thrombus and so should bind pre-formed thrombus in the anti-coagulated recipient. Since it is a small molecule, it can readily penetrate the interstices of a thrombus.

4.11.4 Immunglobulins

Native immunoglobulins have a molecular weight in the range 150–900 kDa. Their half-time of disappearance from the circulation, about 20 days, is even longer than albumin. The immuno-globulins have become very important in nuclear medicine, firstly because of hybridoma technology and production of monoclonal antibodies, and secondly the increasing use of radiolabelled polyclonal human immunoglobulins for localizing infection and inflammation.

4.11.4.1 Monoclonal antibodies

Numerous radiolabelled monoclonal antibodies have been investigated as localizing agents in a variety of pathological processes. Most of the effort has been centred on tumour imaging, principally ovarian, breast and colorectal carcinoma, and teratoma, seminoma and melanoma. Because of the large molecular size of these proteins, a fundamental problem is access to the antigen, which is often on the extravascular side of the endothelium (albeit in neoplasms with malfunctioning endothelium). This has prompted the development of F(ab)s, either divalent or monovalent (**Fig. 4.7**), which in addition to a greater penetration of endothelium, also undergo urinary excretion, thereby contributing to an improved target to background count rate by virtue of a shorter intravascular half-life. Various 'chaser' systems have also been devised to get around the problem of antigen access, including the streptavidin/biotin system, in which unlabelled antibody is given intravenously complexed with streptavidin, followed a few days later by radiolabelled biotin. Biotin is a small diffusible molecule which readily penetrates the endothelium and undergoes almost irreversible binding to streptavidin. It is also excreted rapidly in the urine, thereby improving target to background ratio.

Monoclonal antibodies are available for targeting myosin. This is normally intracellular and completely inaccessible to the antibody. As a result of muscle necrosis, the protein becomes exposed for binding to circulating antibody. These monoclonals may be useful in the diagnosis of myocardial necrosis, the assessment of skeletal muscle trauma and for localizing leiomyosarcomas. Diffusion of the antibody through the continuous endothelium of the myocardium may also be facilitated by ischaemia.

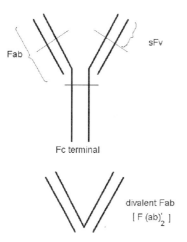

❚ **Fig. 4.7** Structural components of an IgG molecule. The Fab terminal of an antibody is the variable region, especially the sFv which contains the peptide sequences conferring specific antibody targeting. The Fc terminal binds to Fc receptors located on various cells, especially leucocytes and macrophages, thereby allowing the latter to process antibody-antigen complexes. All four components, i.e. whole IgG, F(ab)$'_2$, Fab and sFv, have been used, labelled with radionuclides, in nuclear medicine.

Monoclonal antibodies which target intravascular structures such as blood cells and activated endothelium are particularly attractive because of the range of diseases that could potentially be localized. In general, there is no difficulty with access to the antigen: for instance anti-platelet monoclonal antibodies label circulating platelets within minutes of injection with an *in vivo* labelling efficiency of about 80%. Some anti-platelet monoclonal antibodies are being developed which target activated platelets. Granulocytes and lymphocytes have been labelled *in vivo* with specific monoclonal antibodies, although, with these antibodies, there is the problem of binding to bone marrow precursors, with the result that the labelling efficiency of circulating granulocytes is low, and only about 10% of the circulating radioactivity can be shown to be cell bound. Other monoclonal antibodies with intravascular targets include those against fibrinogen, fibrin and endothelial adhesion molecules. Some antigens, against which labelled antibodies have been explored, are exposed only when the cell is activated, a phenomenon which offers the potential of higher sensitivity. These include firstly, P-selectin, a platelet α particle adhesion molecule which becomes exposed when the α particle membrane fuses with the platelet membrane and secondly, E-selectin, an inducible endothelial adhesion molecule which functions by promoting granulocyte margination at sites of inflammation.

Attempts are being made to reduce the size of immunoreactive agents even further using recombinant techniques of genetic engineering. Thus the region of a monoclonal antibody which is responsible for binding the antigen can be produced separately from the rest of the antibody. A whole monoclonal antibody consists of a complex peptide chain arranged in a Y-shaped structure. The single 'vertical' section of the Y, the Fc fragment, is a single peptide chain with a constant structure, common to its class of antibody, and independent of the antibody's antigen-recognizing ability. The two 'arms' of the Y joined together is the F(ab)'$_2$ fragment. The individual F(ab) component consists of a distal variable portion, which recognizes the antigen, and a proximal portion, which, like the Fc fragment is constant. The terminal end of the Fc fragment binds to Fc receptors on macrophages, thereby bringing antigens bound to the Fab terminals into close proximity with the macrophage. Cleavage of the Fc portion from the whole antibody leaves the $F(ab)'_2$, which in turn can be further cleaved to form the $F(ab)$s. The variable distal portion of the $F(ab)$, called an sFv (single variable chain), can be produced by genetic engineering. It is also possible to encode a short tail of a suitable peptide sequence designed to bind a specific radionuclide, and this has now been achieved successfully with technetium-99m. An sFv has a molecular weight of 27 kDa.

4.11.4.2 Human polyclonal immunoglobulin

Recently human polyclonal immunoglobulin (HIG) has been introduced for imaging inflammation with disputed success. Although specific mechanisms of localization were first put forward, such as binding of cells and proteins to the Fc receptors on the HIG molecule, it is now generally accepted that localization is non-specific and the result of an endothelial leak — predominantly the same mechanism as with gallium-67. Three factors in inflammation contribute to increased uptake; (a) increased blood pool as a result of local vasodilation, (b) expanded extravascular space and (c) increased endothelial permeability. Interestingly, indium-111 labelled HIG appears to perform better than technetium-99m labelled HIG as a result of extravascular dissociation of indium-111 from the HIG and subsequent tight binding to local proteins (**Fig. 4.8**). Technetium-99m labelled HIG, in contrast, tends to diffuse back, intact, into the intravascular space. The logical competitor to indium-111 HIG is not so much labelled leucocytes but rather gallium-67, which, like HIG, performs relatively well in chronic infection and may target tumour, presumably again as a result of an endothelial leak.

4.11.5 Acute phase proteins

The acute phase proteins, which include C-reactive protein and serum amyloid P component (SAP),

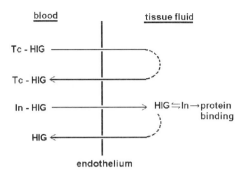

▮ **Fig. 4.8** Different behaviour of In-111 immunoglobulin (HIG) and technetium-99m-HIG. Inflammatory lesions continue to accumulate indium-111 over several days following injection of indium-111 HIG. Technetium-99m is not so avidly retained because of preferential binding to HIG or because of intrinsic instability of technetium-99m binding to extravascular protein.

have been investigated as imaging agents. Radio-iodinated SAP has become established as an effective method for imaging amyloid deposits. Amyloid-bearing organs most clearly seen are the liver, spleen, bone marrow, adrenal glands and kidneys. Tissues with amyloid burden that have not been successfully imaged include the myocardium, skin and Alzheimer's involvement of brain. This would be consistent with the notion that localization depends on this very large molecule (about 300 kDa) crossing the endothelium. The reticulo–endothelial sinusoids have a permeable, fenestrated, endothelium; the adrenal and the kidney also have highly permeable capillaries. The myocardium and skin, on the other hand, have continuous endothelium which is much less permeable. Another, much smaller protein, aprotinin, has recently been used to image amyloid. Labelled with technetium-99m, this agent (about 6000 Da), gives clear images of myocardial amyloidosis, presumably because it is more diffusible through the myocardial endothelium.

5 Scintillation detectors, data processing and quantification

5.1 Scintillation detectors

The radionuclides of interest in nuclear medicine are almost all emitters of gamma photons. Many useful radionuclides also emit beta particles but it is the gamma emissions for which scintillation detectors are generally designed. Positron emitters are also included since, after emission from the nucleus, a positron travels only millimeters before encountering an electron. The two particles annihilate with the conversion of their masses into two gamma photons emitted from the point of annihilation in opposite directions to each other. It is these photons that are detected in positron cameras.

There are several types of gamma detection system used in nuclear medicine: the scintillation well counter, scintillation probe, scintillation camera and positron camera (the scintillation camera may also be referred to as a gamma camera or, after the inventor, the Anger camera; the positron camera may also be called a positron emission tomographic or PET scanner). Well counters are used for measuring the amount of radioactivity in samples of body fluids inserted into a well or hole formed in the crystal. Scintillation probes are used to record the signal from radioactivity within regions of the body. They may be hand held or mounted on a support and include a single cylindrical crystal shielded with lead. Scintillation cameras are used to record an image of the distribution of radioactivity within the body. The two types of imaging device used are the gamma camera and the PET camera. All these detectors depend on the principle that when a photon is absorbed in a transparent crystal, the energy of the photon is converted into light — appearing as a very brief flash or scintillation.

A scintillation detector consists of a single crystal, usually of sodium iodide, 'activated' by atoms of thallium. When a gamma ray photon interacts within the crystal, a scintillation of light is generated. The intensity of this scintillation, which lasts of the order of microseconds, is directly related to the energy

given up by the photon within the crystal. The intensity of the light is too low to be seen directly and the light is therefore first converted to electrons by the photocathode of a photomultiplier tube (PMT), optically coupled to the crystal. The electrons are then amplified within the PMT to produce an electrical pulse that is related to the original energy of the gamma photon. The relationship between the size of the pulse and the energy of the photon is not exact since the conversion process from light to electrical signal is subject to random variations. Rather than a single value for the energy, a range of energies is measured, distributed around a 'photopeak' when a spectrum is acquired. However, since the photopeak is characteristic of a particular radionuclide, the sizes of the pulses issuing from the PMT can still be used to identify gamma emissions and potentially separate individual radionuclides from a mixture. The incoming pulses are sorted according to size using a pulse height analyser which operates by accepting only those pulses which have a size that falls within a 'window' set between selected thresholds. The window control can be calibrated in keV so that, for example, with a lower threshold set at 130 keV and an upper set at 150 keV, the window will accept the photons of technetium-99m, forming a photopeak around a value of 140 keV.

The rate of arrival of photons in the crystal depends on the activity of the source, its proximity to the crystal and the amount of intervening material capable of absorbing or scattering the photons (**Fig. 5.1**). When a photon is deflected (scattered) it loses some energy thereby depositing less energy in the crystal when it is absorbed. If a photon escapes from the crystal before being completely absorbed then a submaximal amount of energy will be deposited, giving a scintillation of correspondingly submaximal brightness. A photon scattered within the crystal can nevertheless be ultimately absorbed in another part of the crystal, in which case the total energy deposited in the crystal will be the same as for

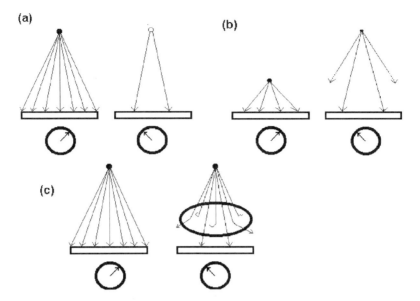

▌ **Fig. 5.1** The rate of arrival of gamma rays on the crystal depends on: (a) the activity of the source — the rate is linearly proportional to the activity; (b) the proximity of the source to the crystal — the inverse square law applies to an uncollimated detector but does not apply when the detector is collimated; (c) the amount and nature of the absorbing or scattering material between source and detector.

photons completely absorbed without prior deflection and will be recorded. Scintillations of energy less than expected from a particular photon source also occur in the crystal if the photon has already undergone scattering before absorption in the crystal and will not be recorded if the energy deposited is above or below the energy window set for the recorder. The process of scattering (called Compton scattering) is particularly important with respect to scintillation cameras since it is essential that gamma rays are imaged directly from their source.

The flashes of light are so brief, and the refractory period of the counting equipment so short, that tens of thousands of photons can be detected per second. If however it so happens that two photons of the same energy were completely absorbed in the crystal effectively simultaneously, then the intensity of the flash would be doubled and interpreted as a single flash from a photon of twice the energy. It is likely to fall outside the energy window that the detector has been set to discriminate. This explains why counters will tend to lose counts and eventually 'saturate' when exposed to very active sources, leading to so called dead-time errors. Clearly, the probability of simultaneous arrival of two photons decreases as the activity of the source decreases, although it remains

possible at lower activities especially with well counters. The relationship between the count rate

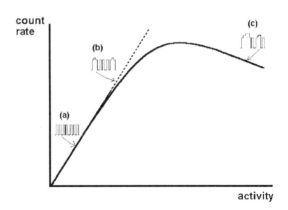

▌ **Fig. 5.2** When the count rate recorded from a detector is plotted against the amount of activity being detected (a) the rate initially increases linearly with increase in activity. (b) As the rate increases there is an increased probability of the individual pluses overlapping in time with the result that multiple counts are recorded as single counts. Because of this, the count rate decreases from the rate predicted from the linear portion of the curve. (c) At very high activity levels the pulses occur so frequently that a significant proportion cannot be resolved; the system is paralysed and the count rate starts to fall from its maximum value.

and counts lost due to dead time is a non-linear characteristic of the detector **(Fig. 5.2)**.

It is important to appreciate that, in general, scintillation probes and cameras are highly inefficient in that the fraction of photons emitted by the activity source that is seen by the detector is very small. This is because of the necessity to define a small region of interest and therefore ignore most of the photons which are emitted in all directions. However the efficiency of the well counter where the sample is almost surrounded by the detector is relatively high.

5.1.1 Scintillation well counter

Well counters are used to measure the concentration of radioactivity within samples, typically of blood or urine. They consist of a single crystal and PMT. The crystal has a hole partially or completely set into it into which the sample can be inserted for counting **(Fig. 5.3)**. The geometry whereby nearly all the emissions are seen by the crystal makes well counters relatively efficient and sensitive and they can count sources undetectable by scintillation probes and cameras. Not surprisingly, they can be easily saturated by samples containing too much radioactivity. This unfortunately precludes direct counting of the normal activity administered to patients and means that a diluted standard with a known relationship to the administered activity (e.g. a dilution of 1: 1000) is usually counted instead. In general, kilobequerel activities are counted rather than activities of megabequerels.

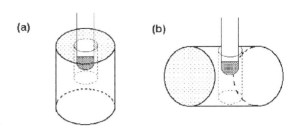

▮ **Fig. 5.3** The crystal detector in a well counter may appear as a solid detector with a 'well' cut into it as shown in (a). A small sample is almost completely surrounded by detector and the efficiency of counting is high. Larger samples may appear above the top of the well and the efficiency decreases. In some counters, as in (b), the sample is placed in a hole bored through the detector, a geometry allowing larger samples to be counted with constant high efficiency.

5.1.2 Scintillation probe

A scintillation probe consists of a single, usually cylindrical, crystal typically 1–5 cm in length and 2–8 cm in diameter coupled to a single PMT **(Fig. 5.4)**. The field of view determining which photons can arrive in the crystal can be limited and a restricted volume of acceptance created by a 'collimator'. In its simplest form it consists of a lead cylinder, with a central hole allowing the gamma photons through, surrounding and overlapping the front face of the crystal. A scintillation probe is unable to distinguish, or resolve, individual activity sources; i.e. it has no spatial resolution and cannot generate an image. Collimated probes can be used to

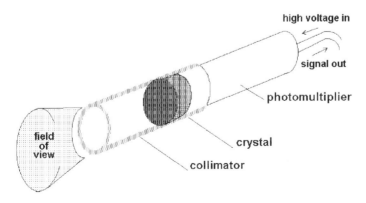

▮ **Fig. 5.4** A scintillation 'probe' consists of a crystal detector viewed by a photomultiplier tube (PMT) in a light tight casing. Lead shielding is placed round the crystal and extends out as shown so that only radiation coming from the limited field of view and entering the collimator is counted. A cable provides the high voltage required by the PMT and also carries the detection signal to the main counting electronics.

monitor, from outside the body, the level of activity of a source in a region within the body. They are generally used in nuclear medicine for dynamic studies of physically constrained sources such as studies of the rate of clearance from a tissue of a locally injected radiopharmaceutical, for example, xenon-133 washout curves following local arterial injection. In order to provide an *image* of the distribution of a source, the gamma camera was developed.

5.1.3 Gamma camera

In a gamma camera there is one large crystal, in the form of a thin rectangular or circular disc, viewed by a large number (50–100) of photomultipliers positioned behind the crystal (**Fig. 5.5**). Clearly, a single source could deposit photons at all locations in the crystal and so some collimating device is required. This is provided by a thick lead disc perforated by several thousand (usually) parallel holes perpendicular to the face of the collimator. The length of these holes is considerably greater than their diameter. Only those photons travelling approximately perpendicular to the face of the collimator will be able to reach the crystal (**Fig. 5.6a**). Those travelling at an angle will be absorbed in the lead of the collimator. A source S will therefore be able to generate scintillations only at one location in the crystal ('S') and there will be a direct relationship between the distance of the source x and the distance of the scintillation x' from the central axis. A scintillation in the crystal is seen by a large number of photomultiplier tubes but generates the largest electrical pulses in the tubes closest to it. The computer to which the tubes are connected can then localize the scintillation from knowledge of the weighted mean of the signals from the PM tubes and their position relative to the edge of the crystal (**Fig. 5.7**). The gamma camera can therefore 'resolve' separate sources of radioactivity and thereby generate an image. The final image is formed from tens of thousands, of detected photons at locations anywhere in the crystal. The same rules governing energy discrimination, scatter and dead-time errors apply to the gamma camera as to the scintillation probe. Energy discrimination, particularly at the lower limit, is more important in the case of the camera. Imagine, for instance, a photon S, initially approaching the face of the camera at an angle, being

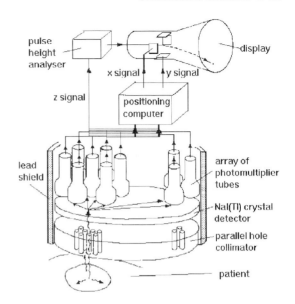

▌ **Fig. 5.5** The component parts of a gamma camera system include a collimator — essentially a lead block pierced by thousands of narrow straight bore holes. The collimator allows only those gamma rays travelling in well defined directions to strike the large diameter, thin crystal detector. Light from each detected scintillation is seen to different extents by a number of PMTs. The distribution of light reaching the PMTs is used in the processing computer to define the x and y co-ordinates of the scintillation in the crystal and its energy (the 'z') signal. For direct display of the scintillation the x and y signals deflect the beam of the display tube while the z signal switches on the beam causing a spot to appear on the display in a position corresponding to its original position in the cyrstal. The accumulation of a large number of displayed spots forms the basis of the image. In a digital camera the signals are processed at the outputs of the PMTs themselves and passed through individual analogue to digital converters. The digital data that result are used directly by the system computer to assign an x and y position and an energy signal which may be accepted or rejected. The display then corresponds to the contents of the computer memory holding the image matrix.

deflected by scatter into a direction perpendicular to the camera face (**Fig. 5.6b**). It could then be deposited in the crystal at a false position, F and would 'degrade' the image if recorded. However, having lost energy as a result of scatter, the scintillation will not be recorded by the camera provided the lower limit of the energy window is appropriately set to reject it. A measure of the ability

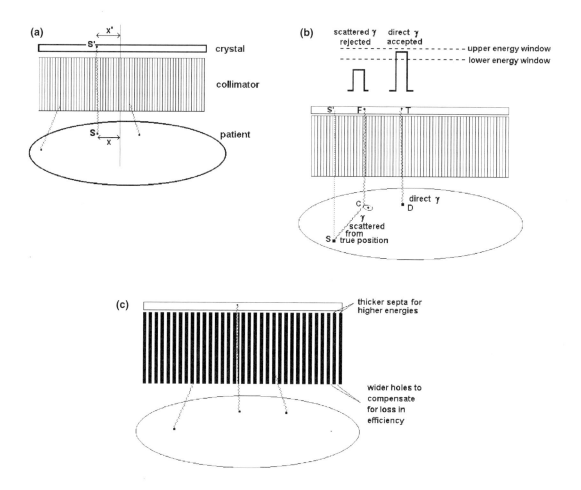

∎ **Fig. 5.6** Characteristics of the collimator used in the gamma camera. (a) Only those gamma rays travelling at right angles to the collimator enter the holes to strike the crystal. A direct relationship between the position of the scintillation in the crystal (*S'*) and the position of the origin of the gamma ray (*S*) is established. (b) A new gamma ray originating at position *S* and scattered at point *C* such that its direction is perpendicular to the collimator can enter and strike the crystal at point *F* rather than at the intended *S'*. This 'false' signal can be rejected by the pulse height analyser as its energy will be less than that of the direct gamma ray because of the energy lost in the scattering process. (c) Collimators used with higher energy gamma emitters require thicker septa (lead inserts between the holes). Because less of the crystal surface is available for detection there will be a loss of sensitivity unless the collimator holes are widened. This widening will however lead to a degradation of resolution.

to discriminate photons of differing energies is called the energy resolution of the camera.

The gamma camera is highly inefficient, recording only a tiny fraction of photons emitted from a source. There are several reasons for this. The collimator absorbs a very large fraction, and a further small fraction goes straight through the crystal without being absorbed since to retain the correspondence between the position of the scintillation in the crystal and the weighted output of the PM tubes, gamma camera crystals are forced to be very thin. This improves resolution since a scintillation taking place at the front of a thick crystal would not be accurately localized. On the other hand, sensitivity is decreased because the probability of absorption within the crystal is decreased. The higher the energy of the radionuclide, the greater will be the probability that the photon traverses the crystal

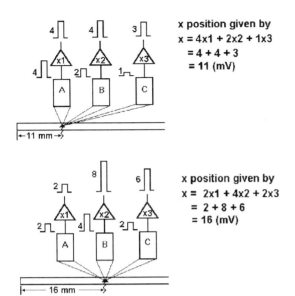

x position given by
x = 4x1 + 2x2 + 1x3
= 4 + 4 + 3
= 11 (mV)

x position given by
x = 2x1 + 4x2 + 2x3
= 2 + 8 + 6
= 16 (mV)

∎ **Fig. 5.7** The principle of positioning a scintillation in the detector from the relative responses of the photo-multiplier tubes. PMTs are positioned above the crystal so that each scintillation is viewed by a number of tubes. Each PMT is given a weight (a particular amplification factor, ×1, ×2, ×3 etc.) according to its distance from a reference point in the crystal and will have an output also dependent on its distance from the scintillation (4, 2, 1 etc.). The weights and outputs are combined to give the total signal. In the example given, a scintillation 11 mm from the edge will have a nominal *x* signal of 11 mV (and an associated *y* signal) while the scintillation 16 mm from the edge will have a nominal *x* signal of 16 mV (and an associated *y* signal).

without detection. So the efficiency of a gamma camera starts to fall appreciably for sources of energy higher than that of technetium-99m (140 keV). Modern cameras are designed around this energy and have crystals of only about one centimeter thickness. These work at efficiencies of about 100% for energies below 80keV, 60% for energies around 200keV and 14% at 511 keV. Higher energy radionuclides also require collimators with thicker septa (i.e. the lead between the holes; **Fig. 5.6c**). They generally give poorer resolution than low-energy collimators because, in order to compensate for the thicker septa (and lower efficiency through greater stopping of the gamma rays), the holes have wider diameters to allow more gamma rays through. This obviously will degrade the image resolution by allowing photons to pass

through the collimator which are not strictly perpendicular to the face of the camera. So for several reasons, gamma camera design is faced with the trade-off of sensitivity versus resolution.

5.1.4 Positron camera

The fourth type of scintillation device is the positron camera. This is designed to detect the so-called coincident photons generated when a positron, which is essentially a positively charged 'antimatter electron', is emitted from the nucleus of a radio-nuclide and reacts with an electron. It does this almost immediately after emission, after travelling up to a few millimetres, with resulting mutual annihilation of the two oppositely charged particles. The two coincident gamma photons leave the point of annihilation effectively at 180° to each other ('back to back'). A basic positron camera consists of a ring of single scintillation probes, any two of which, facing each other, take advantage of the back-to-back emission and simultaneously record the coincident photons assuming that the annihila-tion took place somewhere along a line joining the two probes. Consider a single source as in Fig. 5.8a. This can be identified by counters at A and A' as originating somewhere along the line AA'. When subsequent annihilations take place at the same location, two other opposing probes, such as B and B', will construct other lines which also go through the source. As a result, the positron camera can identify the position and construct a transaxial tomographic image of the source in the plane of the detectors A, A' B and B'. Furthermore, as the detectors are arranged in a series of rings or as sets of opposed two-dimensional arrays, all of which identify the source, its position can be calculated in three dimensions, i.e. multiple tomographic plane images can be depicted as in X-ray CT scanning and MRI. The technique of imaging is known as positron emission tomography (PET). (Because it employs the simultaneous detection of two photons it should be distinguished from the other form of imaging, single photon emission computerized tomography or SPECT which, in one variant, may also be used to image positron emitters.)

An alternative method of detection is to employ two gamma camera heads rather than separate detectors (**Fig. 5.8b**). The camera heads are not fitted with collimators since the back-to-back

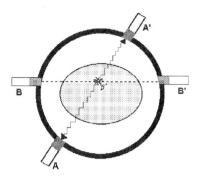

∎ **Fig. 5.8a** Principle of location of a site of positron emission in a positron scanner. A positron annihilates just after creation giving rise to two 'back-to-back' 511 keV gamma rays simultaneously. Detection of both of these by two probes A and A′ indicates that the positron has been emitted somewhere along the line AA′. Other lines of detection such as BB′ will help locate the original source of positrons and also the distribution of positron labelled tracer in the body.

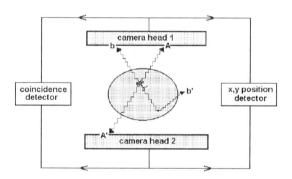

∎ **Fig. 5.8b** Principle of location of a site of positron emission in a positron camera. Two camera heads are set to register a count only when both detect a simultaneous arrival of the 511 keV photons. The positron of points such as A and A′ which define the line of response is given by the conventional camera positioning circuits. A positron emission giving rise to a detected event *b* and a scattered event *b′* which is not recorded by the second camera is not registered. Since the detectors are two-dimensional and the intersections of lines of response give additional depth information, the distribution of positron emitters in the body is determined in three dimensions.

property of coincident photons is used instead of the collimator holes to identify the lines of origin of the radioactive source. The heads are also connected so that coincident events in both heads can be recorded. The positions of two coincident gamma rays such as

A and A′ in the heads are identified in the usual way. So called 'singles' events, such as b, b′, where only one photon is detected and the corresponding photon is scattered do not lead to a coincidence detection and are not recorded. It is apparent that, without physical collimation, count rates are extremely high and the electronic circuits in the camera heads have to be upgraded considerably to cope with them.

The advantages of PET are:

(1) the relatively high levels of sensitivity because no physical collimation restricts the emissions;

(2) the good resolution afforded by the coincidence between small detectors;

(3) the availability of positron-emitting radionuclides of the important elements, carbon, oxygen and nitrogen, and with the ability, e.g. fluorine-18, to label substances of biological interest which are otherwise difficult to label, for example, glucose;

(4) the ability to quantify tissue concentrations of radioactivity in transaxial slices. Positron-emitting radionuclides are often short-lived, with half-times measurable in minutes, and can be incorporated by replacement of a non-radioactive atom, into a wide variety of substances and metabolites of physiological interest, without altering the chemical and physiological properties of the molecule.

5.2 Data

The information generated by a scintillation detector may be handled in several ways. The pulses generated in a scintillation probe expressing, for instance, the level of activity in a source can simply be counted over a set time period in a suitable recording device, or they may be transmitted to a rate meter which records the rate of pulse generation and expresses the level of activity as a count rate. The photons emitted from a source with a continuously changing level of activity, as would be encountered in a dynamic study, can be counted over successive discrete periods of time to produce a digital time record of the data. (NB The *datum* in this context is simply the scintillation itself.) Expressing the data continuously as a count rate, perhaps on a meter, is called analogue recording **(Fig. 5.9)**.

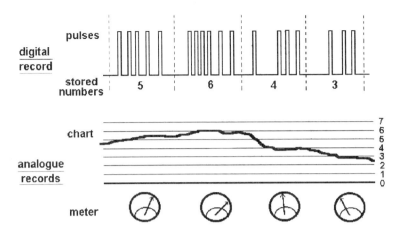

▌ **Fig. 5.9** Illustration of analogue and digital recording. Data from a scintillation counter may be recorded digitally as individual events are counted on a scaler or computer, usually in preset count intervals, or in analogue form as readings on a meter or chart recorder. Counts recorded digitially are often displayed in analogue form, e.g. as a curve, for ease of interpretation.

In the case of the gamma camera, the data, in addition to detection of the scintillation itself, include the location of the scintillation on a two- or three-dimensional display, the energy associated with the scintillation and the time of the detection, sometimes with reference to a physiological signal such as an ECG.

Two types of display are generated — an analogue and a digital display. An analogue image is similar to a photographic image in which the points forming the display are unconstrained so that a continuous two-dimensional display is built up over the exposure time. This may be contrasted with the display being divided up into small square picture elements, or pixels, as in a computer image. The latter is a digital image, which in nuclear medicine is formed by restraining the position of a scintillation to an appropriate pixel of the display in a computer memory matrix. This can be divided up into a set number of pixels ranging from 32×32 to 1024×1024 or more pixels. For dynamic studies, gamma camera data are almost always digitized and each pixel can be thought of a representing a separate tiny scintillation probe. By means of the nuclear medicine computer, regions of interest can be drawn around selected pixels and time–activity curves generated for any chosen portion of the image.

Photon emission is a random event and the statistical certainty with which a count rate, or number of counts recorded, reflects the amount of radioactive material being detected is dependent on the number of counts recorded in a discrete time interval as discussed in Section 1.6.2. This number has a standard deviation (s.d.) which is a measure of the probability of obtaining the same number of counts if the radioactive source was recounted. The s.d. is related to the number of recorded counts N as follows:

$$\text{s.d.} = \sqrt{N} \qquad (5.1)$$

and the relative error.

$$\text{s.d.}/N = \sqrt{N}/N = 1/\sqrt{N}.$$

Thus the larger the number of counts recorded, the smaller will be the relative error in N. For a count rate of 100 the relative error is $(\sqrt{100})/100$ or 10%. For 10 000 counts the relative error is $(\sqrt{10\,000})/10\,000$ or 1%.

As they travel through a material photons are absorbed at random at a rate which is dependent on the density and thickness of the material and the energy of the photon. If material of thickness d is placed between a radioactive source and a detector then the recorded count rate $N_1(d)$ would be less than that, N_0, recorded when no material is interposed between source and detector (**Fig. 5.10**). This is summarized as follows:

$$N_1(d) = N_0 e^{-\mu d} \qquad (5.2)$$

where μ is the linear attenuation coefficient (specific for the material and radionuclide). The expression

$1-e^{-\mu d}$ is the probability of a photon travelling towards the detector undergoing absorption in the material. Analogous to the relationship between half-life and decay constant in radioactive decay, there is a relationship between the half-thickness $d_{1/2}$ and the linear attenuation coefficient μ in radionuclide attenuation:

$$d_{1/2} = \frac{0.693}{\mu} \text{ or } \mu = \frac{0.693}{d_{1/2}}.$$

So $d_{1/2}$ is the linear distance in a material in which half the incident photons are absorbed. Sometimes the tenth value thickness, which is the thickness that reduces the incident flux to 1/10 of its initial value, is quoted. For technetium-99m in tissue $d_{1/2}$ is about 5 cm and $d_{1/10}$ about 18 cm. For iodine-131 in tissue $d_{1/2}$ is about 6 cm and $d_{1/10}$ about 22 cm.

5.2.1 Sources of errors in data

Ideally what is required is a knowledge of the absolute amount of activity at any location in the body at any time. From this data we can estimate the variation in the amounts with time. These variations are compared with models of predicted behaviour for normal and abnormal states so that we can detect and localize abnormalities. Errors in this ideal scenario come about because of several factors:

1. The origins of the counts received by the gamma camera is not known accurately, firstly because of the finite resolution of the camera which worsens at increasing distances from the collimator and secondly because of scattering of the radiation.

2. Movement of the patient or natural motion and distortion of the organ through heartbeat or breathing artifacts also add to the uncertainties in location.

3. The quantity of activity seen is affected by attenuation.

4. Underlying and overlying tissues add background noise to the data originating from a volume of interest.

5. The data are affected by random counting variations.

5.3 Data acquisition

5.3.1 Static acquisition

The simplest form of acquisition is static acquisition. In the case of the gamma camera this consists of a single image of a static source, analogous to a single photograph taken with a light camera. The required exposure times are longer for a radionuclide image than for a photograph but the principle is the same. Positron cameras may also be used to produce static images and this is considered further below. Although scintillation probes are usually used for dynamic studies, they are also occasionally used to record the stable count rate from a static source such as that from an organ within the body; well counters are often used in this mode.

5.3.2 Dynamic acquisition

Scintillation probes are usually used in dynamic mode, as for recording the rate of disappearance of a locally deposited radionuclide. By transmitting the output of pulses from the probe to a rate meter, a continuously varying signal can be recorded to produce a time–activity curve of a quickly changing activity over periods of seconds to hours. Well counters can produce dynamic information about a more slowly varying situation through counting samples taken at different times over periods of minutes to hours. The gamma camera is also frequently used to acquire image data in dynamic

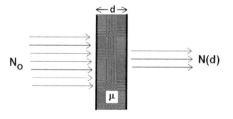

∎ **Fig. 5.10** Illustration of the quantitation of attenuation or absorption by a medium. The absorption of a stream of gamma rays travelling through a medium of linear absorption coefficient μ is given quantitatively by the expression $N(d) = N_0 \, e^{-\mu d}$ where N_0 is the number of gamma rays entering a thickness d of absorber and $N(d)$ the number exiting. The thickness d usually has the units of cm and μ units of cm^{-1} so that the product $\mu \cdot d$ is unitless.

mode. As mentioned above, the data are usually digitized and the computer is programmed to record the number of counts in images or frames in successive time periods. The frame time chosen depends on how fast the measured count rate changes with time. Thus, for a first-pass blood flow study, a frame time of one second (or less) is usually used whereas, say, for a renogram, longer frame times are used, up to one minute per frame. To make a further analogy with light photography, a dynamic gamma camera study is the equivalent of a 'cine' film.

5.3.3 List mode acquisition

The dynamic data recorded from a gamma camera requires pre-selected time frames which may turn out later to be inappropriate. Alternatively therefore the data can be recorded in 'list' or 'histogram' mode, which is a more flexible form of recording, allowing subsequent reformatting of data in any chosen way. In list mode, not only is the position (*x, y* co-ordinates) of each individual scintillation in the crystal recorded by the detector but also its time of occurrence (*t*) and, sometimes, its energy (*Z*) or relation to a physiological signal such as the R wave of an ECG. This gives a greater degree of flexibility and permits analogue display of the data in any

chosen time format but has the disadvantage of requiring a large amount of computer memory.

5.3.4 Gated acquisition

Gated acquisition is used when the radioactive source is associated with an organ such as the heart that is changing position periodically. The movement has to be regular and predictable; for example when imaging the heart, the ECG is first recorded to establish the duration of the cardiac cycle, or more specifically the R–R interval. The computer then divides the cycle into a number of equal time segments – 16 or 32, for example. The detector records data from many cycles, each new cycle being signalled by the R wave through an on-line ECG monitor. All the counts recorded during the first time segment are added together, and so on (**Fig. 5.11**). The computer then repetitively displays one complete composite cycle, from which, in the case of the heart, chamber emptying and filling can be visualized. Another example of a moving organ is the lung which, of course, moves with respiration. Lung imaging can also be gated. In practice however gated acquisition is applied almost exclusively to cardiac imaging. It is an important mode of acquisition from a quantitative point of view providing, for example, a useful non-invasive technique for measurement of ejection fraction.

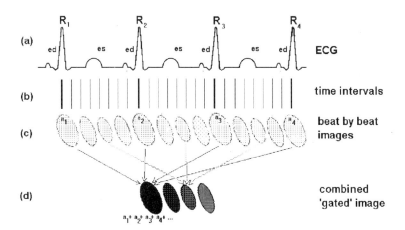

▌ **Fig. 5.11** Images from multiple gated acquisition of images of the left ventricle. Dynamic images of the beating heart may be made to resemble a closed loop cine film giving rise to a repeated sequence of images. The sequence runs in conjunction with the ECG trace (a) and the starting point of each sequence can be fixed to the *R* wave of the ECG. The RR interval is split into 16–50 time intervals to define the time of each image (b). Out of the sequence of images the end systolic and end diastolic images are important for determining the ejection fraction of the heart (c). The indistinct individual beat by beat images are added in sequence (a_1 to a_2 to a_3 etc.) to form an interpretable combined 'gated' image sequence (d).

5.3.5 Single photon emission computerized tomography

As with CT, PET and MRI, single photon radio-nuclide images (to distinguish from the dual coincident photon imaging of PET) can be generated as 'slices' and viewed in three dimensions; the technique is called single photon emission compu-terized tomography (SPECT). SPECT is rather time consuming compared with the other forms of three dimensional imaging because the gamma camera has to move around the patient and take 60–100 discrete static images at regular angular intervals over 180° to 360° ('step and shoot'). Imaging time can be reduced if a detector with more than one head is used, or alternatively multiple detectors may be fixed around the source. SPECT is essentially a technique for the generation of images and, at least at present, cannot be used for quantification because of difficulties in correcting for attenuation.

Gamma cameras can also perform dynamic SPECT. The rapidity of the dynamic acquisition; i.e. the maximum frame rate that can be achieved, depends on how fast the camera can rotate. With 'slipring' technology, this may be 4 times per minute which, if the camera has two heads, gives a frame rate of 8 per minute. Although not quite fast enough for blood flow studies, it is fast enough for, say, renography, including the second phase (see Chapter 11). Gated 3-D images can also be produced though there is usually too little data to allow, for example, more than perhaps 16 images per heart period.

5.3.6 Positron emission tomography

The datum in PET is a pair of scintillations simultaneously recorded in two opposing probes facing each other along the pathway taken by the two annihilation photons. *No valid datum is recorded* if only one of the pair of emitted annihilation photons succeeds in reaching its corresponding probe. It is because of this constraint that quantifica-tion, in terms of tissue radioactivity, is possible with PET. Imagine looking through the edge of a transaxial slice of the body (**Fig. 5.12**). The probability of either of the two annihilation photons reaching its corresponding crystal can be stated as $e^{-\mu d_1}$ or $e^{-\mu d_2}$ where μ is the linear attenuation coefficient of the photon in tissue and d_1 and d_2 the

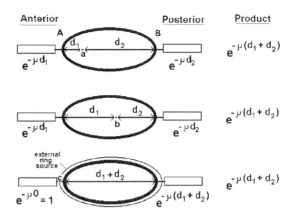

▮ **Fig. 5.12** Attenuation correction in Positron Emission Tomography. Unlike the case of single photon tomogra-phy accurate attenuation correction is possible because of the existence of the two annihilation gamma rays travelling the whole length of the body AB. The attenuation for the line AB is the same ($e^{-\mu(d_1+d_2)}$) for any source of positron emissions on the line, e.g. 'a' and 'b', or even outside the body, 'c'. The attenuation can therefore be determined from outside the body using an external (ring) source.

distances travelled in tissue (see equation 5.2). The probability of *both* photons simultaneously reaching their corresponding probes will be equal to the *product* of their two respective probabilities; $e^{-\mu d_1} \cdot e^{-\mu d_2}$, which is equal to $e^{-\mu(d_1+d_2)}$. It follows that wherever two equally active positron sources existed in the slice, the count rate recorded by the PET camera from them would be the same, since $d_1 + d_2$ is a constant equal to the diameter of the slice. The total count rate is composed of:

(1) true, unscattered, coincidence counts; these are the 'correct' counts which enable the origin of the photons to be located;
(2) true scattered coincidence counts which do not give good imaging information because of the misplacement of the origin of the scattered photons;
(3) random coincidences between two quite in-dependent events;
(4) unrelated single photon events occurring in each of the detectors which are not counted as coincidence events but essentially block up the counting circuits and degrade count rate performance.

If the patient is surrounded by a ring source of a known tracer concentration, then the probability of simultaneous detection in two coaxial probes would still be $e^{-\mu(d_1+d_2)}$. The image then generated will be one showing the effects of attenuation which can be used to correct for attenuation of photons arising from within the patient. The camera can therefore be calibrated and the count rate recorded from the slice of patient, and expressed in MBq/ml. The factor of ml here depends on the volume resolved by the camera, i.e. on the slice width and resolution in the slice.

As with gamma camera acquisition, PET can be performed in static or dynamic mode. Since there is a complete ring of detectors, rotation is not required. A cost-limiting development in PET is the use of two opposing two-dimensional arrays of a limited number of single detectors, rather than a complete ring. This however does require the arrays to rotate in order to compensate for the 'absent' detectors and limits dynamic acquisition to a maximum frame rate of about 30 per minute.

Because of the availability of useful, short-lived positron-emitting radionuclides such as oxygen-15 (half-life, 2 min) and rubidium-82 (half-life, 75 sec), static acquisition can be combined with continuous administration of the positron labelled tracer. A dynamic equilibrium is then established in which the administration rate into an organ can be equated with the sum of outflow rate plus the physical decay rate. Examples include oxygen-15 labelled water and rubidium-82, both for measuring tissue perfusion (Sections 7.1.1.3 and 7.1.1.4).

It is important to recognize that positron emitters do not require to be detected exclusively by positron cameras. The 511 keV energy of the annihilation photons is generally too high for the gamma camera, with their thin crystals and shielding, though with special extra high-energy collimation, relatively crude images can be acquired. Most present day cameras can be fitted with these collimators which achieve a resolution of up to 20 mm and a sensitivity of about 2% of a PET scanner. A specially adapted double-headed camera may also be operated in coincidence without a collimator **(Fig. 5.8b)**. The adaptation involves increasing the count rate capability to 2 million counts per second and adding coincidence circuitry. The resolution of such cameras approaches that of a PET scanner but the sensitivity still remains low unless a thicker crystal is used when the efficiency increases to about 3%. The field of view of the camera is reduced by the need to have coincidences occurring between the two heads.

An energy of 511 keV is not necessarily too high for scintillation probes, which, because they are not required to resolve spatially, can have much thicker crystals. The limitation facing probes for positron detection is the thickness of the lead collimator and the lead shielding for the back and sides of the probe housing to prevent scattered radiation from reaching the crystal from the rear. This results in a very heavy detection system.

5.4 Quantification

Generally, *quantification* in nuclear medicine is based on three fundamental variables: time (min), volume (ml) and quantity (mg or MBq). These three variables are related to each other by three fundamental equations of great importance in nuclear medicine (see Chapter 2):

(1) $T = V/Q$;   (5.3)

(2) $C = M/V$;   (5.4)

(3) rate of change of mass in an organ = influx rate − outflux rate,   (5.5)

e.g., for tracer uptake in an organ with loss only via venous outflow;

$$\mathrm{d}M/\mathrm{d}t = Q(C_a - C_v);$$

where T is mean transit time, Q is blood flow, M is the quantity and C the concentration in volume V and C_a and C_v the concentrations in arterial and venous blood draining the organ, respectively. Equation 5.5 is a statement of the Fick principle.

Many physiological variables are simply times or volumes, such as mean intravascular transit time or blood volume, or combinations of them, such as blood flow and clearance. Others are based on quantities, such as the amount of sodium present in the body, or quantities combined with time, as in flux rates like solute transfer across a capillary membrane, or the cerebral utilization rate of glucose. Although primarily based on one or more of these three fundamental units, physiological variables are sometimes more usefully expressed, in a unitless form, as a fraction of another variable with the same units. Examples are expressing renal blood flow as a fraction of cardiac output or organ clearance as a fraction (i.e. the extraction fraction) of organ blood flow.

5.4.1 Time

We are usually concerned here with the direct measurement of mean transit or residue time, or of its reciprocal which is known as a rate constant. Other measurements, like that of cardiac output derived from a radionuclide dilution curve, are also based on time. Measurement of transit time can be combined with volume to give a measure of flow (e.g. cerebral blood flow measurement with labelled red cells) or with flow to give a measure of volume (as in the measurement of extra-cellular fluid volume).

There are two possible approaches to the direct measurement of the transit time of a tracer through a tissue or organ: monitoring the residue following injection of tracer into the tissue or organ (residue detection) or monitoring the concentration of tracer in effluent blood (outflow detection). Outflow detection is usually mandatory for non-radioactive substances. It may be performed by arterial sampling following intravenous injection, as in the measurement of cardiac output, or by venous sampling following arterial injection, as in the measurement of organ blood flow.

Consider an injection by a perfect bolus input (i.e. with instantaneous deposition) of a radioactive tracer into an organ. The time–activity curves respectively recorded by residue and outflow detection will resemble those shown in **Fig. 5.13**. In residue detection, the minimum transit time is the duration of the plateau, while in outflow detection it is the period up to the time at which tracer is first detected in effluent blood. In residue detection, the units of the *y*-axis are effectively those of quantity while in outflow detection they are those of concentration. The curve in outflow detection is actually a histogram of transit times, while in residue detection it is a retention function curve (see Section 1.5). The mean transit time of the tracer in residue detection is the ratio of the area under the curve to the zero-time (i.e. plateau) height. A curve recorded from outflow detection can be converted to the corresponding curve that would be recorded by residue detection by imagining it to be integrated backwards; i.e. from time infinity instead of from time zero. Conversely a

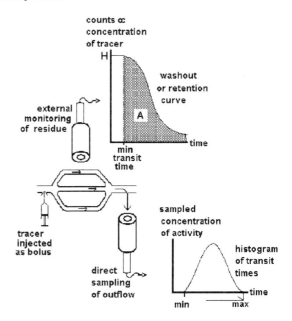

▌ **Fig. 5.13** Time–activity curves recorded by residue and outflow detectors. A bolus injection results in a washout curve (retention function) with a height *H* and area under the curve *A*, the ratio of which (*A/H*) is the mean transit time. The minimum transit time corresponds to the end of the initial plateau. The same bolus also gives the histogram of transit times from the external sampling of outflow. The gradient of the washout curve at any time gives the value of the outflow curve at the corresponding time.

residue curve can be converted to the corresponding outflow curve by plotting its derivative as a function of time. The residue curve that would have been recorded following a sharp bolus input may be generated by deconvolution analysis when the tracer is not deposited instantaneously. One can imagine that if the input was not an instantaneous pulse but 'smeared', as it would be for the case of a detector over the left ventricle and an injection given intravenously, then the residue curve would also be smeared. It would in fact be the summation of individual small residue curves displaced in time, each the result of one of a series of small bolus inputs also displaced in time and the summation of which gives the actual input function (Section 1.5).

5.4.1.1 Measurements of rate constants

Measurement of rate constants provides an indication of the speed of disappearance of a tracer from the system being monitored, such as an organ or distribution volume. In nuclear medicine where the tracer is labelled with a decaying radionuclide the disappearance of tracer associated with a biological process such as excretion or metabolism is always combined with the disappearance of tracer due to decay. This may be expressed by saying that the measured rate constant is the sum of the rate constants associated with the biological and physical processes. If α_{eff} is the measured overall rate constant, α_{biol} the rate constant of the biological process and α_{phys} the rate constant of radioactive decay then

$$\alpha_{eff} = \alpha_{biol} + \alpha_{phys} \qquad (5.6)$$

Since the rate constant α can be expressed in terms of the half-life $T_{1/2}$ of the disappearance curve by the relationship $\alpha = 0.693/T_{1/2}$ then equation 5.6 can be reformulated as

$$\frac{0.6930}{T_{eff}} = \frac{0.693}{T_{biol}} + \frac{0.693}{T_{phys}}$$

or

$$\frac{1}{T_{eff}} = \frac{1}{T_{biol}} + \frac{1}{T_{phys}} \qquad (5.7)$$

where T_{eff}, T_{biol} and T_{phys} correspond to the rate constants above.

Measurements of α from experimental curves have thus to be corrected for the physical decay though the correction is more or less important depending on the half-life of the radionuclide used. In some cases where the physical half-life is much greater than the biological half-life of the biological process involved then the measured effective half-life or rate constant is close to the biological half-life or rate constant. Thus if indium-111 with a half-life of 67 hours ($\alpha_{phys} = 0.01$ h^{-1}) is used to measure a fast process with a rate constant of, say, 1 h^{-1} then only a 1% correction would have to be made which is probably not necessary. In the more usual case when technetium-99m ($T_{1/2} = 6$ hrs, $\alpha_{phys} = 0.116$ h^{-1}) is employed in the measurement of biological half-lives of between 0.1 and 0.01 h^{-1} then such a correction is always necessary. In later discussions of measurement of rate constants from experimental curves it is assumed that physical decay has been taken into account by subtraction from the measured rate constant.

5.4.2 Volume

Physiological volumes are usually measured using the dilution principle. For example, measurement of plasma volume involves the injection of a known amount of tracer which remains confined to plasma. After the tracer has been allowed time to mix completely throughout the blood, the plasma concentration is measured from a blood sample. Then the initial concentration is equal to the sampled concentration or

$$\frac{\text{total injected activity}}{\text{total volume}} = \frac{\text{sample activity}}{\text{sample volume}}.$$

Blood flow (like clearance) represents a 'moving' *volume* and so its measurement usually also involves measurement of dilution. Look at the equation for cardiac output (CO) measurement (Section 3.2):

$$CO = \frac{\text{injected activity}}{\text{area}} \qquad (5.8)$$

where area is total area under the recirculation-corrected arterial time–concentration curve. This is a combination of a volume measurement by dilution (note that the units of the ordinate of the time activity curve are those of concentration) and a transit time measurement (which may be by residue detection over the left ventricle or outflow detection by arterial sampling). Because of the relationship between volume, flow and mean transit time (equation 5.3), volume can also be obtained from separate measurements of transit time and flow, as in the measurement of extra-cellular fluid volume. Note however that this also involves dilution measurement by virtue of measurement of flow (i.e. glomerular filtration rate in the case of extracellular fluid volume).

5.4.3 Quantity or mass

There is an important distinction to be made between *quantitative* measurements and *numerical* or *digital* measurements. Absolute quantitation gives the amount of material as an activity in a volume of tissue expressed in, say, MBq. A numerical count gives simply a number, say 400 counts per second associated with but not equal to or even perhaps not directly related to the amount of material. Thus a standard digital whole body scan will give an image based on the numbers of counts detected from the liver, lungs spleen etc, that does not have a direct relation to the total activity in MBq in those organs unless an elaborate system of correction is applied. The principal reasons for the disparity between numerical and absolute quantitation are attenuation and scattering from the body itself and the inclusion of background activity which depends on the imaging process used. Tissue absorption or attenuation and scattering from the field of view reduces the number of photons reaching the detector. The reduction will be a function of the density and amount of interposed material. Photons scattered into the field of view from areas outside will tend to increase the count. Depending on the method of imaging (2-D projections or 3-D reconstructions of the 3-D distribution), the counts from the volume of interest can be increased by contributions from overlying and underlying tissues, the actual contribution depending on how well the volumes involved are resolved.

Often what is required is a simple assessment of *relative* changes compared with an initial distribution. Here a numerical approach without correction for the factors outlined above is often quite sufficient. A quantitative measurement of activity is to be preferred since absolute changes over time can be assessed on a scale and significant changes dealt with quickly. Although a quantitative measurement is achievable it may not be very accurate firstly because of the random nature of the counting process and secondly, because we are always interested in the spatial–temporal distribution as well as the amount of activity. Any measurement of the volume or area or time increment over which the measured activity extends is prone to errors because of the finite resolution of nuclear medicine imaging devices.

Although not so easily conceptualised as a physiological variable, mass (activity) is frequently directly measured in nuclear medicine. For example, quantitative scanning is performed to identify the whole body distribution of a particular radiopharmaceutical although, strictly speaking, this is not usually a physiological measurement. An example of quantitative scanning which *is* a physiological measurement is the quantification of the content of labelled platelets in the spleen as a measurement of the capacity of the splenic platelet pool. Measurement of flux rates also involves measurement of mass, such as in the determination

of solute transfer rates across a capillary bed or glucose utilization by the brain. Since any record of the count rate from activity in the body is affected by tissue attenuation, a correction for the attenuation must be applied for the count rate to equate to activity or quantity. There are several approaches to the measurement of the quantity of a radiopharmaceutical in an organ.

5.4.3.1 Simple depth correction

This form of correction for a gamma camera is based on the fact that when a *parallel* collimator is used, the count rate from a small source *in air* does not vary as the source moves away from the collimator face (over a wide range of distances). This is because the inverse square law that normally operates with a detected source and dictates a *decrease* in counts as the square of the distance is compensated exactly by the area of detector seen which *increases* as the square of the distance. The fall-off in count rate for a source in d cm of of medium of linear attenuation coefficient μ cm^{-1} is therefore dependent only on the relation $C = C_0 \, e^{-\mu d}$. If C, μ and d are known or are measured then the required C_0 may be found. The value of μ may vary somewhat with the degree of scatter in a particular situation but at a nominal energy is sufficiently constant for the relationship to work in practice. It is most readily applicable to a small compact organ with a reasonably regular shape, such as the kidney. For a probe, where a single hole rather than a multiple hole collimator is used both the inverse square law and the exponential fall of in counts must be applied.

For depth correction using the gamma camera, a region of interest is drawn around the image of the organ acquired over a known period of time. The total number of counts recorded in the region of interest can then be compared with the in-air counting sensitivity of the camera (which has units of counts/min/MBq). Since many of the photons emitted from the radionuclide within the organ are absorbed in the interjascent tissues and never leave the body, a correction based on the depth of the organ needs to be made. A reasonable approximation for the depth of the organ d is obtained by measuring the distance from its centre to the body surface on a calibrated lateral projection (**Fig. 5.14**). If M is the activity in the organ, N is the recorded count rate and γ the sensitivity of the camera (in units of MBq/

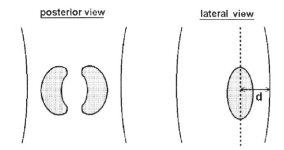

▌ Fig. 5.14 Simple method of attenuation correction by assessing the depth of a source. A lateral view of the source gives an approximate value for the distance of intervening attenuating material on which the correction ($e^{+\mu d}$) may be based.

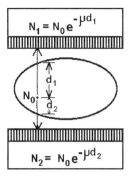

▌ Fig. 5.15 Method of attenuation correction based on the geometric mean of anterior and posterior counts. A source giving N_0 count in air will give counts $N_1 = N_0$ $e^{-\mu d_1}$ and $N_2 = N_0$ $e^{-\mu d_2}$ on the anterior and posterior views respectively. The geometric mean of these gives $N_0 = \sqrt{(N_1 N_2)} \cdot (e^{+\mu(d_1+d_2)/2})$.

counts/min) in air (i.e., without any intervening absorbing material), then

$$M = N\gamma. \tag{5.9}$$

In order to correct for depth, we use

$$M = (N\gamma) \cdot e^{+\mu d}. \tag{5.10}$$

5.4.3.2 Geometric mean

The geometric mean of two numbers, in contrast to their arithmetic mean, is the square root of their product. Depth correction can be made by taking the geometric mean of the numbers of counts respectively recorded from the organ in anterior and posterior projections. It has been found in practice that the whole of the activity dispersed throughout the organ may be treated as approximating to a point source at particular distances, d_1 and d_2, from anterior and posterior surfaces of the body, respectively (**Fig. 5.15**) giving count rates, N_1 and N_2.

Then

$$N_1 = N_0 \, e^{-\mu d_1} \tag{5.11}$$

and

$$N_2 = N_o \, e^{-\mu d_2} \tag{5.12}$$

where N_0 is the count rate recorded that would be recorded if there were no photon attenuation.

Multiplying together equations 5.11 and 5.12,

$$N_1 \cdot N_2 = N_0^2 \cdot e^{-(d_1+d_2)\mu}. \tag{5.13}$$

If $(d_1 + d_2) =$ body thickness D then

$$N_0 = \sqrt{(N_1 N_2 / e^{-\mu D})}$$
$$= \sqrt{(N_1 N_2)} \cdot e^{+\mu D/2}. \tag{5.14}$$

In addition to measuring the count rate from the organ from anterior and posterior projections, it can be seen from equation 5.14 that the lateral view is also required to measure body thickness. When only a change in activity over time is required, as for example in the measurement by whole body counting of whole body losses of a substance, the distribution of which changes in the body, then only the geometric mean of anterior and posterior counts is required and not body thickness.

5.4.3.3 Comparison with a phantom

Phantoms made of tissue equivalent materials such as acrylic and filled with water have been made to simulate several organs and also the whole body. The counts rates emitted from the phantoms after adding a known amount of the same radionuclide to the water to act as background are then compared with the count rates from the patient. Small corrections may be made for the fact that the size of the organ and the whole body do not correspond.

5.4.3.4 Comparison with another radiopharmaceutical

If one could be certain that all of an administered dose of a radiopharmaceutical were essentially uniformly distributed throughout an organ, then the amount of another radiopharmaceutical, labelled with

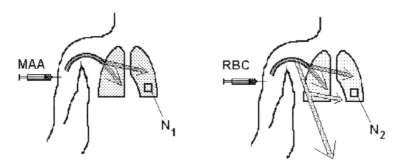

▌ **Fig. 5.16** Correction for attenuation by comparison with a radionuclide with known distribution. In the example, an injection of technetium-99m labelled macroaggregated albumin distributes completely in the lung, giving essentially a calibration factor relating counts in the lung to the known injected activity. The counts can be compared with those resulting from an injection of technetium-99m labelled red blood cells, only part of which distributes in the lung. The ratio of count rates will be proportional to the activities of each radiopharmaceutical and since the activity of MAA is known that of the RBC can be determined.

the same radionuclide, which may vary with time but with the same distribution in that organ, can be quantified by comparison of the count rates emitted from the organ by the two radiopharmaceuticals. This essentially represents calibration of the count rate **(Fig. 5.16)**. Take the lung as an example. Essentially all of an intravenously injected dose of technetium-99m macroaggregates (MAA) is deposited in the lungs and produces a count rate in a region of interest (ROI) over the lung of N_1 counts per minute. If the MAA is then followed by an injection of, say, technetium-99m labelled red cells, and the net count rate in the ROI is now N_2 counts per minute (after subtraction of the preceding N_1 counts per minute from the MAA), then the quantity, M_{RBC}, of red cells in the lungs (*not the ROI*) in MBq is given in terms of M_{MAA}, the activity attached to the MAA, by

$$M_{RBC} = M_{MAA} \times \frac{N_1}{N_2}. \qquad (5.15)$$

It has been assumed that the two agents have the same distribution in the lungs. The approach is greatly simplified if the same radionuclide is used for RBC and MAA, otherwise corrections for different soft-tissue attenuations, gamma emission rates, collimator and crystal penetration etc. become necessary.

5.4.3.5 Correction for attenuation in SPECT imaging

A number of solutions have been suggested for attenuation correction leading to quantitative imaging. These include:

1. Assuming that all linear absorption coefficients in an image have the same value and that the shape of the patient can be determined by external means (e.g. by a system of light beams and sensors). This 'broad beam' value is generally less than the theoretical 'narrow beam' attenuation coefficient. Thus for technetium-99m a value of 0.12 cm^{-1} would be used rather than the theoretical value of 0.15 cm^{-1}.

2. Using an iterative technique in which an image of each section is produced and, treating this image as a rough approximation of the attenuation-free image, estimating the absorption factors involved. This is done by considering the distribution of activity and the geometry of the absorbing medium around it for each section. Applying these estimated correction factors to the original data produces sectional images that are closer to the ideal and a basis for another, better, estimation of the absorption correction factors involved. The iteration may continue until the images are judged not to be significantly improved by the process.

3. Using a separate external source to produce a transmission image that is the equivalent of the emission image for each section. The transmission image is essentially a map of the correction factors to be applied to the emission image to correct for attenuation. The transmission imaging may be carried out simultaneously with the emission imaging, in which case it would need to have a distinguishable energy (e.g. technetium-99m transmission with thallium-201 emission) or could be done separately (e.g. before the patient is injected).

5.5 Image analysis

Much data in nuclear medicine come from the analysis of images. These images may be single static images or sets of dynamic or tomographic images; or they may be 'parametric' images which are indirect images of a derived mathematical function rather than of sampled count rates. Some information comes from analysing the curves derived from those images. A succession of questions is then asked about each image or curve; is it normal? what is abnormal about it? How abnormal is it? What the brain does in answering these questions and what a computer may be able to do in analysing the information is to identify and sort the features characterizing the image or curve. These features are compared with a 'library' of stored (remembered) features or accepted normal variants. Due weight is given perhaps to the effects of how the information was obtained and to modifying features of the information e.g. the data is from an oblique rather than a lateral view or comes from a paediatric rather than an adult patient.

A useful approach to simplifying the problem of analysing the data is to consider the given images or curves as a normal example on which perhaps a small pathological feature is superimposed. Subtracting what is standard from this would thus reveal the presence of the abnormality. Alternatively some simple features are extracted from the given image or curve and displayed as a separate image or curve (a 'parametric' or 'functional' image) useful for further analysis. How this is done depends on the way the features are analysed and a complicated image or curve may be simplified by decomposing it into a set of simpler features in various ways. In factor or principal component analysis the image or curve can be decomposed into a series of shapes that can then be separated into those that are expected or treated as normal and those that are suspicious. The above approaches are different from, though perhaps additional to the treatment of images and curves in order to detect or verify the presence of an abnormality. Thus an image may be smoothed or viewed in colour or on a non-linear scale or certain filters may be applied in order to accentuate features and make abnormalities more apparent. What we are concerned with here however is extraction of usually quantitative information rather than detection of abnormalities.

The starting point for these treatments is the digital image that represents the activity distribution in a region of the body at a particular time as projected onto the detector or the gamma camera. This is stored in the computer as a two-dimensional array of numbers. To display the numbers they are coded with an analogue colour or grey scale to form a recognizable picture. They may also be used as numerical input data to form curves and other images from which the physiological data is derived. In conventional static imaging a two-dimensional (x and y) image is formed of the three-dimensional (x, y and z) original distribution. In SPECT a series of 2-D images of contiguous planes gives information about the 3-D distribution. In dynamic imaging a fourth dimension is added, time, so that 3-D (x, y, t) or 4-D (x, y, z and t) images are acquired. These images can be examined in detail so that the time course of the tracer can be derived as a function of time in any one 2-D or 3-D element (pixel or voxel). The smallest size of the element that can be *reliably* distinguished is determined mainly by the spatial resolution of the detection system and the random variation in the number of counts captured within the element. The smallest significant time interval into which a dynamic study can be decomposed is also determined by the number of counts within each element.

It can be seen that a very large amount of data may be acquired and it is the aim of the mathematical image analysis to condense this data to produce a manageable amount from which useful information can be obtained more efficiently and economically: i.e. we want a useful data compression technique that will reduce the large number of images to perhaps a single easily interpreted image. In some cases however only a global estimate is required. Thus for a conventional ejection fraction measurement the whole of the left ventricle is examined.

For the more advanced mathematical treatments (data compression techniques, functional/parametric imaging, phase amplitude imaging, principal component analysis) a regional dynamic map is required. Each frame of a dynamic or gated study is divided into a large number of picture elements and the time course of counts in each is used to derive the final 'condensed' image.

5.5.1 Parametric analysis

In parametric analysis or parametric imaging, instead of displaying an image of the counts (or activity) distribution in the patient, the image of a 'parameter' is generated; i.e. each pixel has a number that is associated with a mathematical function rather than with an activity.

A relatively simple parametric image can be generated from a dynamic study by plotting the time course of the counts in each pixel of each frame of the study. A 64×64 pixel image may thus yield up to 4000 different curves. If each is treated as, say, a mono-exponential decay curve and for each curve a decay constant is calculated and displayed, the $64 \times 64 \times n$ time intervals may be represented by a single image in which each pixel shows a number representing the decay constant: i.e. the display is a map of the rates of decay over the image. Regions in the body where the process takes place abnormally rapidly or slowly are immediately visible and physiological interpretations such as high oxygen metabolism in certain regions can be made. A common application is to generate a volume curve for each pixel covering the left ventricle in a multiple gated acquisition study described in Section 5.3.4. A figure for the ejection fraction can then be calculated for each curve and used to produce a parametric image of the regional ejection fraction that shows how ejection varies over the organ. Other parameters from the curves associated with each pixel can be generated, such as the mean transit time, a colour coded time of arrival of activity at a particular location or an attenuation corrected geometric mean count. The essence of the parametric image is to produce a picture where any of the parameters, indices or mathematical functions discussed in this book are represented for each pixel as a visually coded element of the display. The addition of these visual cues can aid the interpretation of the bare distribution of count information available from the standard images.

5.5.2 Phase and amplitude analysis

This technique has been applied most often to the heart because of the periodic nature of the beating organ but could also be applied to lung and perhaps to the kidney. For the first study the data analysed are the sets of frames built up over the heart cycle from a large number of beats (300–500) as described in Section 5.3.4 and Fig. 5.11. The computer is triggered at the start of the heart cycle to acquire a new set of images of the heart. The sets of images are overlaid to form a single set with enough total counts in each frame to produce a useful count in individual pixels. As an example of this constraint imposed by the limited activity able to be administered and the resulting count rates can be given we can consider a gated study over a period of 5–10 minutes where a typical activity of 550 MBq might lead to a total of 500 000 counts in each of 32 frames. The counts may be distributed over 25% of a 128×128 image and therefore occupy about 2000 pixels with an average count per pixel of 250 leading to an acceptable $\pm 6\%$ statistical error.

Two different images are derived from the 20–50 images making up the dynamic ventriculogram. The first, called a phase image, is a dynamic image with a time scale over the whole cardiac cycle. It shows the sequence of emptying of parts of each heart element relative to other parts of the heart (it may also be related to the waves of electrical signals travelling over the heart). This sequence can be visualized by a colour map showing the stages of emptying; these are colour coded on the heart image and by a curve showing the number of heart elements. It appears as a wave front that sweeps through the heart. Sites of tachycardia and delayed emptying can be visualized. A simple curve plotting the number of heart elements involved at each stage of the cycle can be generated. This curve usually exhibits two peaks in the atrial and ventricular phases; these are distorted in the case of cardiac pathologies.

The second image derived from the original acquisition is the amplitude image which shows the individual stroke volume of each element of the heart. This can show up areas of dyskinesis.

The method of generating these images is to derive an emptying and filling curve for each pixel of the cardiac image. This curve resembles a cosine curve and indeed a cosine wave is fitted to the pixel count data. The amplitude and phase of this cosine wave is noted. Essentially a set of simple cosine waves is found each with its own phase (starting time relative to the start of the cycle) and its own amplitude (baseline-to-peak height). Each element is then coded with a colour corresponding either to the value of the phase or the value of the amplitude to form the final two images. Cycling a colour

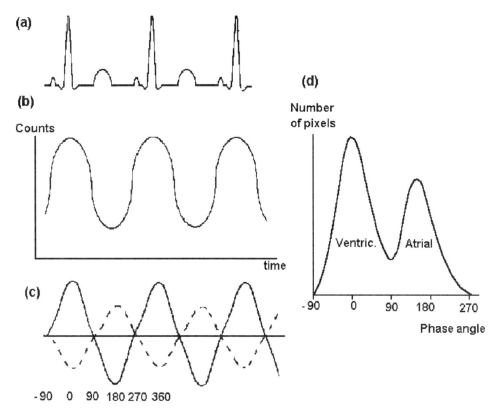

▌**Fig. 5.17** Illustration of phase–amplitude cardiac analysis. A gated volume curve (b) is generated using trigger signals from the ECG (a) for each pixel making up the cardiac image. The periodic volume curves are approximated to cosine curves (c) and amplitude and 'phase angle' (i.e. time difference from curve to curve) are each recorded on separate images. The amplitudes and phase angles are colour coded. In addition, a histogram of the number of pixels with a particular phase angle is produced (d). This shows two peaks corresponding to the ventricular and atrial segments of the heart image.

corresponding to the phase angle through the range of phase angles generates a dynamic image of heart electrical activity (**Fig. 5.17**).

5.5.3 Principal components and factor analysis

These approaches attempt to simplify images and reduce the amount of information available to manageable quantities. A complicated image or time–activity curve may generally be thought to be made up of a number of simpler components — images as regular simple shapes and curves as simple waves patterns such as sine waves.

In principal components and factor analysis the variation of counts recorded in each pixel of an image over the study is used to generate a set of time–activity curves. Instead of matching a simple mathematical function to this curve it is assumed that the complex shape of the curve is a combination of time–activity curves resulting from a number of independent physiological factors. These factors or principal components are similar to the compartments used in compartmental analysis but are capable of dealing with more than one compartment at a time (equivalent to the sampling of overlapping compartments) and just as a solution may be associated with an infinite number of compartments so an infinite number of combinations of factors could explain the time–activity curves. The art of using principal components factor analysis is in the methods used to constrain and reduce the number of solutions.

The practical compartmental approach has been seen (Section 1.3.3) to lead to the decomposition of multi-exponential curves into the various mono-

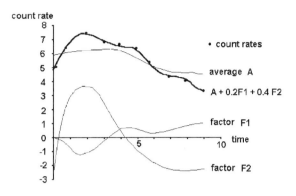

▌ **Fig. 5.18** Illustration of factor analysis to generate a good approximation of an experimental count rate curve from an 'average' curve and two different degrees of contribution from two other 'factor curves'. Thus, for example, the response curve may be a combination of a normal curve plus varying amounts of arterial contribution and a venous contribution.

exponential functions from which the different relative compartmental sizes involved and their rate constants can be derived. This principle appears in factor analysis when an experimental curve can be expressed as a number of other curves. One of these curves may be the 'average' curve obtained from a number of subjects. To this curve is added various amounts of different factor curves (**Fig. 5.18**) through a series of computer iterations until a good fit is made to the original data. In gross terms what is being done is either to add to the 'normal' curve various degrees of 'abnormal' curves each associated with a different pathology or to an average curve various degrees of a physiological component such as an arterial contribution or a venous contribution. The final result might indicate the size of the different contributions. Since the process involves simply adding small stored variations to a stored standardized average curve it is a relatively efficient process.

5.6 Measurement of affinity and dissociation constants

Tracers which bind reversibly to their receptors display the phenomenon of saturable binding. In

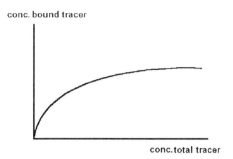

▌ **Fig. 5.19** Binding of a ligand by its receptor gives rise to the phenomenon of saturable binding.

other words, the more tracer (often known in this context as ligand) made available to the receptor, the more becomes bound until, in the presence of an excess of tracer, all the available receptors are occupied and no more tracer can be bound. By adding increasing amounts of ligand (for example, a radiolabelled monoclonal antibody) to a suspension *in vitro* containing the receptor (for example, an antigen on a blood cell), a graph of cell-bound tracer (*y*-axis) versus total tracer (*x*-axis) can be constructed. If the monoclonal antibody displays saturable binding to its antigen on the blood cell, the graph will be curved, convex upwards, and reach a plateau when all the receptors are bound (**Fig. 5.19**). The height of the plateau indicates the total number of available receptors, or, in this example, antibody-binding sites. The affinity of the binding, as well as the total number of available receptors, can be measured by a graphical technique called Scatchard analysis.

Thus, if we call the ligand concentration $[L]$, the receptor concentration $[R]$ and the concentration of bound ligand $[L–R]$, then the dissociation constant K_d can be defined as

$$K_d = \frac{[L] \times [R]}{[L - R]}. \qquad (5.16)$$

Here $[R]$ is the difference between the bound receptor concentration $[L–R]$ and the total number available $[R]_{max}$, i.e.

$$[R] = [R]_{max} - [L - R]. \qquad (5.17)$$

Therefore, substituting for $[R]$ in equation 5.16

$$K_d = \frac{([R]_{max} - [L - R]) \times [L]}{[L - R]} \qquad (5.18)$$

rearranging,

$$[L - R] = [R]_{max} - \frac{K_d[L - R]}{[L]}. \qquad (5.17)$$

Therefore a plot of the bound antibody concentration $[L–R]$ against the ratio of the bound to free antibody concentrations $[L–R]/[L]$ should produce a straight line if the system is displaying saturable binding, with a y-axis intercept equal to $[R]_{max}$ and a gradient K_d equal to the dissociation constant (**Fig. 5.20**). Note that the units of K_d are expressed as a molar concentration and the value of K_d is usually, for a monoclonal antibody, a very small number. Alternatively, the bound to free ratio is plotted on the y-axis against bound concentration on the x-axis. The gradient in this case is then the affinity constant.

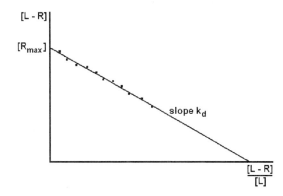

∎ **Fig. 5.20** Scatchard plot. The plot of bound ligand against the ratio of bound to free ligand generates a straight line with a negative slope which represents the dissociation constant of the receptor–ligand complex and a y-axis intercept which represents the maximum number of receptors available for binding the ligand. The linearity of the plot proves that the system is showing saturable binding.

6 The peripheral circulation and microvascular solute transfer

6.1 Peripheral circulation

6.1.1 Skin blood flow

Blood flow to the skin serves two purposes:

(1) supporting the metabolism of the skin itself;
(2) regulating heat loss.

The blood flow requirements for the second function are several times those for the first. Metabolically determined blood flow exhibits reactive hyperaemia and autoregulation, both of which are under local nervous control, whereas blood flow for the purpose of heat regulation is under the control of central neuronal regulation and influenced by temperature changes elsewhere. Local warming produces local vasodilatation of resistance vessels and arteriovenous anastomoses but, as core temperature rises, vasodilatation in skin occurs elsewhere.

Because of the structure of skin, its blood flow is difficult to measure and usually expressed as perfusion rather than total blood flow. Skin perfusion can be measured by inert gas clearance (Lassen *et al.* 1983). Local intradermal injection is necessary since it is difficult to resolve skin clearance from clearance from underlying muscle following intra-arterial injection. However counting the beta emissions from krypton-85 is well suited to skin perfusion because the depth of tissue from which beta particles emerge is only a few mm, so a detector applied to the skin records only dermal tracer clearance following arterial injection of the gas. Local direct injection has the appeal of being non-invasive. Perfusion may be temporarily disturbed however as a result of trauma, local disturbance to the micro-vessels and diffusion limitations within the depot of injected tracer. Skin perfusion in moderate ambient temperature is similar to that of resting muscle, about 5 ml/100 g/min. By comparing xenon-133 washout rates following respective injection into skin folds devoid of subcutaneous tissue and skin with abundant subcutaneous tissue, it has been shown that cutaneous perfusion is much higher than subcutaneous perfusion (Sejrsen 1969).

6.1.2 Muscle blood flow

Resting skeletal muscle blood flow is about 5 ml/min/100 ml. It increases markedly with exercise. At rest, most muscle capillaries are closed as a result of pre-capillary vaso-constriction. This situation is not static and capillaries open and close cyclically, with about 80% closed at any one time. Exercising muscle meets increasing oxygen demands by two mechanisms:

(1) recruitment of a considerable capillary reserve;
(2) increase in the oxygen extraction efficiency.

It is difficult clinically to measure muscle blood flow exclusively, although limb blood flow is a close approximation to it. Limb blood flow becomes more specifically muscle blood flow if measured during exercise. Muscle blood flow can also be measured with microspheres administered via the left ventricle or, based on the same principle of cardiac output fractionation, with thallium-201, which is a potassium analogue rapidly taken up into the intracellular potassium pool of skeletal muscle. Technetium-99m labelled isonitriles are based on the same principle. Local injection of inert gas has also been employed (Lowy *et al.* 1976), as for measurement of skin perfusion.

6.1.3 Limb blood flow

6.1.3.1 Plethysmography

Limb blood flow can be measured by plethysmography. For a brief period following rapid application of an external pressure just above the venous pressure, the arterial inflow into the limb remains unchanged while venous outflow is occluded. The rate of increase in volume of the limb during this period, which is equal to blood inflow, can be measured by several techniques, including strain gauge plethysmography or more simply by observing the rate at which water is displaced from a vessel in which the limb is immersed. Following injection of a radiotracer that remains in the blood volume, the rate of increase of limb volume after application of the external pressure can be measured from the rate of increase in count rate recorded over the limb by a probe. By taking a blood sample, this rate of increase in count rate can then be equated with the rate of increase in volume; i.e. flow.

Plethysmography based on *arterial* occlusion has also been developed as a radionuclide technique for measurement of limb blood flow (Parkin *et al.* 1991). The blood flow to the limb is first occluded by application of an external pressure higher than systolic blood pressure. An intravascular tracer, such as technetium-99m labelled human serum albumin, is then injected intravenously and allowed to mix within the blood volume, so that arterial and venous concentration equalise; i.e. $C_a = C_v$. A venous blood sample is then taken. After about two minutes of occlusion, the external pressure is released. The rate at which the count rate in the previously occluded limb increases *immediately* after release is proportional to the rate of inflowing radioactive blood. Absolute blood flow Q can be calculated from the immediate upslope gradient dN/dt of the time–activity curve recorded over the limb and the venous concentration C_v (**Fig. 6.1**)

Thus

$$\frac{dM}{dt} = Q \cdot C_a = Q \cdot C_v \qquad (6.1)$$

where M is the quantity of radioactivity in the limb. The units are

$$\frac{MBq}{min} = \frac{ml}{min} \times \frac{MBq}{ml}.$$

If γ is a constant relating radioactivity in the limb to N, the count rate recorded by the detector (with units of MBq/counts/min), then

$$\gamma \frac{dN}{dt} = \frac{dM}{dt} \qquad (6.2)$$

so

$$Q = \frac{dN}{dt} \times \frac{\gamma}{C_v} \qquad (6.3)$$

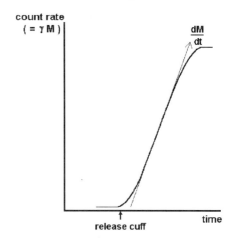

▌ **Fig. 6.1** Measurement of limb blood flow using an intravascular tracer. Following occlusion of the arterial inflow of the limb by means of an inflatable cuff, technetium-99m human serum albumin is injected intravenously. The tracer is allowed to mix within the circulation and then a blood sample is obtained. With subsequent instantaneous release of the occlusion, circulation though the limb is re-established resulting in a sharp increase in limb radioactivity recorded with an external detector. The slope dM/dt of the recorded curve depends on the concentration of tracer in the blood and on the limb blood flow immediately following release of the cuff. It should be noted that the flow measured is not resting or basal flow but the flow of reactive hyperaemia. This is an advantage since resting flow is poor in the distinction of the diseased from the normal limb.

The units are

$$\frac{counts}{min^2} \times \frac{MBq\ min}{counts} \times \frac{ml}{MBq} = \frac{ml}{min}.$$

The constant γ incorporates values for photon attenuation and camera sensitivity. A potential problem arises in the derivation of γ as a result of a varying attenuation correction factor. Thus attenuation will decrease as the radioactivity moves from the central artery (popliteal or femoral) towards the periphery of the limb. In other words, the upslope gradient on the time–activity curve is due partly to the inflow of blood and partly to its centripetal movement. Nevertheless the technique is non-invasive, simple to perform and is able to distinguish between limb pain due to ischaemia and pain due to other causes, unrelated to ischaemia. It should be noted that Q is measured at reactive hyperaemia but, for the clinical application of the technique, this is an advantage because resting blood flow may be normal in peripheral vascular disease.

6.1.3.2 Inert gas washout

A more invasive technique for measuring limb blood flow, but one which could be adopted for use in the angiography theatre, is inert gas washout following injection into the femoral artery. A detector positioned over the calf will record both skin and muscle blood flow. The proximity of the skin to the detector weights the signal towards skin flow while, conversely, the greater bulk of muscle weights it towards muscle flow, particularly if plantar and dorsiflexion against resistance is employed in order to increase flow as a result of exercise. Because xenon-133 can be administered on two or three occasions without significant accumulation in tissue fat, the response of perfusion to an intervention, such as peripheral arterial angioplasty, can be studied. The perfusion of resting muscle, about 5 ml/min/100 ml, corresponds to a half-time of clearance of about ten minutes, necessitating rather long periods between injections. Nevertheless, one can record the effect of an intervention such as limb exercise on washout already in progress **(Fig. 6.2)**.

6.1.4 Peripheral arterio–venous shunting

Peripheral arterio–venous shunting may be the result of congenital arterio–venous malformations (AVMs)

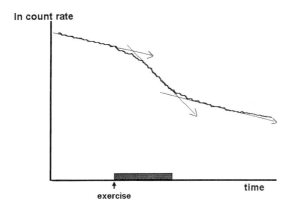

In count rate

exercise

time

▮ **Fig. 6.2** Xenon-133 washout from the resting limb is very slow. The effect of exercise can be evaluated by recording a change in readout gradient already in progress from an earlier xenon-133 administration via the artery supplying the limb.

or may be acquired, such as the transhepatic shunts of hepatic cirrhosis, or following trauma, or iatrogenic, such as the implanted shunts of patients receiving haemodialysis.

The quantification of peripheral arterio–venous (A–V) shunting in arterio–venous malformations is of potential value to the interventional radiologist as a guide to successful embolization. A simple semi-quantitative approach is to inject a tight bolus of any recirculating radioactive tracer intravenously and record first-pass curves over the arterio–venous malformation, so-called radionuclide angiography. If the AVM is situated peripherally in a limb, then measurement of its flow can be assessed by comparing a time–activity curve from a region of interest placed over the AVM with that from a similar sized region of interest over the corresponding site in the contralateral limb. Alternatively flow, as a fraction of cardiac output, can be measured using the technique described in Sections 3.3 and 11.1.1.3, which, in essence, reproduces cardiac output fractionation. This technique is also applicable to more proximally situated A–V shunts, provided that a reasonably accurate estimation of photon attenuation is possible, for example from measurements in phantoms of similar shapes.

Measurement of iatrogenic A–V shunt patency in patients on chronic dialysis may be helpful to establish that such shunts remain patent. In one such technique, a bolus is injected *proximal* to the shunt (Seo *et al.* 1984). Dynamic imaging over the shunt reveals an immediate peak, the size of which represents the injected activity, and a delayed smaller curve representing recirculation of the tracer to the shunt. The area under the second curve expressed as a fraction of the area under the immediate curve is a measure of shunt flow which is essentially a variant of the cardiac output fractionation technique. A patient with a large peripheral A–V shunt usually has an increased cardiac output, measurement of which, before and after therapeutic embolization, will give some indication of the success of the procedure.

More accurate measurements of systemic A–V shunt flow require arterial cannulation and injection of radiolabelled microspheres which are trapped in the pulmonary vascular bed if they traverse the shunt, or are trapped in the vascular bed distal to the shunt if they do not traverse the shunt. The proportion of the injected microspheres embolizing in the lungs is equal to the proportion of blood flow *at the tip of the catheter* which passes through the shunt (**Fig. 6.3**). Clearly the closer the catheter is advanced towards the shunt, such that it is increasingly placed beyond branching arteries, the greater will be the fraction of tracer passing through the shunt. This fraction can be quantified by comparing the count rate N_{ia} recorded over any part of the lung following injection into an artery supplying the shunt with N_{iv} recorded following intravenous injection of the same amount of tracer. The intravenous dose, which represents 100% shunting, is used to calibrate the count rate recorded over the lung.

Then

$$\frac{\text{shunt flow}}{\text{total flow}} = \frac{N_{ia}}{N_{iv}}. \qquad (6.4)$$

The use of radio-labelled microspheres in this setting has two drawbacks:

(1) an increasing lung radioactivity signal is produced with each injection;

(2) it is difficult to standardize the injected dose as a result of the 'stickiness' of the microspheres. In order to measure dose accurately, counting of the residual activity in injection lines and syringes is necessary.

An alternative tracer, which behaves rather like radio-labelled microspheres, is xenon-133 (Kennedy *et al.* 1995). Thus shunted xenon-133 is trapped in the lung as a result of rapid diffusion into alveolar gas and can be retained during a period of breath-holding. Non-shunted xenon-133 has a relatively long transit time through muscle and skin and is effectively trapped there long enough for the spike of shunted activity to be clearly identified. This circumvents both of the drawbacks of microspheres; xenon-133 can be given repeatedly, and is dispensed by the manufacturer in injection cartridges containing a standard dose. It is thus particularly suited to repeated measurements in the angiography theatre for the assessment of the efficacy of therapeutic

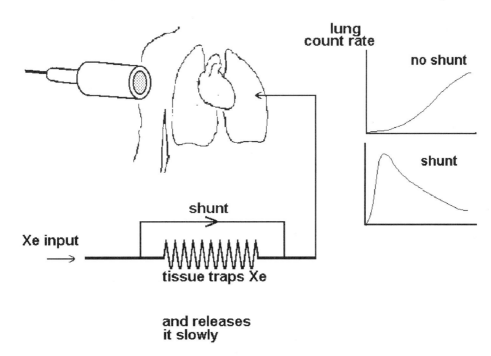

▌ **Fig. 6.3** Principle of measurement of systemic arteriovenous vascular shunting using xenon-133. In the presence of a shunt, a proportion of xenon-133 bypasses the capillary bed distal to the shunt and arrives in the lung rapidly where it enters alveolar gas and can be recorded by an external scintillation probe as a 'spike' of activity during a brief period of breath holding. The xenon-133 entering the distal vascular bed is delayed and arrives in the lung later and more gradually. The amplitude of the initial lung activity is proportional to the blood flow through the vascular shunt and can be calibrated by an intravenous injection of xenon-133 which represents 100% shunting.

embolization, provided the tip of the catheter is replaced at exactly the same location for each injection. The technique does not work as well for shunts in vascular territories with a high perfusion, such as the carotid, because the non-shunted tracer has a relatively short transit time and appears early in the lung, thereby interfering with the detection of shunted activity.

6.2 Microvascular water and solute transfer

In order to reach cells from the plasma, water and solutes are required to pass through the endothelial lining and basement membrane of blood vessels and the interstitial fluid surrounding the cells. Different tissues and organs have different microvascular and interstitial anatomy, with the result that the kinetics of water and solute transfer are highly variable. For example the kinetics of solute transfer across the endothelium are highly dependent on whether the endothelium is continuous, as in muscle and skin, or fenestrated, as in the liver and bone marrow.

6.2.1 Water

Water continuously exchanges between the interstitial fluid and plasma by two processes: filtration and diffusion.

6.2.1.1 Filtration

Starling's law states that *net* water transfer is proportional to the hydrostatic and osmotic pressure gradients across the capillary. An osmotic pressure gradient exists because the endothelium is essentially impermeable to protein. At the arterial end of a capillary, the hydrostatic pressure gradient is opposite to and exceeds the osmotic gradient and there is net water movement into the interstitial space whereas, at the venous end, the osmotic pressure exceeds the hydrostatic pressure, and there is net water movement towards plasma. It is important to realize that although this process of filtration results in the *net* transfer of a relatively small amount of water at either end of the capillary, there is, as a result of *diffusion*, transfer of almost 100% of water molecules between plasma and interstitial fluid during one pass through a capillary.

Microvascular net water transfer (J_w) from plasma to interstitial fluid is described by the Starling equation as follows:

$$J_w = P_w S[(p_i - p_e) - \sigma(\pi_i - \pi_e)] \qquad (6.5)$$

where P_w is the water permeability coefficient of the capillary, p is the hydrostatic pressure, S is the surface area of the capillary and the subscripts i and e refer to intravascular and extravascular respectively. The parameter σ is called the osmotic reflection coefficient and has a value which depends on the capillary's permeability to protein; π is oncotic pressure (due to protein). Normally, the capillary is essentially impermeable to protein and so σ has a value of unity. In the presence of a protein leak the value of σ lies between 0 (free permeability to protein) and 1, and the effect of the oncotic pressure gradient is modified accordingly. The filtration coefficient, $P_w S$, has units of ml/min/mm Hg/100 ml tissue and incorporates the capillary surface area available for exchange. The interstitial fluid normally contains some protein and so π_e is not negligible. In muscle and skin, intravascular protein concentration is 5–10 times higher than interstitial concentration.

Water transfer by filtration is important from the point of view of nuclear medicine in the glomerular capillary where it can be imaged as the glomerular filtration rate. Water transfer by diffusion is of more general importance especially in relation to measurement of tissue perfusion.

6.2.1.2 Diffusion

It is important to realise that although the process of filtration results in the net transfer of a relatively small amount of water at either end of the capillary the process of *diffusion* results in transfer of almost 100% of water molecules between plasma and interstitial fluid during one pass through a capillary. This can be demonstrated with labelled water, which effectively behaves like a lipophilic inert gas (e.g. xenon-133) in that it completely equilibrates throughout the water of a tissue (including intracellular water) and as such can be used to measure tissue perfusion in the same way as an inert gas (Section 3.1.1).

6.2.2 Solutes

Like water, lipophilic solutes, such as inert gases, carbon dioxide and oxygen, diffuse rapidly across the endothelium, directly through the endothelial cells as well as between them through the inter-endothelial pores, and have an extraction efficiency across the endothelium during one pass through a capillary which is almost 100% (**Fig. 6.4**). Indeed, unless perfusion is very high, these solutes equilibrate between tissue fluid and plasma well before the distal end of the capillary, and this forms the basis of their use for measuring tissue perfusion. Water behaves similarly, with almost complete equilibra-

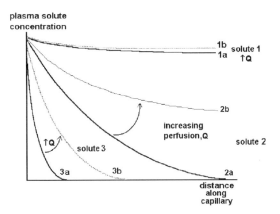

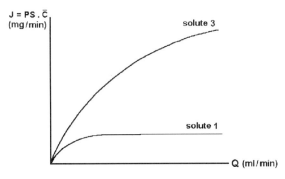

▮ **Fig. 6.4** Principle of diffusion-limited and perfusion-limited solute diffusion across the vascular endothelium illustrated by a curve of capillary solute concentration versus distance along the capillary. For two levels of perfusion *Q* solute 1 gives curves 1a and 1b while solute 3 gives curves 3a and 3b. Since less than 10% of solute 1 is extracted, increasing *Q* from the lower to the higher value would not result in a significant increase in the tissue uptake and so solute 1 is said to undergo diffusion limited uptake. On the other hand, more of solute 3 would be taken up with an increase in *Q* and so solute 3 displays perfusion-limited uptake. Solute 2 gives rise to curves 2a and 2b. It would have diffusion limited uptake at the higher level of perfusion and perfusion-limited uptake at the lower level of perfusion.

tion in one pass. Hydrophilic solutes however, because of their polarity, are unable to penetrate cells and must transit the endothelium via the inter-endothelial pores. Provided the pores are large enough relative to the diameter of the solute, the diffusion rate through the pores is governed mainly by solute size; i.e. by the free diffusion coefficient of the solute in aqueous solution at 37 °C. The free diffusion coefficient of a solute is broadly proportional to the cube root of its molecular weight which is proportional to its linear dimension. Small solutes like technetium-99m DTPA (molecular weight 492 Da; cube root ~7.9) and chromium-51 EDTA (molecular weight 390 Da; cube root ~7.3) diffuse relatively rapidly while large hydrophilic solutes, such as inulin (molecular weight 6000 Da; cube root ~18), diffuse more slowly. If, on the other hand, a solute diffuses across the endothelium at a rate slower than expected from its free diffusion coefficient, its diffusion through the endothelium is said to be restricted. The molecular weight at which diffusion starts to be restricted in continuous endothelium, such as in muscle and skin, is about 6000 Da, a diameter which is about 10-fold less than pore diameter in these vessels.

The unidirectional extraction fraction *E* of DTPA in one pass through a capillary in resting muscle is about 0.5 whereas for inulin it is about 0.2. Endothelium in skin and muscle is relatively impermeable (or restricted) to hydrophilic substances of molecular weight greater than about 6000. Tissues with fenestrated endothelium, such as liver and bone marrow, are relatively permeable to high molecular weight substances, and this is essential for their functions. Fenestrated endothelium is also present in salivary and endocrine glands and in the peritubular capillaries of the kidney, which display high degrees of permeability to hydrophilic solutes (Table 6.1).

6.2.2.1 Permeability surface area (*PS*) product for solutes

This section will concentrate on the small hydrophilic solutes, the endothelial permeability to which, in tissues like skin and muscle with continuous endothelium, is quantified in terms of a variable called the permeability surface area (*PS*) product (Crone & Levitt 1984).

The rate of solute transfer J (mg/min) across the endothelium from plasma into the extra-vascular space is proportional to the average concentration C (g/cm³) of solute within the capillary, the surface area S (cm²) of the capillary available for exchange, and the permeability coefficient P (cm/min) of the capillary endothelium for that solute. Assuming that the extravascular concentration of the solute is zero (i.e. considering transfer only from plasma to interstitial space), then

$$J = PS \cdot C_p \qquad (6.6)$$

where C_p is mean capillary concentration. Now, according to the Fick principle.

$$J = Q(C_a - C_v) \qquad (6.7)$$

where Q is the tissue blood flow and C_a and C_v are the solute concentrations of incoming (arteriolar) and outgoing (venular) blood respectively.
So

$$PS = \frac{Q(C_a - C_v)}{C_p}. \qquad (6.8)$$

It can be seen that PS product has units of ml/min or cm³/min; i.e. flow. Since the units of surface area are cm², those of permeability itself must be cm/min; i.e. velocity.

Fixing C_a as unity (**Fig. 6.5**).

$$C_v = 1 - E \qquad (6.9)$$

and

$$C_a - C_v = E. \qquad (6.10)$$

The mean concentration C_p is defined as that concentration, which if it were constant along the capillary, would enclose an area under the concentration–capillary distance graph equal to the actual area (**Fig. 6.5**). Thus, assuming that the concentration falls exponentially along the capillary, i.e. $C_v = e^{-kd}$, it can be seen from Fig. 6.5 that

$$\begin{aligned} C_p \cdot d &= \frac{1}{k} - \frac{(1-E)}{k} = \frac{E}{k} \\ &= \frac{C_a - C_v}{k} \end{aligned} \qquad (6.11)$$

Where k is the rate constant with which the concentration decreases with respect to distance along the capillary (analogous to rate constant of decay) and d is distance along the capillary.

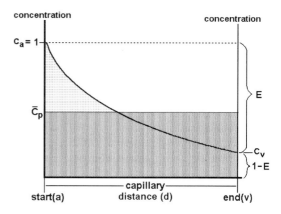

▌ Fig. 6.5 Kinetic basis for the quantitative definition of PS product (the solute transfer rate per unit solute concentration gradient). The incoming arteriolar tracer concentration C_a is normalized to unity. Extraction fraction, E, is then $1 - C_v$. Mean concentration C_p, is the vertical height of the rectangle which has an area equal to that under the capillary time–concentration curve.

From equations 6.8 and 6.11

$$kd = \frac{C_v - C_a}{C_p} = PS/Q \qquad (6.12)$$

but

$$\ln C_v = -kd$$

So

$$C_v = e^{-PS/Q}. \qquad (6.13)$$

From equation 6.9

$$C_v = 1 - E \qquad (6.14)$$

So that

$$E = 1 - C_v \qquad (6.15)$$

and

$$E = 1 - e^{-PS/Q}. \qquad (6.16)$$

This is an important expression relating extraction fraction to PS product and blood flow.
Then since

$$\begin{aligned} e^{-PS/Q} &= 1 - E \\ -PS/Q &= \ln(1 - E) \end{aligned} \qquad (6.17)$$

and

$$PS = -Q \cdot \ln(1 - E). \qquad (6.18)$$

By analogy with tissue perfusion, it is convenient to express PS product in terms of tissue volume V in which case tissue perfusion Q/V rather than absolute

Vascular bed	PS product		
	EDTA/DTPA MW ~ 400	Inulin ~ 6000	Sodium 23
Myocardium	30	12	120
Skeletal muscle	5	1	15
Peri-tubular capillaries		1200	
Brain	0.02	0.0014	0.23
Lung	40	20	
Salivary gland	800	180	

Modified from Crone and Levitt (1984).

▌ **Table 6.1** Endothelial *PS* product (ml/min/100 g tissue) in some tissues

blood flow Q would be measured, i.e.

$$\frac{PS}{V} = -\frac{Q \cdot \ln(1 - E)}{V}. \qquad (6.19)$$

Note that the minus sign in front of Q appears because $\ln(1 - E)$ is always negative.

Thus PS product is essentially a variant of clearance. It is the clearance that would exist if the capillary concentration was maintained at the same level as arterial instead of decreasing along the capillary. This is why it has the same units as clearance. Clearance may refer to plasma or to whole blood, so the same is true of *PS* product, although, as with clearance, plasma is the fluid of reference if the tracer is confined to plasma and Q refers to plasma flow rather than blood flow. Tracers that exchange between red cells and plasma, or are partially protein bound, are generally avoided in endothelial permeability studies since they introduce ambiguity in the meaning of Q (see Section 2.4.1). The *PS* product per unit of tissue volume for the unidirectional endothelial transfer of a particular solute varies enormously from one tissue to another. It is about 5 ml/min/100 ml for technetium-99m DTPA in muscle and skin, rising to about 800 in the salivary gland and to over 1200 in the peritubular capillary plexus of the kidney (Table 6.1).

6.2.2.2 Diffusion restriction

According to the pore theory of solute permeability, solutes diffuse through inter-endothelial pores or clefts at the junction of endothelial cells. The free diffusion coefficient of a solute in water at 37°C is roughly proportional to the cube root of molecular weight and determines how rapidly the solute diffuses through the inter-endothelial pores. Provided the diameter of the pore is at least ten times the molecular diameter of the solute, the diffusion rate of the solute across the endothelium is commensurate with its free diffusion, and permeability is said to be unrestricted. Above a molecular weight of 6000 Da, solute diffusion across continuous endothelium, such as in muscle and skin, becomes restricted. In the absence of diffusion restriction, the ratio of endothelial diffusion rates of two solutes of different size is approximately equal to the ratio of their free diffusion coefficients and thereby inversely proportional to the ratio of the cube roots of their molecular weights. If the ratio of endothelial transfer rates of the two solutes (large to small) is less than their free diffusion coefficient ratio, then diffusion of *at least one of the solutes* is likely to be restricted. Diffusion restriction can therefore be assessed by the simultaneous use of two solutes, since

$$\frac{P_1 S}{P_2 S} = \frac{-Q \cdot \ln(1 - E_1)}{-Q \cdot \ln(1 - E_2)} \qquad (6.20)$$

and therefore

$$\frac{P_1}{P_2} = \frac{\ln(1 - E_1)}{\ln(1 - E_2)}. \qquad (6.21)$$

Thus the effects of capillary surface area and perfusion on solute transfer cancel out and the ratio of permeabilities can be obtained from measurement of the respective solute extraction fractions. There has been very little clinical exploitation of this technique.

6.2.2.3 Relation between *PS* and clearance

The *PS* product is essentially a clearance measurement or an index of clearance; it is the clearance that could be achieved if the intra-capillary concentration (i.e. the 'driving' concentration) was maintained at the arterial value throughout the length of the capillary, as for example by increasing blood flow. For solutes with low extraction fractions, this is in fact the case and for them clearance and *PS* product are almost the same at the prevailing level of perfusion. Thus, substituting Z/E for Q in equation 6.16,

$$PS = -Z\frac{\ln(1 - E)}{E}. \qquad (6.22)$$

At low values of E, the term $-\ln(1 - E)/E$ approaches unity. Therefore *PS* approaches clearance and becomes independent of flow. The transfer of solute is then said to be diffusion dependent. When E is high, on the other hand, *PS* exceeds Q because more solute *could* be transferred across the endothelium if the concentration gradient between the capillary and tissue fluid was not allowed to fall before the distal end of the capillary. Also when E is high the capillary solute concentration approaches the interstitial fluid concentration before the end of the capillary. Solute transfer rate can therefore be increased by increasing the blood flow and is said to be perfusion dependent. This is the basis of blood flow measurement with labelled water and lipophilic agents like the inert gases. It is worth noting that the ratio C_p/C_a is equal to the ratio, Z/PS because the solute transfer rate is $C_p \cdot PS$ or, according to the definition of clearance, $Z \cdot C_a$.

Although originally applied to the unidirectional transfer of substances across the endothelium, *PS* products can also be specified for transfer of compounds at other interfaces, such as inter-compartmental transfer in a compartmental model (see Section 3.1.3.4). For example, consider the uptake of MDP by bone. The unidirectional clearance and extraction fraction from plasma to bone interstitial fluid is determined by the *PS* product of the endothelium and bone blood flow.

The steady state extraction fraction of MDP from plasma to bone crystal (within which the MDP is essentially fixed) is the product of the extraction fractions from plasma to bone fluid and from bone fluid to bone crystal. A *PS* product will therefore exist for net bone crystal uptake from plasma which will depend on steady state extraction fraction and steady state clearance. It is important to realize that fluid in a space other than plasma can be *cleared* of tracer, and that equation 6.6 can be applied to such a space (with C_p substituted by the tracer concentration within the space). A *PS* product therefore exists for tracer movement out of that space.

6.2.2.4 Measurement of *PS* product of endothelium

In general, if clearance and extraction fraction are known for the transfer of a substance across an interface, or system of interfaces, then *PS* product can be calculated. The system may be thallium uptake by the myocardium (involving endothelial transfer and uptake by the myocyte) or transfer of a solute from interstitial fluid to plasma (involving one interface). This section concentrates on measurement of *PS* product for endothelial solute transfer. In general, the solutes that have been used to measure endothelial *PS* product are hydrophilic, thereby able to cross only through interendothelial junctions, metabolically inert and not actively retained in the tissue being studied.

There are several approaches to the measurement of endothelial *PS* product with respect to hydrophilic solutes, including:

(1) indicator dilution, in which the disappearance of solute from blood to tissues is monitored by venous blood sampling following local injection into an artery;
(2) residue detection in which the rate of disappearance of radioactive solute from tissue to blood is recorded following direct tissue or local arterial injection of tracer;
(3) tissue uptake measurements in which the appearance of radioactive solute in the tissues from blood is monitored;
(4) measurement of the disappearance rate of solute from plasma and the subsequent rate of equilibration of solute between intravascular and extravascular spaces.

6.2.2.4.1 Indicator dilution

Indicator dilution methods were first used many years ago, and do not require the exclusive use of radionuclide tracers (Trap-Jensen 1970, Trap-Jensen and Lassen 1968, Sejrsen 1979). A diffusible solute is injected as a compact bolus into an artery supplying the vascular bed. In man, the exercising forearm has been studied with brachial arterial injection, although many different vascular beds have been studied in experimental animals. The tracer concentration downstream in venous blood is then measured in blood samples taken at frequent intervals from the vein draining the vascular bed (for example, the antecubital vein in man following brachial arterial injection). A non-diffusible reference tracer which remains within the intravascular space, such as indocyanine green or Evan's blue, or radio-labelled protein, is injected with the diffusible tracer. For the first few seconds after injection, the venous concentration–time curves for the two tracers

(diffusible and non-diffusible) diverge as the diffusible tracer enters the extravascular space. At about 30 seconds after injection, diffusion of the diffusible tracer back into the blood causes its plasma concentration curve to fall less rapidly and eventually to cross the reference tracer curve (**Fig. 6.6**). The unidirectional extraction fraction of diffusible tracer into the vascular bed is equal to the ratio of the areas under the two curves, or their heights, before back-diffusion of tracer commences. Blood flow can be simultaneously measured by the indicator dilution technique (Section 3.2), thereby allowing measurement of the *PS* product (from equation 6.18). The *PS* product that is measured can be heavily weighted towards skeletal muscle by hand grip exercise, which increases muscle blood flow. Although conceptually a constant, *PS* product may increase during exercise as a result of capillary recruitment and a consequent increase in capillary surface area.

This technique was first applied, at a clinical level, to diabetics with micro-angiopathy, in whom it was shown that the *PS* product for iodide, bromide, sucrose and chromium-51 EDTA were all elevated. The technique has the disadvantages of being cumbersome and invasive. It can be reproduced by residue detection with a scintillation probe and radioactive diffusible and reference tracers, thereby circumventing venous sampling but not arterial injection. The extraction fraction is equal to the ratio of the difference between the two curves and the difference between the reference curve and its maximum height (**Fig. 6.7**) at a time before back diffusion. A single venous blood sample obtained after complete mixing of the reference tracer in the circulation can be used to calibrate the reference and solute curves in units of MBq/ml.

6.2.2.4.2 Tissue uptake measurements of *PS* product

The rate of uptake of solute in the extravascular space of a tissue is a function of capillary permeability with respect to the solute and has been used extensively to measure *PS* product in the experimental animal. However, whereas in the animal, tissue can be removed for sampling at specified times after injection of the tracer for direct measurement of tracer concentration, this is usually not possible in man. Some measurements based on direct tissue sampling have been attempted in man, such as muscle biopsy after intravenous injection of

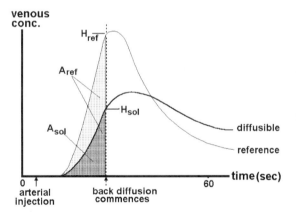

▌ **Fig. 6.6** Measurement of *PS* product using the indicator dilution technique. The test solute and a reference solute which does not cross the endothelium (such as a labelled protein) are injected simultaneously into the brachial artery. Frequent venous sampling generates two simultaneous time–concentration curves. The curve for the test solute is flatter than for the reference solute, reaching a height of only H_{sol} as a result of diffusion into the interstitial space of the forearm. The fraction of test solute extracted into the interstitial space is $[H_{ref} - H_{sol}]/H_{ref}$ or, since the surves have an identical shape up to the time of back diffusion, $[A_{ref} - A_{sol}]/A_{ref}$. The curves soon cross as a result of test solute re-entering plasma from the interstitial space. Blood flow can be measured for the reference curve using the indicator dilution technique.

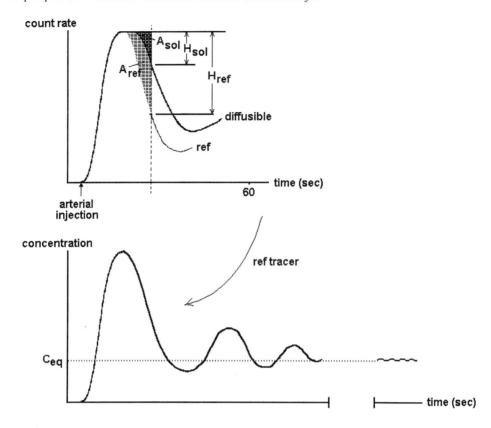

▎ **Fig. 6.7** Measurement of *PS* product for residue detection reproducing the indicator dilution technique without the need for multiple blood sampling. The fraction of test solute extracted is $[H_{ref} - H_{sol}]/H_{ref}$. An intravenous sample obtained after mixing of the reference tracer throughout the circulation can be used to calibrate the reference solute curve and thereby to measure forearm blood flow (cf. measurement of cardiac output by external scintigraphy — Section 7.2.1).

fluoroscein, a low molecular weight hydrophilic dye of about 400 Da used for microangiography. Because of the tissue sampling limitation, external detection of radiolabelled solute accumulation offers the potential for measuring *PS* product non-invasively in man.

In principle, the technique measures the clearance of solute into the extravascular space by uptake measurement, analogously to measurement of organ clearance described in Section 2.2.1.3. Thus the count rate detected over tissue at a site such as the forearm, remote from the kidney, following intravenous injection of, say, technetium-99m DTPA, results from the sum of intravascular M_i and extravascular M_e radioactivity. If, for a short period of time after intravenous injection, it can be assumed that there is negligible back-diffusion, then the rate of accumulation of extravascular activity will be proportional to the arterial plasma concentration C_a

so

$$\frac{dM_e}{dt} = Z \cdot C_a \tag{6.23}$$

where Z, the constant of proportionality, is clearance of tracer from intravascular to extravascular spaces. Integrating,

$$M_e = Z \int C_a(t) \cdot dt \tag{6.24}$$

and

$$Z = \frac{M_e}{\int C_a(t) \cdot dt} \tag{6.25}$$

with units

$$MBq \times \frac{ml}{MBq \cdot min} = ml/min.$$

So Z can be obtained if M_e can be measured separately from M_i.

E	ln $(1-E)/E$	Difference (%)	Significance
0.1	1.05	5%	not significant
0.2	1.12	12%	
0.25	1.15	15%	significant
0.3	1.19	19%	significant

▌ **Table 6.2** From equation 6.22, $PS = -Z \ln (1 - E)/E$. If the extraction fraction of the solute is relatively low, say less than 0.2 then $\ln (1 - E)/E \approx 1$ and Z is close to the PS product. However, for an extraction fraction greater than about 0.2, the transfer rate of tracer becomes significantly blood flow dependent and Q is required to convert Z to PS product. The impact of the value of E can be seen from the Table 6.2.

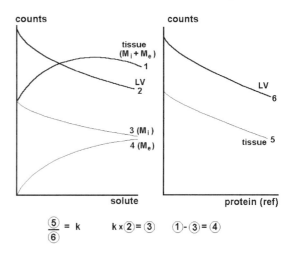

$$\frac{\text{⑤}}{\text{⑥}} = k \qquad k \times \text{②} = \text{③} \qquad \text{①} - \text{③} = \text{④}$$

▌ **Fig. 6.8** Procedure for measuring the extravascular concentration of diffusible solute. The reference tracer (a labelled protein) establishes the relationship (with constant of proportionality k) between the vascular signal in the tissue (curve 5) and the intracardiac signal (curve 6). Multiplication by k of the left ventricular signal from the diffusible solute (curve 2) defines the tissue intravascular signal (curve 3), subtraction of which from the total tissue signal (curve 1) gives the *extravascular* signal (curve 4).

It is clear from equation 6.24 that, in addition to monitoring a tissue region of interest for M_e, it is also necessary to monitor C_a, the concentration of arterial plasma activity of the diffusible solute. This can be obtained from a region of interest over the cardiac blood pool, although correction for extra-vascular activity in the chest wall is required. Note that C_a cannot be based on venous blood sampling because, initially, during the period of minimal backflow, there is an arterio–venous concentration difference for the solute in forearm blood.

The radioactivity signal detected in the tissue region of interest also includes a quantity M_i of tracer in plasma. This can be subtracted by administering a radio-labelled protein which, be-cause it does not undergo any significant extra-vascular clearance, can be used as a reference plasma marker. By comparing the activities of the two markers (reference and diffusible) in sampled plasma (after the diffusible solute has equilibrated between intravascular and extravascular spaces), with the corresponding cardiac blood pool signals, it is possible to subtract the component of the signal in the tissue region that is due to intravascular activity **(Fig. 6.8)**. The plasma concentration of the diffusible solute can be used to convert the continuously recorded cardiac plasma curve from units of camera counts to absolute units of MBq/ml. This is necessary in order to measure Z in ml/min, which also requires that the units of M_e be converted from detector count rate into absolute units of MBq by calibration with a known source. This is not an approach that would be recommended but it serves to illustrate the complexity avoided by the following modified approach which exploits Patlak–Rutland graphical analysis and which can be developed to show that a radiolabelled protein is not necessary to subtract the intravascular signal from the total signal (although a plasma sample would still be necessary to express Z in absolute units).

We can say that M_i is some fraction f of the activity recorded over the cardiac blood pool, which in turn is taken to represent a pure blood pool signal. The actual radioactivity signal recorded over the tissue is $M_i + M_e$. Then

$$M_i + M_e = Z \int C_a(t) \cdot dt + f \cdot C_a. \qquad (6.26)$$

Dividing through by $C_a(t)$

$$\frac{M_i + M_e}{C_a} = \frac{Z \int C_a(t) \cdot dt}{C_a} + f. \qquad (6.27)$$

Thus we have a linear regression equation of $(M_e + M_i)/C_a$ on $\int C(t) \cdot dt/C_a$ in which the slope is Z and the intercept f. This graphical approach, generally known as the Patlak plot but first developed by Rutland for nuclear medicine applications, has widespread applicability in quantitative nuclear medicine, and has been used not only to measure vascular permeability in skin and muscle but also to measure glucose utilization rates in the myocardium and brain, protein transfer from plasma into the pulmonary interstitial space (as a measure of pulmonary endothelial permeability), fluorine-18 uptake into bone, and gallium-68 EDTA transfer from intravascular to extravascular space in cerebral tumours using positron emission tomography.

The early part of the regression curve (up to about 2 min) defined in equation 6.27 is almost linear, indicating that backflow into the intravascular space is probably negligible compared with outflow into the extravascular space (Peters 1990). By about 2–3 minutes however, as backflow increases, the gradient for a solute like technetium-99m DTPA decreases, and by about 20 minutes, the gradient is almost horizontal (**Fig. 6.9**). The information required to obtain Z and f in absolute units is, as stated above, a timed blood sample with which to calibrate the plasma curve in units of MBq/ml, and detector sensitivity γ to convert $(M_i + M_e)$ to MBq. However, in a location such as the forearm, and especially when using a scintillation probe, the latter

conversion is difficult for geometric reasons, and it is better to find a valid way of expressing the PS product in terms of tissue volume, analogously to tissue perfusion. Since the y-axis of this regression essentially represents the distribution volume of the solute, which at time infinity is the extracellular fluid volume $(V_{ecf})^{\dagger}$ within the tissue region of interest, the gradient of the regression Z can be expressed in relation to the plateau, reached by about 20 min, thereby giving the ratio PS/V_{ecf} (Cousins *et al.* 1995).

A note of caution, generally applicable to the Patlak–Rutland plot, is necessary regarding the assumption that M_i is proportional to C_a. Early after injection, when non-radioactive plasma in capillaries is being replaced by radioactive plasma, C_a is out of proportion to M_i. This results in a small positive gradient, even when the technique is applied to labelled protein, and the process is known as vascular dispersion.

6.2.2.4.3 Residue detection

Following injection into a tissue by local arterial injection, the subsequent clearance of a small hydrophilic solute is bi-exponential over a period of

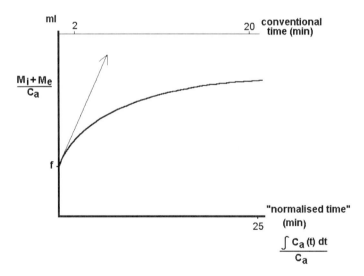

▮ **Fig. 6.9** Patlak–Rutland plot based on a tissue radioactivity signal (output) and arterial or cardiac pool signal. Relative to the duration of the plot, back-diffusion occurs early so there is only a short initial linear segment followed by a curve (convex upwards) as a result of increasing back diffusion. The plot becomes horizontal when the tracer equilibrates throughout the regional extracellular fluid space. The initial slope reflects unidirectional solute transfer while the y-axis intercept represents the distribution volume at zero time; i.e. plasma volume. The x-axis has units of so-called 'normalized time'. When C_a is falling, normalized time 'exceeds' 'clock' time (shown on the upper axis).

$\dagger$Because of the eventual existence of a concentration gradient between intravascular and extravascular spaces, this is not quite equal to the distribution volume, unless the plasma clearance of the tracer is very low (see Sections 11.1.2.1 and 13.1.1).

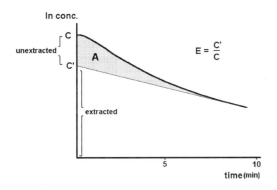

∎ **Fig. 6.10** Measurement of PS product from residue detection following intrarterial injection of a diffusible radiolabelled solute. The residue curve displays an early exponential (shaded) which represents intravascular transit of solute that does not enter the interstitial space. The solute entering the interstitial space immediately following injection is subsequently cleared (washed out) at a rate depending on the PS product of the endothelium and tissue perfusion and defines the gradient of the later exponential. The gradient is also equal to the clearance rate of tracer Z divided by its extravascular volume of distribution. Since $PS = -Z \ln(1 - E)/E$, PS can be calculated from the gradient and the value of E. Alternatively, as performed in the experimental animal, Q can be measured from the first exponential if the blood volume V of the region is known or assumed since $Q = V/T$ where T is the mean intravascular transit time, and $PS = -Q \cdot \ln(1 - E)$.

about 20 minutes (**Fig. 6.10**). The first exponential corresponds to washout of tracer that remains intravascular and is therefore brief. The second exponential represents clearance of tracer initially extracted into the interstitial space. When the second exponential is extrapolated towards zero time, the difference between its value at the time of the peak and the peak itself represents unextracted tracer. The amplitude of the extrapolated exponential at the time of the peak divided by the peak is equal to the extraction fraction E so the value $1 - E$ is the fraction of tracer that remains intravascular and leaves the tissue rapidly.

The rate at which the extracted solute is subsequently cleared from the interstitial space is proportional to the local perfusion and to the PS product. The washout rate constant α of a hydrophilic solute with a distribution volume V_{ecf} and partition coefficient λ is proportional to Q/V_{ecf}. If for a hydrophilic solute λ is taken as unity, the value of α is then clearance divided by volume of distribution (cf. xenon washout); i.e.

$$\alpha = \frac{Q \cdot E}{V_{ecf}} \qquad (6.28)$$

$$= \frac{Z}{V_{ecf}}. \qquad (6.29)$$

Note that clearance in this context is clearance from a static volume. Since

$$PS = -Z \cdot [\ln(1 - E)]/E,$$
$$PS/V_{ecf} = \alpha \cdot [\ln(1 - E)]/E$$

assuming P is the same in both directions across the endothelium.

Although it is conventional to express PS in relation to total tissue volume, ECF volume is an alternative that carries some validity in view of the fact that the relevant solutes have a distribution volume which is the ECF rather than total tissue volume. Correcting for recirculation by recording over the opposite limb, Z/V_{ecf} has been measured for technetium-99m DTPA in man following femoral arterial injection and shown to agree well with Z/V_{ecf} measured from tissue uptake and Patlak–Rutland graphical analysis following intravenous injection (Cousins *et al.* 1995). Another technique to obtain Z/V_{ecf} based on intravenous injection is deconvolution analysis applied to the limb time–activity curve using arterial samples as the input function. The values of Z/V_{ecf} by this approach also agreed with values based on femoral arterial injection.

As an alternative to local arterial injection, solute may be injected directly into skin or muscle for the measurement of endothelial permeability by residue detection. The solute should be accompanied by xenon-133 as a marker of tissue perfusion, otherwise there is no way of relating clearance to permeability. In order to accelerate clearance, the injection can be given during reactive hyperaemia, induced by a period of ischaemia, or during the ischaemia itself before release of the arterial occlusion. Solutes investigated in this way in man include bromium-77 (Lowy *et al.* 1976) and radiosodium (Veall and Vetter 1958). Concerns about the validity of this form of administration include local haemodynamic disturbance to the tissue and diffusion limitations within the depot. Thus it is difficult to accept that the distribution volumes of locally injected solutes are the physiological distribution volumes achieved after intra-arterial injection (ECF for bromium and total tissue volume for xenon). If the injection is given during arterial occlusion, then a period will ensue, before release of the occlusion, during which the deposited solutes will have the opportunity to diffuse locally, thereby promoting access to their physiological distribution volumes. In the case of bromide and sodium, the subsequent clearance curve is interrupted by recirculation, but for well-collimated detectors, this is minimal.

Notwithstanding these limitations, the ratio of clearance half-times of bromium-77 to xenon-133 range from about 0.8 at a tissue *plasma* perfusion of about 8 ml/min/100 ml (corresponding to a xenon clearance constant of 0.2 min^{-1}) to about 0.3 at a perfusion of about 30 ml/min/100 ml (Lowy *et al.* 1976). Because of different volumes of distribution, both within the tissue and the effluent capillary blood, these ratios are difficult to translate to a *PS* product for bromium-77 but illustrate the effect of perfusion on solute clearance. Nevertheless, for a xenon clearance of 0.2 min^{-1}, the clearance rate constant for bromium, 0.16 min^{-1} (0.8 × 0.2), corresponds to a clearance of 16 ml/min/100 ml ECF, or about 4 ml/min/100 ml tissue — an extraction fraction of 0.5 at a perfusion of 8 ml/min/100 ml, corresponding to a *PS* product of 5.5. Likewise, at the higher perfusion level, *PS* product is about 6.5 ml/min/100 ml tissue. This fits well for a molecule of 77 Da (cube root ~4) compared with technetium-99m DTPA (cube root ~8), which has a *PS* product in resting muscle of about 2.5.

Residue detection has been used extensively in the experimental animal to measure *PS* product with a somewhat different theoretical approach (Paaske 1977, Sejrsen 1979). Recirculation is eliminated by the experimental set-up, in which venous return is diverted. Instead of measuring the rate constant of the second exponential, *PS* is based on *E* measured by the extrapolation of the second exponential, as described above. Flow *Q* is measured from the transit time equation, $Q = T/V$, using the first exponential to determine *T* and a value for *V*, local blood volume, established from previous experiments in the same experimental preparation.

A variant of local arterial injection, applicable only to the experimental animal, is continuous arterial infusion of tracer such that the arterial concentration is constant. The concentration of tracer in the tissue bed supplied by the artery then increases exponentially with a rate constant which is proportional to *PS* product. The curve of tissue activity

versus time so recorded is known as a saturation curve, and it is mentioned here only because this technique for measuring *PS* product is in principle identical to the classical technique for measuring cerebral perfusion by continuous carotid arterial infusion of nitrous oxide, discussed in Section 12.1.1.2. Nitrous oxide is freely diffusible and completely extracted and the equation for measuring perfusion is shown in Section 12.1.1.2 to be

$$C_\tau = C_a(1 - e^{-[Q/\lambda V]t}). \qquad (6.30)$$

Rewriting this for incompletely extracted tracers:

$$C_\tau = C_a(1 - e^{-[QE/\lambda V]t}). \qquad (6.31)$$

So, if Q/V is known, *PS* product can be measured from the rate constant of disappearance or uptake. [Note that this is the same as the rate constant of disappearance of locally deposited tracer in which C_a is zero **(Fig. 6.11)**]

6.2.2.4.4 Measurement of solute disappearance from plasma — the whole body *PS* product

The initial rate at which a hydrophilic solute disappears from the plasma is the sum of its plasma clearance rates.

(a) into the interstitial space;

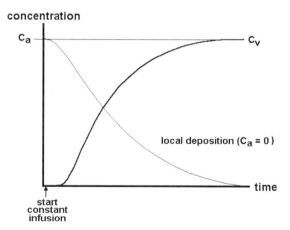

∎ **Fig. 6.11**   A tissue saturation curve obtained following commencement of arterial infusion of solute at a constant rate. If $C_a = 0$ in equation 6.31, then the curve becomes a washout curve of locally deposited tracer (i.e. following bolus arterial injection). The rate constant of uptake is the same as the rate constant of disappearance and equal to $(Q \cdot E)/\lambda V$.

(b) resulting from glomerular filtration (assuming it is not irreversibly removed elsewhere.)

Subtraction of glomerular clearance from total clearance yields clearance into the interstitial space, which, for solutes with blood flow-independent microvascular transfer, is the average whole body endothelial *PS* product for the solute (Henriksen 1985, Neilsen 1985).

In order to understand the technique for measuring whole body *PS* product, it is necessary to distinguish between sojourn time and residence time of a tracer. Imagine a solute diffusing bi-directionally between plasma and interstitial fluid. Sojourn time is the average time it spends in either compartment before returning to the other. Residence time in either compartment is the *total* time spent in that compartment before irreversible removal from plasma (by glomerular filtration). The *sum* of the residence times in plasma and interstitial fluid is the residence time in the ECF. For systems in which the tracer is confined to plasma and disappears uni-directionally, such as colloid uptake into the liver, sojourn and residence times (in plasma) are identical.

If, using the transit time equation, clearance is based on the relationship between plasma volume V_p and plasma sojourn time T_p^s then a solute molecule is treated, upon entering the interstitial space, as though it leaves the intravascular space for good, and so the clearance (which, according to the transit time equation, is V_p/T_p^s) is the sum of renal clearance and unidirectional clearance into the extravascular space. This is the basis of whole body clearance measurement. As shown above, for perfusion-independent solute transfer (i.e. when E is small), extravascular clearance is equal to *PS* product, which can therefore be calculated if GFR is known. Both GFR and sojourn time in plasma can be calculated from the solute plasma clearance curve (for GFR, see Section 11.1.2.1). The entire plasma disappearance curve is needed for calculation of sojourn time, which, for a bi-exponential plasma clearance curve, is

$$T_p^s = \frac{A+B}{A\alpha_1 + B\alpha_2} \qquad (6.32)$$

with units
$$\frac{MBq \cdot ml^{-1}}{MBq \cdot ml^{-1} \cdot min^{-1}} = min$$

and where A and B are the zero time intercepts of the two exponentials and α_1 and α_2 their corresponding

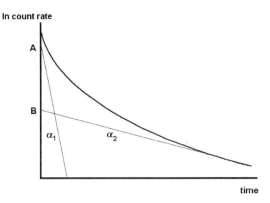

▮ **Fig. 6.12** Bi-exponential plasma clearance curve in which the rate constant of the fast exponential with intercept A is α_1 and of the slow exponential with intercept B, α_2. The sum of the concentrations A and B is the concentration at zero time when theoretically all of the activity is within the plasma compartment. Plasma volume would then be equal to injected activity/$[A + B]$.

rate constants (**Fig. 6.12**). [Note the residence time in plasma, T_p^r = area under curve/initial height = $(A/\alpha_1 + B/\alpha_2)/(A + B)$. Also note the equation for residence time in the extracellular fluid volume (Section 13.1.1.).]

Since it is essentially the initial slope of the plasma clearance curve that is important, it is clear that any early exponentials of the plasma clearance curve are important. It is well described that for solutes used for the measurement of GFR from plasma clearance (e.g. chromium-51 EDTA and technetium-99m DTPA) the clearance curve does not become mono-exponential until 1.5–2 hours after injection, and this is explained as the time required for equilibration of tracer between the intravascular and extravascular spaces of the ECF. However, the presence of an early exponential can be appreciated by taking the sum of the zero-time intercepts, A and B, of the conventional exponentials of the DTPA clearance curve (i.e. the total initial concentration) and comparing it with the injected dose. This ratio should be equal to the plasma volume. However, performing this for a bi-exponential DTPA plasma clearance curve, recorded between 10 min and 4 hr, gives a plasma volume of about 8 litres, clearly an overestimate of the true volume and a reflection of an additional space of about 5 litres in which DTPA exchanges rapidly.

Using the unidirectional extraction fraction for EDTA (or DTPA) into the tissues and a rough estimate of whole body clearance, it is possible to estimate roughly the time constant of the first exponential. Thus the extraction fraction of EDTA/DTPA into the interstitial space of skin and muscle, which represents most of the extracellular extravascular space, is about 0.5. Postulating a total plasma flow of 800 ml/min to muscles and skin (see Table 3.1), an extraction fraction of 0.5 corresponds to a clearance of 400 ml/min. The fractional rate constant α_{pe} of transport of tracer from plasma to extravascular space will then be the clearance divided by the distribution volume. Although at first sight the distribution volume might appear to be plasma volume, it is higher than this because tissues like the liver, lung and kidney have a relatively small extravascular ECF and a relatively high endothelial permeability and therefore a rapid rate of equilibration, and so their combined interstitial fluid volumes, say about 2 litres, should more appropriately be added to plasma volume, a total of about 5 litres.[†]

Therefore,

$$\alpha_{pe} = 0.5 \times \frac{800}{5000} \sim 0.08 \text{ min}^{-1}. \quad (6.33)$$

Recall from Chapter 1 that the rate constant of equilibration in a two compartmental model is equal to the sum of the two opposite transport rate constants. So α_{ep}, the fractional transport rate constant in the reverse direction, assuming a muscle and skin interstitial fluid volume of 6 litres, would be[‡]

$$\alpha_{ep} = 0.5 \times \frac{800}{6000} \sim 0.07 \text{ min}^{-1}. \quad (6.34)$$

The sum of rate constants in both directions gives a rate constant of equilibration of 0.15 min^{-1}, from which the time to 95% of equilibration can be calculated from

$$y(t) = y(0) \cdot e^{-\alpha t} \quad (6.35)$$

where, at 95% equilibration, $y(t)/y(0) = 0.05$ and therefore $y(0)/y(t) = 20 = e^{-0.15t}$.
Thus

$$t = \frac{\ln 20}{0.15 \text{ min}^{-1}} \sim 20 \text{ min}. \quad (6.36)$$

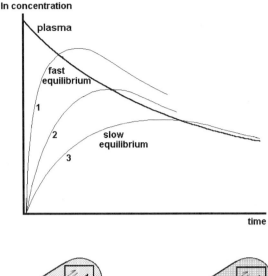

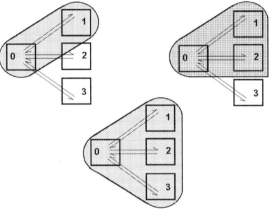

∎ **Fig. 6.13** Plasma solute disappearance curve progressively 'picking up' solute accumulation curves in individual compartments with which the plasma equilibrates. The rate of equilibration between compartment 0 (plasma) and compartment 1 is dependent on the volume of the two compartments. Once equilibrium is achieved between 0 and 1, the effective volume of distribution determining the fractional transfer constant leading to equilibrium with further spaces, is the sum of the volumes of plasma and compartment 1, and so on. The rate of equilibration between plasma and compartment 2 is consequently slower than it would be if compartment 1 did not exist. This is of relevance to DTPA which will equilibrate rapidly with, say, liver and lung but slowly with muscle.

[†]When tracer equilibrates simultaneously between plasma and several parallel compartments, the volume of distribution, which is initially the plasma volume, steadily rises as each compartment equilibrates with plasma. This results in a rate constant of equilibration which becomes disproportionately slower as the more rapidly exchanging compartments equilibrate (**Fig. 6.13**).
[‡]This value is consistent with the experimentally observed clearance rate constant of technetium-99m DTPA from the human calf following intra-femoral arterial injection (Cousins *et al.* 1995) (**Fig. 6.10**).

A rough estimate of 20 minutes, remembering renal clearance has been ignored, is consistent firstly with the finding that the arterio–venous gradient in the forearm equalises by about 20 minutes after intravenous injection of DTPA (Cousins *et al.* 1998) and secondly with the tissue uptake curves over the arm or leg of the type determined by the Patlak plot, as described by equation 6.22 and illustrated in Fig. 6.9, since this plot becomes almost horizontal by the same time.

Although not visible on venous sampling because of the effects of solute exchange in the tissue drained by the antecubital vein, this early exponential can be well defined on arterial sampling after DTPA injection, is separate from intravascular dispersion, and lasts for about 20 min. Although it clearly corresponds to equilibration in skin and muscle, as shown by a Patlak plot, the morphological equivalent of the second exponential (conventionally described in the literature as the first) is not clear. It probably represents solute exchange in less accessible regions of the extravascular space which, if they were in muscle and skin, would imply a three-compartmental model in series. This would fit with the concept proposed by Katz (1980) of a gel meshwork within the interstitial space consisting of huge molecules from which interstitial macromolecules the size of proteins are excluded but which small solutes can slowly permeate (**Fig 6.14**). Support for this model comes from the residue detection method for measuring *PS* product in skeletal muscle in the experimental animal in which recirculation is abolished (Lassen and Sejrsen 1971). By recording for up to 90 minutes following intra-arterial injection of chromium-51 EDTA, a curve is obtained which, after exclusion of the transit of intravascular unextracted tracer, is clearly bi-exponential, with the terminal exponential identifiable from about 30 minutes. This experimental finding is entirely consistent with a two-compartmental model with run-off and therefore a three-compartmental model for the ECF (**Fig. 6.15**).

Ignoring the early exponential, whilst making little difference to the measurement of GFR, produces a large error in whole body *PS* product. In order to measure whole body *PS* product for DTPA and other hydrophilic solutes, all three exponentials of the plasma disappearance curve are required. The first exponential is too rapid to be measured by venous blood sampling and can only be

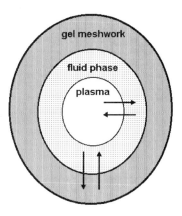

∎ **Fig. 6.14** Plasma DTPA disappearance curve in which the zero-time concentration is 'fixed' to the injected activity/plasma volume (PV), PV having been separately measured with a radiolabelled protein. The sum [A + B] falls well short of this activity /PV, indicating the presence of an earlier exponential with intercept C = [activity/PV] −(A + B]. This early exponential is not clearly seen with antecubital venus sampling because it is obscured by tracer exchange across the vascular endothelium of the forearm vascular bed.

defined by arterial sampling. Alternatively, it can be quantified by separately measuring plasma volume with labelled albumin. The plasma volume and injected dose then 'fix' the sum of the zero time intercepts; i.e. A + B + C. The rapid exponential (with rate constant α_{fast}) can be identified from a sample at 10–15 min (**Fig. 6.16**). The fast exponential is then inserted into a modified version of equation 6.32:

$$T_p^s = \frac{A\alpha_1 + B\alpha_2 + C\alpha_{fast}}{A + B + C} \quad (6.37)$$

Then

$$PS_{\text{whole body}} = (V_p/T_p^s) - \text{GFR}. \quad (6.38)$$

As stated above, it is whole body clearance that is measured, and this is only equal to *PS* product for molecules of molecular weight greater than about 5000 Da.

A somewhat cruder method of quantifying whole body *PS* product is to measure the rate at which an intravenously injected solute equilibrates throughout the extracellular fluid; i.e. to measure the time at which the multi-exponential clearance curve reaches the terminal exponential. One way of expressing this is the time to 95% equilibration (Peters and Myers

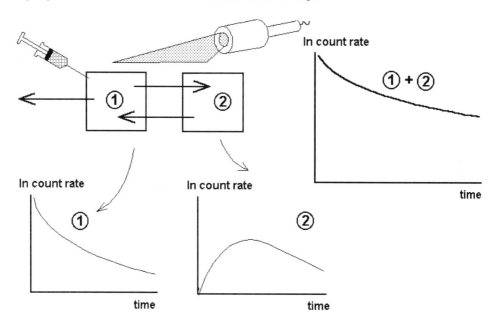

▮ **Fig. 6.15** Two-compartment model with run-off representing the experimental preparation of skeletal muscle in which solute is instantaneously deposited in the interstitial fluid space. Run-off is into plasma. The two compartments represent fluid phase and gel meshwork, as in Fig. 6.14. The model predicts a bi-exponential curve for the muscle.

1989). This time depends on diffusion across the barrier within the interstitial space, as well as the endothelium itself, and is therefore only an *index* of whole body *PS* product rather than a physiologically

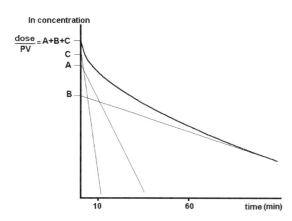

▮ **Fig. 6.16** Extracellular fluid space represented by a three-compartmental model. Small hydrophillic solutes exchange rapidly between plasma and the fluid phase of the extravascular space, but more slowly between the latter and the gel meshwork in which very large macromolecules tend to 'crowd'. Proteins exchange very slowly between the fluid phase and the gel meshwork, at a rate which may determine the value of the 'transcapillary escape rate' (TER).

definable entity. Nevertheless it correlates with *PS* product measured from tissue uptake (Section 6.2.2.4.2).

6.2.2 Microvascular protein transfer

Peripheral capillaries are much less permeable to protein compared with small solutes. Protein transfer is more rapid across fenestrated capillaries such as liver and bone marrow sinusoids and certain other vascular beds, including the adrenal gland and spleen. In sites outside these specialized vascular beds, it is likely that proteins cross the endothelium via relatively large pores. Although small solutes can also cross via these large pores, the majority cross via small pores which greatly outnumber the large ones. This explains why under some circumstances, such as histamine-induced microvascular 'leakiness', there may be increased permeability to protein but not to small solutes (Rippe and Grega 1978). Histamine increases the number of large pores but not small pores and by doing so reduces the restriction to diffusion of proteins imposed by the endothelium.

Most clinical studies on abnormalities of microvascular permeability have been based on radiolabelled proteins rather than small solutes (Parving

& Gyntelberg 1973) and employ a variable called the transcapillary exchange rate (TER, Fleck *et al.* 1985). This is the rate constant of radiolabelled protein disappearance from plasma between 10 and 60 min after injection and in the normal subject is about 5% per hour (or 0.0008 min^{-1}), compared with DTPA for which it is about 1% per minute. This approach represents an attempt to measure average whole body *PS* product for protein, analogous to whole body *PS* product for small solutes. As with small solutes, there is a rapid early exponential in the plasma disappearance curve (Bent-Hansen 1991), which should be taken into account for whole body *PS* product measurements. There are grounds for believing that the first exponential (up to 10 minutes) represents transfer across the endothelium while the second (up to 60 minutes) is more a reflection of the rate at which protein penetrates the gel meshwork of the interstitial space from the fluid phase (Katz 1980) **(Fig. 6.14)**. Indeed, because of possible misinterpretation of the plasma protein clearance curve between 10 and 60 minutes, the importance of recognising the three-compartmental ECF model is perhaps more relevant to the measurement of permeability to protein than small solutes. It is not known to what extent abnormal *endothelial* permeability may influence solute exchange, especially of macromolecules, between the two compartments of the extravascular ECF.

Plasma albumin has a metabolic turnover rate measurable in days, although its turnover between plasma and interstitial fluid (via transcapillary exchange and the lymphatics) is measurable in hours. In other words, an albumin molecule circulates between plasma and lymphatics several times before metabolic destruction. Radio-iodinated albumin is stable and can be used to measure TER by recording the rate at which it leaves plasma over the first few hours before it returns via the lymphatics. Evans blue, which is a dye tightly bound by albumin in plasma, has also been used for this purpose (Brown *et al.* 1989). Technetium-99m human serum albumin is not reliable because of instability of the label, such that the plasma clearance of radioactivity is influenced by the clearance of the much smaller technetium-99m. An area of clinical research which has received little attention is the relationship between abnormal permeability to macromolecules and changes in *PS* product of small solutes.

References

Bent-Hansen L. Whole body capillary exchange of albumin. *Acta Physiologica Scandinavica* 1991, **143**: (Suppl 603): 5–10.

Brown A, Zammit VC and Lowe SA. Capillary permeability and extracellular fluid volumes in pregnancy-induced hypertension. *Clinical Science* 1989, **77**: 599–604.

Cousins C, Jonker ND, Banks LM, Mohammadtaghi S, Myers MJ and Peters AM. Non-invasive measurement of microvascular permeability to a small solute in man. Validation of the technique. *Clinical Science* 1995; **89**: 191–200.

Cousins C, Gunasekera RD, Mubashar M, Mohammadtaghi S, Strong R, Myers MJ and Peters AM. Comparative kinetics of microvascular inulin and Tc-99m-DTPA exchange. *Clinical Science* (in press).

Crone C and Levitt DG. Capillary permeability to small solutes. In: Renkin EM and Michel CC (eds) *Handbook of physiology* section 2: The cardiovascular system IV. American Physiological Society, Bethesda, Maryland: 1984, 375–409.

Fleck A, Raines G, Hawker F, Trotter J, Wallace PI, Ledingham McA and Calman KC. Increased vascular permeability: a major cause of hypoalbuminaemia in disease and injury. *Lancet* 1985, **1**: 781–3.

Henriksen JH. Whole-body microvascular permeability of small molecules in man: clinical aspects, basic concepts and limitations of the single injection technique. *Scandinavian Journal of Clinical and Laboratory Investigation* 1985, **45**: 509–13.

Katz MA. Interstitial space — the forgotten organ. *Medical Hypotheses* 1980, **6**: 885–98.

Kennedy AM, Banks LM, MacSweeney JE, Myers MJ, Peters AM and Allison DJ. The use of xenon-133 for measurement of blood flow through systemic arteriovenous malformations before and after therapeutic embolization. *British Journal of Radiology* 1995, **68**: 844–9.

Lassen NA and Sejrsen P. Monoexponential extrapolation of tracer clearance curves in kinetic analysis. *Circulation Research* 1971, **19**: 76–87.

Lassen NA, Henriksen O and Sejrsen P. Indicator methods for measurement of organ and tissue blood flow. In: Shepherd JT and Abboud FM (eds) *Handbook of physiology* section 2: The cardiovascular system IV. American Physiological Society, Bethesda, Maryland: 1983, 21–63.

Lowy C, Arnot RN and Fraser TR. Measurement of an index of muscle capillary permeability and its correlation with serum insulin values in maturity-onset diabetic subjects. *Clinical Science & Molecular Medicine* 1976; **50**: 131–8.

Neilsen OM. Extracelluar volume, renal clearance and whole body permeability-surface area product in man measured after a single injection of polyfructosan. *Scandinavian Journal of Clinical and Laboratory Investigation* 1985; **45**: 217–22.

Paaske WP. Capillary permeability in skeletal muscle. *Acta Physiologica Scandinavia* 1977, **101**: 1–14.

Parkin A, Robinson PJ, Martinez D, Wilkinson D and Kester RC. Radionuclide limb blood flow in peripheral vascular disease: a review of 1100 measurements. *Nuclear Medicine Communications* 1991, **12**: 835–51.

Parving H and Gyntelberg F. Transcapillary escape rate of albumin and plasma volume in essential hypertension. *Circulation Research* 1973, **32**: 643–51.

Peters AM. Measurement of microvascular permeability to small solutes in man. Limitations of the technique. *Cardiovascular Research* 1990, **24** 504–59.

Peters AM and Myers MJ. Solute transfer into the extravascular space: comparison of two non-invasive measurement techniques. *Cardiovascular Research* 1989, **23**: 639–45.

Rippe B and Grega GJ. Effects of isoprenaline and cooling on histamine induced changes of capillary permeability in the rat hindquarter vascular bed. *Acta Physiologica Scandinavica* 1978, **103**: 252–62.

Sejrsen P. Blood flow in cutaneous tissue in man studied by washout of radioactive xenon. *Circulation Research* 1969, **24**: 215–29.

Sejrsen P. Capillary permeability measured by bolus injection, residue and venous detection. *Acta Physiologica Scandinavica* 1979, **105**: 73–92.

Seo IS, Sy WM, Heneghan W, Manoli A and Gozum M. Radionuclide fistulogram in hemodialysis patients (abstract). *Journal of Nuclear Medicine* 1984, **25**: P48.

Trap-Jensen J. Increased capillary permeability to 131–I and 51-Cr -EDTA in the exercising forearm of long term diabetics. *Clinical Science and Molecular Medicine* 1970, **39**: 39–49.

Trap-Jensen J and Lassen NA. Increased capillary diffusion capacity for small ions in skeletal muscle in long term diabetics. *Scandinavian Journal of Clinical and Laboratory Investigation* 1968, **21**: 116–22.

Veall N and Vetter H. *Radioisotope techniques in clinical research and diagnosis.* Butterworth, London, 1958; 350–84.

7 The heart

7.1 Myocardial haemodynamics

7.1.1 Myocardial blood flow

Blood flow through the left coronary artery is unique in that it is maximal during diastole. This is because of the mechanical effects of ventricular contraction. Increasing abruptly at the onset of diastole, blood flow gradually falls during the remainder of diastole and the direction of flow may actually reverse. The time-dependent profile of flow through the *right* coronary artery depends upon whether this vessel is dominant. If not, it demonstrates a flow profile similar to other arteries, with maximal flow during systole. Although this pattern is displayed by total myocardial blood flow, the transmural flow profiles are different. Thus, in the sub-endocardium, which is close to the effects of systolic compression, the effect is maximal, whereas in the sub-epicardium, the flow profile is more like that of any other artery. Because the sub-endocarium relies on diastolic blood pressure for its flow, its vascular bed is closer to its maximum vasodilatory capacity than that of the sub-epicardium. Indeed, under normal circumstances, sub-endocardial perfusion slightly exceeds sub-epicardial perfusion, probably because the sub-endocardium performs more work, which in turn is due to the higher wall tension developed in this region. This also reduces the sub-endocardial vasodilatory reserve. For these two reasons, the sub-endocardium is more at risk in the presence of coronary stenosis than the sub-epicardium, particularly during exercise, when myocardial oxygen requirements increase and also, importantly, the relative duration of diastole decreases.

Like the cerebral and renal vascular beds, coronary blood flow displays the phenomenon of autoregulation, as can be shown in the isolated perfused organ. Thus, within the physiologically encountered perfusion pressure range, coronary blood flow remains relatively constant, implying that coronary resistance varies directly with coronary perfusion pressure. Below 60 mm Hg, autoregulation fails; i.e. at this perfusion pressure, the autoregulatory capacity is maximal and no further vasodilatation can occur. This point of maximal coronary vasodilatation is important, in relation not only to the transmural distribution of myocardial blood flow, but also to regional blood flow distribution in coronary artery stenosis.

Normally myocardial oxygen extraction is nearly complete and coronary venous oxygen tension is low. The major determinant of myocardial blood flow is the myocardial oxygen requirement and so myocardial blood flow shows a nearly linear correlation with myocardial oxygen consumption. Several factors determine the myocardial oxygen requirement, the most important of which are the preload, the afterload, the heart rate and the inotropic state of the heart.

1. *Preload* The preload is the force extending the cardiac muscle prior to contraction. It determines the degree of stretch and tension in the muscle fibres before they contract. Most readers will be familiar, as physiology students, with the isolated muscle preparations from which weights were suspended to apply preload. Muscle contraction is initially isometric; i.e. muscle contracts with an increase in tension but without a change in fibre length. When the load is 'taken up', the fibre contracts isotonically; i.e. it contracts with reduction in length but without further change in tension. In the intact beating heart, ventricular preload is determined by the diastolic pressure and by the degree of dilatation of the ventricular chamber.

2. *Afterload* When the aortic and pulmonary valves are opened by ventricular contraction, the ventricle is exposed to pulmonary arterial or aortic pressure and is required to move blood against this pressure. Before the valves open, the ventricles must be contracting isometrically, but after they open they contract isotonically while being exposed to the afterload. As far as the left ventricle is concerned,

therefore, the oxygen requirement per beat is proportional to ventricular dilatation, diastolic ventricular pressure and systolic (or aortic) pressure.

3. *Heart rate* With each heart beat, this cycle repeats itself and so it is easy to appreciate that another determinant of oxygen requirement is the heart rate. Any intervention which changes heart rate is said to have a chronotropic effect.

4. *Inotropic state* In addition to chronotropic changes, the inotropic state of the heart may change. The inotropic state of cardiac muscle refers to the force with which the myocardium contracts, independently of the other determinants — preload, afterload and heart rate. The contractility of the heart depends on its biochemical milieu, for example on calcium fluxes. An increase in the inotropic state or, in other words, exposure to a positive inotropic influence, increases myocardial oxygen requirements and therefore increases myocardial blood flow.

The importance of varying the myocardial oxygen requirements by these mechanisms within a nuclear medicine context lies in the field of myocardial perfusion imaging and multiple gated (MUGA) blood pool imaging, and the effects of stress. In myocardial perfusion imaging, for example, increases in myocardial blood flow in healthy regions of the heart may outstrip increases in regions supplied by stenosed vessels, resulting in the accentuation of regional defects of uptake of perfusion agents in ischaemic zones. Exercise is the most physiological way to stress the myocardium. Normal myocardial perfusion at rest is about 100 ml/min/100 ml, rising to levels of about 400 ml/min/100 ml during maximal exercise. However exercising the patient is not always possible; for example, when pain (either peripheral or anginal) may limit tolerance, or the patient may have arthritis. Alternatively, therefore, any of the four specific factors which increase myocardial oxygen requirements can be increased either individually, or more usually in combination. *Exercise* increases heart rate, workload and inotropic state in broadly equal proportions. *Electrical pacing* obviously increases oxygen consumption by increasing the heart rate but it also has a positive inotropic influence. The heart can also be stressed pharmacologically either by *dipyridamole* or by *dobutamine*. The best known agent is dipyridamole. However the mechanism whereby this drug changes myocardial blood flow distribution is different from those interventions which stress the heart by increasing oxygen requirements. Thus dipyridamole is a coronary vasodilator and promotes a redistribution of blood flow to non-ischaemic zones because the ischaemic zones have already exceeded their autoregulatory capacity and are fully vasodilated downstream from an arterial stenosis. Another agent used for pharmacological intervention is dobutamine, which increases oxygen requirements by increasing the inotropic state of the myocardium.

7.1.1.1 Xenon-133

Myocardial blood flow (MBF) can be measured using intra-arterial xenon-133 at the time of coronary angiography. The principle is the same as for measurement of perfusion in other organs such as liver, kidney and brain. The washout curve is dominated by a single exponential (Bassingthwaite *et al.* 1968, L'Abbate & Maseri 1980). Because of the proximity of the myocardium to the lungs, it is necessary to record the washout curve with a gamma camera rather than a scintillation probe so that the xenon-133 injected into myocardial vascular territory can be clearly delineated from the intra-alveolar xenon-133 in the lungs.

7.1.1.2 Cardiac output fractionation — radiolabelled microspheres

Following the principles outlined in Section 3.3., myocardial blood flow can be measured with radiolabelled microspheres. This has been done in man using left atrial injection of technetium-99m labelled microspheres followed by absolute quantification of myocardial activity by quantitative scanning, thereby giving myocardial blood flow as a fraction of cardiac output. The theoretical requirement of this technique for complete mixing of the radio-labelled microspheres proximal to the supplying artery may not be so easily met with respect to the myocardium because of the proximity of the coronary arteries to the outflow tract of the left ventricle.

Microspheres can be labelled with positron-emitting radionuclides (gallium-68 or carbon-11), and myocardial blood flow measured in absolute units using PET to quantify tissue concentration of radioactivity (Section 3.1.2.). In order to obtain myocardial blood flow in units of ml/min/ml, the

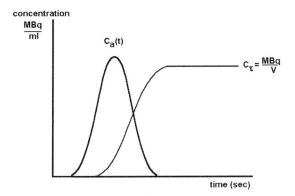

∎ **Fig. 7.1** Arterial time–concentration curve and time–activity curve recorded from myocardium following injection of labelled microspheres into the left side of the heart. If M_τ is in units of MBq then M_τ/injected activity is equal to myocardial blood flow/cardiac output. If C_a and C_τ are measured (such as by PET) in units of MBq/ml then myocardial tissue perfusion Q/V is equal to $C_\tau / \int C_a(t) \cdot dt$.

measurement of arterial concentration of radiolabelled microspheres, prior to their removal from blood, is also required (Weisenberg *et al.* 1981). The technique is essentially the same as measurement of clearance from organ uptake measurement, as outlined in Section 2.2.1.3. Myocardial blood flow is generated because the extraction fraction of microspheres is unity; i.e. myocardial microsphere clearance is equal to myocardial blood flow (**Fig. 7.1**). Thus

$$Q = \frac{M_\tau}{\int C_a(t) \cdot dt} \qquad (7.1)$$

where M_τ is myocardial tissue activity and C_a is arterial tracer concentration.

The integral $\int C_a(t) \cdot dt$ is given by total counts in an arterial sample drawn over a period encompassing injection and microembolisation of the particles (Section 3.3). Substituting for M_τ

$$Q = \frac{C_\tau \cdot V}{\int C_a(t) \cdot dt} \qquad (7.2)$$

where C_τ is myocardial tissue concentration and V is tissue volume.
Re-arranging,

$$\frac{Q}{V} = \frac{C_\tau}{\int C_a(t) \cdot dt}. \qquad (7.3)$$

It is desirable to allow the myocardium to complete its uptake; i.e. wait until C_a is zero, so that the timing

of t is not critical and $C_\tau(\infty)$ is not influenced by blood pool activity within the myocardial chambers. Alternatively, the area under the arterial time activity curve can be obtained from imaging the myocardial blood pool offering the advantage that neither C_τ nor C_a need be measured in concentration units of MBq/ml, but can be expressed instead as PET counts (per minute for C_τ at time t, and total counts up to t for $\int C_a(t)dt$) (see Section 3.1.3.1).

The microsphere principle can be adopted for a recirculating tracer using first-pass kinetics as described in Section 3.3. The principle is that any tracer can be regarded as a microsphere during the period of the minimum myocardial intravascular transit time (Mullani & Gould 1983). Equation 7.3 is again the fundamental equation but now, instead of infinity, data are acquired only up to the minimum intravascular transit time. For a deposited microsphere, the minimum intravascular transit time *is* infinity.

Taking derivatives of numerator and denominator in equation 7.3,

$$\frac{Q}{V} = \frac{dC_\tau}{dt} \times \frac{1}{C_a(\text{peak})}. \qquad (7.4)$$

If dC_τ/dt is the maximum gradient of the tissue uptake curve then $C_a(\text{peak})$ is the peak height of the arterial curve (**Fig. 7.2**). Note that with this approach the time interval between arterial and tissue curves is not critical. The principle of the technique

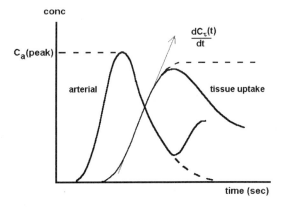

∎ **Fig. 7.2** Measurement of myocardial tissue perfusion using a recirculating tracer (analogous to Fig. 3.3) and either PET or dynamic CT. Tissue perfusion Q/V is equal to the maximum slope of the tissue curve $dC_\tau(t)/dt$ divided by the peak height $C_a(t)$ of the arterial concentration time curve determined from a region of interest over a major artery or left ventricular cavity.

is essentially the same as for measurement of organ blood flow as a fraction of cardiac output using a single photon tracer but, because of blood background, the technique works better as applied to the myocardium using PET since carbon-11 monoxide labelled red blood cells can be used for subtraction of blood background.

Radio-labelled microspheres form the theoretical basis for the use of the so-called 'chemical' microspheres, rubidium-82m (Mullani and Gould 1983, Goldstein *et al.* 1983 a & b) and nitrogen-13 labelled ammonia (Schelbert *et al.* 1981), which are positron-emitting radionuclides and which can be given intravenously instead of into the left ventricular cavity. They have the additional advantage that, as the result of intravenous injection, they mix better than microspheres and their myocardial distribution more accurately reflects the distribution of blood flow. However the myocardial clearances of ammonia, and particularly of rubidium-82, are less than myocardial blood flow, particularly at high flow rates. In cardiological nuclear medicine, the relationship between myocardial tracer extraction fraction and myocardial blood flow has received considerable attention, and it is well recognized that at increasing flow rates, tracer uptake progressively underestimates flow. The relationship between uptake and flow is a characteristic feature of a myocardial perfusion tracer and is dependent on the Crone–Renkin constant for that tracer (i.e. permeability–surface area product) (Crone & Levitt 1984). Therefore, in order to measure myocardial blood flow using these tracers without having to assume an extraction of unity, it is necessary to know the *PS* product of the myocardium for the tracer. Recall from Section 6.2.2.1 that the *PS* product for endothelial transfer, is given by

$$PS = -Q \ln(1 - E) \qquad (7.5)$$

which, re-arranged, gives

$$E = 1 - e^{-PS/Q}. \qquad (7.6)$$

Using *PS* in its more general sense; i.e. in the situation in which *E* is the steady-state extraction fraction of the tracer by the myocardium, and rewriting equation 7.3 for clearance instead of blood flow,

$$E \cdot \frac{Q}{V} = \frac{C_\tau}{\int C_a(t) \cdot dt} \qquad (7.7)$$

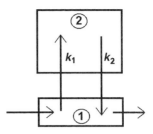

▌ **Fig. 7.3** Two-compartmental model illustrating the kinetics of the 'chemical microspheres' rubidium and ammonium ion. Compartment 1 represents tissue fluid and plasma compartments (combined) between which it is assumed that the tracer exchanges freely, while compartment 2 represents the myocyte in which tracer is considered to be 'irreversibly trapped' (i.e. $k_2 \cong 0$).

we can combine equations 7.6 and 7.7 to calculate *Q/V*, provided *PS/V* for the tracer is known:

$$\frac{Q}{V} = \frac{C_\tau}{\int C_a(t) \cdot dt \cdot [1 - e^{-PS/V/Q/V}]}. \qquad (7.8)$$

Alternatively, the two-compartment model, with exchange rate constants k_1 and k_2, described in Section 3.1.3.2, can be used with non-linear regression analysis (**Fig. 7.3**). For both rubidium-82 and ammonia, k_2 is assumed to be equal to zero. In order to meet this assumption, especially for ammonia, dynamic acquisition is limited to 90 sec after injection, after which nitrogen-13 labelled metabolites of ammonia return to the circulation. Rubidium-82, as a potassium analogue, diffuses out of the myocardium slowly, so for a rapid dynamic study, k_2 is also zero. Assuming free diffusion between vascular and interstitial spaces,

$$\frac{dM_f}{dt} = Q \cdot C_a - (k_1 \cdot C_f + Q \cdot C_f) \qquad (7.9)$$

where C_f is concentration of free tracer in compartment 1; the units are:

$$\frac{MBq}{min} = \frac{ml \cdot MBq}{min \cdot ml} - min^{-1} \cdot MBq - \frac{MBq}{min}.$$

Dividing equation 7.9 by the volume of compartment 1, V_1, to convert M_f to C_f, and then multiplying by V_1/V, where *V* is tissue volume,

$$\frac{V_1}{V} \frac{dC_f}{dt} = \frac{Q}{V} \cdot C_a - C_f(\frac{Q}{V} + \frac{k_1}{V}). \qquad (7.10)$$

The term V_1/V scales concentration in compartment 1 to concentration with respect to total tissue volume, which is the concentration measured by PET. Likewise for compartment 2, where the tracer is bound or 'trapped'):

$$\frac{V_2}{V_1} \cdot \frac{dC_\chi}{dt} = \frac{k_1}{V} \cdot C_f \qquad (7.11)$$

where V_2 is the volume of compartment 2.

The tissue concentration C_τ recorded by PET is the sum of concentrations C_χ and C_f. However C_χ and C_f are concentrations with respect to the volumes of their respective compartments. Since PET records the tracer concentration with respect to *total* tissue volume C_χ and C_f must be scaled down according to the proportion that these volumes occupy of total tissue volume, i.e.

$$C_\tau = (V_1/V) \cdot C_f + (1 - V_1/V) \cdot C_\chi. \qquad (7.12)$$

Although C_a can be measured and V_1/V assumed, there are still four unknowns, Q/V, k_1/V, C_χ and C_f, but only three equations. However two further equations involving E can be introduced:

$$E = \frac{k_1/V}{k_1/V + Q/V} \qquad (7.13)$$

and

$$Q \cdot E = \frac{M_\tau}{\int C_a(t) \cdot dt}. \qquad (7.14)$$

Only one further unknown (E) has been introduced, but now we have five unknowns and five equations, from which both E and Q can be calculated.

7.1.1.3 Rubidium-82 continuous infusion

Since it has a short half-life (75 seconds), rubidium-82 offers another approach for measuring perfusion, which, in principle, is similar to that for continuously infused oxygen-15 labelled water or krypton-81m. With a continuous infusion, a steady state is reached which is the result of equality of inflow and outflow rates *plus* radionuclide decay rate; i.e.

$$\frac{dM_\tau}{dt} = QC_a - (QC_v + C_\tau V\delta) \qquad (7.15)$$

where Q is myocardial blood flow (ml/min), C_a and C_v are arterial and venous tracer concentrations respectively, V is tissue volume and δ is the rubidium-82 physical decay constant.

At steady state,

$$dM_\tau/dt = 0. \qquad (7.16)$$

Therefore

$$Q \cdot C_a = Q \cdot C_v + C_\tau \cdot V \cdot \delta. \qquad (7.17)$$

The first feature of this equation that differs from its application with respect to water and krypton-81m is that extraction fraction of rubidium-82 by the myocardium is not 100%, especially at high flow rates. We should therefore introduce the term extraction fraction (E) into equation 7.19:

$$E \cdot QC_a = QC_v + C_\tau V\delta. \qquad (7.18)$$

As with continuous infusion of labelled water (Araujo *et al.* 1991) or krypton-81m (Selwyn *et al.* 1978), *extracted* rubidium-82 can diffuse out of the myocardium back into the blood, and so at equilibrium the term λ for partition coefficient has to be introduced; i.e.

$$C_\tau = C_v \lambda. \qquad (7.19)$$

Substituting for C_v in equation 7.18 and rearranging we arrive at an equation with which the reader should now be familiar

$$\frac{C_\tau}{C_a} = \frac{E \cdot [Q/V]}{\frac{Q}{\lambda V} + \delta}. \qquad (7.20)$$

Another feature of equation 7.20 is that λ is very high (because the blood concentration is very low). The term $Q/\lambda V$ is therefore effectively negligible in comparison with δ, even for tissues with very high perfusion. Thus

$$\frac{C_\tau}{C_a} = \frac{E \cdot Q}{\delta \cdot V}. \qquad (7.21)$$

So the dependence of C_τ on Q is fundamentally different with rubidium-82 compared with both labelled water and krypton-81m in that their relationship is, at least in theory, linear. In practice however it remains non-linear because extraction fraction falls with increasing flow rates. Nevertheless, this feature of rubidium-82 does allow its use to be extended to tissues with high rates of perfusion, particularly the kidney, for which continuous infusion of labelled water is too insensitive to distinguish between regions of varying, although high, perfusion.

7.1.1.4 Oxygen-15 labelled water

This technique, and its variation between bolus injection (Bergmann *et al.* 1981) and continuous infusion, (Araujo *et al.* 1991) is described in Section 3.1.3.1. When applied to myocardial perfusion, it has the advantage that the arterial input concentration can readily be measured in the same slice from blood within the left ventricle. Because of its diffusibility, labelled water clearance into the myocardium remains almost equal to myocardial blood flow over a wide range of flow values. At high flow rates, as already noted in Section 3.1.3.1, bolus injection, in contrast to continuous infusion, is preferable.

7.1.2 Distribution of myocardial perfusion

Imaging the distribution of radiolabelled microspheres throughout the myocardium following left ventricular injection provides an image of the distribution of myocardial blood flow. This is analogous to the intravenous injection of radiolabelled microspheres as a measure of the distribution of pulmonary blood flow. For routine use, this is too invasive. It is reproduced, however, using intravenously injected potassium analogues as described above and in Section 4.6.1. Sapirstein (1958) described how the early distribution of potassium analogues reflects the organ distribution of cardiac output, and pointed out that this is not necessarily the result of an extraction fraction in peripheral tissues of 100%, but is because the extraction fraction in many organs is the same as whole body extraction fraction. So the principle of the chemical microspheres is still valid even if it takes more than one circulation to achieve complete extraction.

The measurement of the distribution of myocardial perfusion using potassium analogues as a substitute for microspheres is a widely practised, clinically useful, investigation. Thallium-201 is the analogue usually employed with gamma cameras, although, for PET, rubidium-82 is used. Areas of reduced activity, visualized within a few minutes of injection, indicate reduced blood flow. Increasing myocardial oxygen requirements, such as by exercising the patient at the time of injection, increases the sensitivity of detecting ischaemic regions since the myocardium supplied by stenosed vessels is already close to its vasodilatory capacity and the

effect of stress is to divert the radioactivity towards regions supplied by normal vessels. The regional distribution of activity in the myocardium is actually proportional to regional tracer clearance, and so faithfully reflects the distribution of blood flow only if the extraction efficiency of the tracer is constant throughout the myocardium or, from a more practical viewpoint, is the same in ischaemic and non-ischaemic regions.

With the passage of time after injection, potassium analogues redistribute to regions of viable myocardium in proportion to the tissue potassium 'volume'. In other words, immediately after injection, the distribution is flow-dependent whilst some hours later it is potassium pool (or tissue volume)-dependent. The sequential appearances in ischaemic heart disease are characteristic. Following injection under stress, a region of hypoperfused, but viable, myocardium appears as a defect on early imaging but 'fills in' on later imaging, whereas a region of infarcted (i.e. non-viable) myocardium appears as a defect at all times (i.e. is a 'fixed' defect). It is important to realize that, at rest, a partially occluded coronary artery may furnish a sufficient blood supply to a region of myocardium, and so appear normal if the patient is injected at rest. As well as exercise, the myocardium may be stressed by electrical pacing or pharmacologically with agents, such as dipyridamole, which cause coronary vasodilatation. The effect is the same, namely the 'stealing' of radioactivity by the normally perfused myocardium at the expense of hypoperfused regions, unable to achieve any further vasodilatation.

It is now well recognized that redistribution of thallium-201 from normal to ischaemic regions may take several hours and that ischaemic but viable myocardium may require considerably longer than 3 hours to accumulate sufficient activity to fill in on delayed imaging (Dilsizian *et al.* 1990). Unless sufficient time has been allowed, viable myocardium may be misinterpreted as infarcted. The rate of equilibration of thallium-201 between a region of ischaemic myocardium and the rest of the body throughout which thallium-201 is distributed is dependent on the fractional rate constants respectively governing the input into, k_1[†], and the output from (the thallium-201 washout rate constant k_2), the

---

[†]Note the small case k_1 to indicate a fractional rate constant; i.e. fraction of whole body tracer entering the myocardium in unit time; and to distinguish from the *PS* product K_1.

ischaemic myocardium. Note that k_2 is very low, in fact considered to be negligible over the course of a relatively short dynamic study (see above and estimated from experimental canine studies to be between 0.01 and 0.03 min^{-1} (Budinger 1992).

The value of k_2 is also very low for all other tissues, resulting in a low plasma concentration. Given the relatively enormous pool of thallium-201 throughout the body, the low plasma concentration (almost zero) and the low rate of resting blood flow into the ischaemic myocardium, k_1 (the fraction of total body thallium entering the myocardium in unit time), is also very small, in fact much smaller than k_2. The rate constant of equilibration is equal to the sum of k_1 and k_2; if we assume this to be essentially equal to k_2, then 95% equilibration would require ln 20/0.01 min for a k_2 of 0.01 min^{-1}; i.e. 5 hr, or for a k_2 of 0.001 min^{-1}, 50 hr.

Since at equilibrium, the thallium-201 flux rate into and from the myocardium is equal,

$$K_1 \cdot C_p = K_2 \cdot C_\tau \qquad (7.22)$$

where K_1 and K_2 are *PS* products, and subscripts p, and τ refer to capillary and intramyocyte concentrations. The final distribution of thallium-201 between normal and ischaemic myocardium depends on the ratio K_1/K_2. This ratio has been estimated to be about 30, but significantly is essentially the same for normal and ischaemic myocardium (Budinger 1992), explaining why viable ischaemic myocardium appears normal when equilibrium is finally achieved. One way of promoting equilibration is to give the thallium-201 with the patient at rest. This effectively puts ischaemic myocardium on a higher point on the equilibration curve, since it receives more tracer immediately after injection. It is now well recognized that severely ischaemic but viable myocardium may only be seen to accumulate thallium-201 following an injection at rest. Non-functioning ischaemic myocardium which is nevertheless viable is called hibernating myocardium. It is important to identify hibernating myocardium since unless it is revascularized it will continue not to function, and to compromise the patient's overall cardiac function. It can be distinguished from 'stunned' myocardium which although also non-functioning will sponta-neously regain function. Stunned myocardium, in contrast to hibernating myocardium, is an acute entity, usually sustained following myocardial infarction. Since thallium-201 is a potassium analogue and therefore subject to the cellular sodium–potassium pump mechanism, it is important to realize that it is not only a marker of myocardial perfusion but also of metabolism.

A new class of agents has recently been developed for imaging myocardial perfusion, the technetium-99m labelled isonitriles of which the best known is MIBI or sestamibi. Like rubidium-82, thallium-201 and nitrogen-13 labelled ammonia, but unlike labelled water, the extraction efficiency of sestamibi decreases with increasing perfusion. The steady-state *PS* product of sestamibi is somewhat less than that of thallium-201; i.e. for any level of myocardial blood flow its steady-state extraction efficiency is slightly less than that of thallium-201. Although technetium-99m labelling is an advantage over thallium-201, sestamibi does not redistribute like thallium-201 and therefore, in order to distin-guish viable from non-viable myocardium, has to be given as two separate injections, one at exercise and one at rest. It is more a marker of perfusion than of metabolism compared with thallium-201 since even when injected at rest may fail to show severely ischaemic but viable muscle. There are therefore, four types of image available in myocardial per-fusion imaging:

(1) early imaging after injection under stress (thallium or sestamibi):
(2) delayed imaging after injection under stress (thallium);
(3) early imaging after injection at rest (thallium or sestamibi);
(4) delayed imaging after injection at rest (thallium).

With thallium, all four may differ.

Thallium-201 and technetium-99m sestamibi give comparable information for the detection of cor-onary artery disease. For the detection of viable myocardium, however, thallium-201 has an advan-tage on account of its ability to redistribute, especially into regions that appear as defects even on images obtained immediately after injection at rest. Perhaps the best protocols are those which combine an injection of sestamibi under stress and an injection of thallium at rest, thereby exploiting the superior imaging properties of technetium-99m and the functional information of thallium.

7.2 Extrinsic parameters of cardiac performance

The three critical variables concerned in the maintenance of a circulation are cardiac contraction (producing the cardiac output which is the product of heart rate and stroke volume), blood volume and blood pressure. Control of the latter involves both arterial and venous vasoconstriction. The mechanisms controlling these three variables are closely related and involve neuronal and humoral activity. The afferent connections in the short-term neuronal control of cardiac output and blood pressure are from the baroreceptors, which respond to stretch, and chemoreceptors, which respond to blood gas tensions.

Baroreceptors are located in the arterial walls of the carotids (at the carotid sinus) and the aortic arch. They are sensitive not only to mean arterial pressure but also to the rate of change of pressure and therefore to pulse pressure. Chemoreceptors are located in the carotid arteries at their bifurcation (the carotid bodies) and in the intrathoracic aorta; they exert less influence on blood pressure control than baroreceptors. Interestingly, the carotid body has an extremely high perfusion, about 2000 ml/ 100 g/min, some 20–30 times higher than, for example, resting myocardial perfusion.

The efferent neuronal connections mediating blood pressure control are relayed through the cerebral cortex and hypothalamus to the heart and peripheral blood vessels via the sympathetic and parasympathetic autonomic nervous systems. A positive inotropic stimulus to the heart generally equates with an increase in stroke volume while a positive chronotropic stimulus equates with an increase in heart rate. The response to an acute increase in arterial blood pressure, which stimulates the baroreceptors, is a reduction in sympathetic tone of the peripheral vasculature, including the venous capacitance vessels, and an increase in the parasympathetic (vagal) tone to the heart. A decrease in blood pressure causes an increase in sympathetic tone both to peripheral vessels and to the heart, with both positive inotropic and chronotropic effects. The peripheral vasculature is largely under the control of vasoconstrictor tone, with vasodilation resulting from removal of this tone. The existence of fibres which actively induce vasodilatation is doubtful in man, although they may be present to induce vasodilatation as a result of cerebral cortical activity, such as the anticipation of exercise.

The long-term control of blood pressure is closely linked to the control of blood volume and is predominantly humoral. The sensors controlling blood volume include:

(a) osmoreceptors in the hypothalamus which influence thirst and control the secretion of anti-diuretic hormone (ADH) from the posterior pituitary;

(b) stretch receptors in the wall of the cardiac chambers, predominantly atrial, which respond to increased intravascular pressure by secreting the peptide, atrial natriuretic factor (ANF or ANP) and decreasing ADH secretion via central neuronal links;

(c) the juxtaglomerular apparatus of the kidney which secretes renin in response to a reduction in the renal tubular sodium delivery to the macula densa.

ADH reduces water excretion, ANP promotes the urinary excretion of sodium, while renin acts enzymatically on angiotensinogen to produce first angiotensin-1 and then, through angiotensin converting enzyme, angiotensin-2 (A-2). A-2 is a powerful local renal and more widespread vasoconstrictor, increases thirst and stimulates the production of aldosterone from the zona glomerulosa of the adrenal cortex, which in turn acts on the renal tubule to promote reabsorption of sodium. GFR and aldosterone used to be considered the two factors governing the urinary excretion of sodium until it was demonstrated that even when they were both controlled, the kidney could excrete increased amounts of sodium in response to sodium loading, implicating the presence of a third factor. This turned out to be ANP, which is not only natriuretic but also tends to lower blood pressure and blood volume by respectively opposing the vasoconstrictor effect of A-2 and increasing post-capillary resistance relative to pre-capillary resistance, thereby promoting fluid shift to the tissues. Changes in sympathetic tone mediated through stretch receptors in the circulation also contribute to blood volume regulation through renal sympathetic vasoconstrictor activity.

Whereas the roles of all these mediators, especially hormonal, are reasonably well understood in the aetiology of renovascular hypertension, their roles in essential hypertension are obscure, with other factors being involved, and cannot be further discussed here. Similarly, haemodynamic control in heart failure is abnormal and complex, with amongst many other changes, abnormalities in renal control of blood volume, disturbed baroreceptor control and depletion of myocardial neurotransmitter stores. The last-mentioned has recently been exploited by imaging with iodine-123-metaiodobenzylguanidine (MIBG).

7.2.1 Cardiac output

Cardiac output (CO) is most accurately measured by rapid bolus injection of tracer into the right atrium followed by continuous measurement of the concentration in an artery. In the absence of blood flow shunting this may be the pulmonary artery or a systemic artery

Then

$$CO = \frac{\text{injected activity}}{\text{area under time-concentration curve}} \quad (7.23)$$

with units

$$\text{ml/min} = \text{MBq}/(\text{MBq} \cdot \text{ml}^{-1} \cdot \text{min}) = \text{ml} \cdot \text{min}^{-1}.$$

This is the Stewart–Hamilton equation, the principle of which can be understood by examining its units, and also by multiplying the numerator and denominator of the transit time equation, $Q = V/T$, by the arterial tracer concentration C_a.

Thus

$$Q = \frac{V \cdot C_a}{T \cdot C_a} \quad (7.24)$$

The product $V \cdot C_a$ is a mass and, with respect to blood being ejected from the left ventricle, is the injected dose, while $T \cdot C_a$ is the area under the time concentration curve recorded in any artery. In other words, equation 7.23 is an example of the general equation, $Q = \text{mass/area}$.

Before all the tracer has entered the systemic circulation for the first time, the decreasing arterial concentration curve is interrupted by recirculation. In order to obtain the area under the curve, therefore,

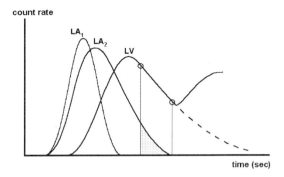

count rate

time (sec)

▌ **Fig. 7.4** Exponential fit to downslope of left ventricular time–activity curve. Since the left ventricle (LV) ejects a constant fraction of its contained radioactivity, an exponential fit would be mathematically appropriate provided all first pass activity had entered the left ventricle, as in the case where left atrial activity is represented by LA_1. In the case where left atrial activity is represented by LA_2, activity is still entering the left ventricle at the first time of the period for which the exponential is fitted, and the system approaches that in Fig. 7.5.

the first-pass curve has to be corrected for this recirculation. This can be achieved by assuming that the downslope of the arterial curve is exponential and fitting it with an exponential function. This exponential is then extrapolated forwards, from time t, just before recirculation, to infinity. The area under the curve from t is then $C_a(t)/\alpha$ where α is the rate constant of the exponential. The area, $C_a(t)/\alpha$, is then added to the area under the curve up to time t. Alternatively, recirculation can be eliminated by fitting a gamma function to the first-pass curve (Section 2.1.2.1).

Fitting an exponential function to the downslope of the arterial curve would be appropriate if all the injected activity had arrived in the left ventricle by the time of the first of the two time points between which the exponential function is fitted (**Fig. 7.4**), since, with stable left ventricular function, the left ventricle ejects a constant fraction of the tracer within it. Indeed

$$\alpha = \frac{\text{ejection fraction} \times \text{LV volume} \times \text{pulse rate}}{\text{LV volume}}$$

$$(7.25)$$

i.e. α is the product of ejection fraction and pulse rate. However, most of the bolus spreading between the right atrium and arterial sampling point takes

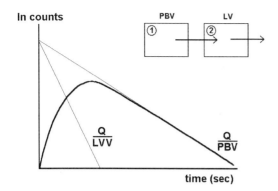

In counts

PBV   LV

Q
––
LVV

Q
––
PBV

time (sec)

∎ **Fig. 7.5**   If there is negligible bolus spreading in the left atrium, then the time course of the concentration of a tracer in the left ventricle following bolus intravenous injection would reflect an input function dependent on the histogram of pulmonary transit times and an output function depending on the fraction of blood ejected from the ventricle per unit of time. Assuming tracer leaves the lung exponentially, then the two compartments, lung and left ventricle, will effectively be in series producing a curve convex upwards which is the difference of two exponentials. The curve under these circumstances approaches the slower rate constant which would correspond to Q/pulmonary blood volume rather than Q/left ventricular volume because pulmonary blood volume is greater than left ventricular volume.

place within the pulmonary vascular bed and the downslope on the arterial curve is more a reflection of the distribution of intravascular transit times within the pulmonary vascular bed. Recall the compartmental model for two compartments in series (Section 1.4), in which tracer leaves the first exponentially, with rate constant α_1 and enters the second. It then leaves the second exponentially with rate constant α_2. The signal from the second compartment therefore rises to a peak and then falls with a rate constant equal to whichever is the lower of α_1 and α_2. The lung can be considered as compartment 1 and the left ventricle as compartment 2 (ignoring the transit through the left ventricle). Now α_1 in this setting is Q/pulmonary blood volume and α_2 is Q/left ventricular volume. Pulmonary blood volume exceeds left ventricular volume so the downslope of the left ventricular curve should reflect Q/pulmonary blood volume. In other words, the left ventricular downslope and, therefore also that in a systemic artery, should reflect the distribution of pulmonary intravascular transit times, which would be expected to be almost exponential (**Fig. 7.5**).

In practice, the downslope is close to being exponential and is well fitted as such. Alternatively a gamma function fit can be fitted to the entire first-pass curve between take off point and the time of recirculation. The area under the curve based on gamma function fitting is slightly smaller than that based on exponential fitting to the downslope. The difference in area between the two fitting procedures varies with the width of the curve (i.e. its area/peak height ratio) but is generally not more than about 10%.

The tracers used to measure cardiac output by arterial sampling include the dyes indocyanine green and Evan's blue (dye dilution), and heat (thermodilution). With this latter approach cold saline can be injected intravenously and the temperature of arterial blood monitored continuously with a thermistor placed in the artery. The assumption has to be made that there is no heat exchange between injection and sampling points. In fact significant heat is transferred during transit through the lung, and so it is preferable to inject the cold saline into the pulmonary vein. This measurement is usually made in the Intensive Care Unit, where access is already available. An advantage of thermodilution is the ability to perform repeated measurements without build-up of tracer.

Radiolabelled intravascular markers, such as labelled red cells or human serum albumin, can be used to measure cardiac output non-invasively. Instead of sampling arterial blood, a detector placed over the right lung or heart is used to continuously monitor the first-pass time–activity curve through the pulmonary vascular bed or heart. After about 5 minutes, the count rate stabilizes, even though the tracer has not completely mixed within the circulation. By taking an intravenous blood sample at 5 minutes for counting in a well counter, the concentration in blood in absolute units (MBq/ml) can be related to the count rate recorded by the detector at the time of sampling, thereby converting the first pass curve into absolute units.

Then

$$\text{cardiac output} = \frac{\text{dose}}{\Gamma \cdot \int N(t)\mathrm{d}t} \qquad (7.26)$$

where N(t) is the recirculation-corrected first-pass time–activity curve and Γ is the proportionality constant relating the concentration of radioactivity in blood to the count rate recorded by the detector and is given by

$$\Gamma = C_{eq}/N_{eq} = \frac{MBq}{ml} \times \frac{min}{counts}$$

where C_{eq} at N_{eq} are the concentration and count rate respectively recorded at 5 minutes when the count rate is relatively stable.

This is not as accurate as arterial sampling because whereas activity is confined to the lungs on first pass, the equilibrium count rate (N_{eq}) includes activity in chest wall blood. Although the volume of blood in the chest wall is small compared with the underlying cardiac chambers, it is closer to the detector than cardiac or pulmonary blood. A less important error is caused by free tracer which adds to the chest wall signal by diffusing into the extra-vascular space of the chest wall. This latter consideration explains why one cannot use diffusible tracers, like technetium-99 m DTPA, for measuring cardiac output.

If it is placed over the left ventricle, the region of interest may also include counts from the right ventricle. In addition, some activity from the lung may be detected, particularly from a posterior projection, because some of the left lower lobe intervenes between the left ventricle and posterior chest wall. The first-pass time–activity curve will then be a composite of curves from the ventricles and lung, all separated in time as the tracer moves through them. However this does not matter since it can be imagined that we have 2 (or 3) separate curve areas each with its own corresponding equilibrium count rate (i.e. N_{eq}) but all with the same injected dose. In effect, the area under the curve and N_{eq} of equation 7.26 represent these separate components, all summated. Placement of the region of interest over the cardiac chambers does however disqualify the use of a gamma function fit, which requires a single smooth curve, and necessitates the use of an exponential fit to the downslope for the correction of recirculation. To use a gamma function fit requires that the curve is based on a lung region of interest which is an adequate alternative to the left ventricle.

The clinical value of measuring cardiac output is limited and performed only in a setting (for example in the intensive care unit) in which the patient is likely to have an arterial line anyway. The radio-nuclide technique therefore has minimal clinical value. It may have value however when it accompanies the measurement of other physiological variables. For example, renal blood flow can be measured non-invasively as a fraction of cardiac output (Section 11.1.1.3) and can then be converted to absolute units if cardiac output is measured. If an intravascular tracer is used, then this can be from the same dose of radionuclide. Also, if cardiac output is known, then other indices of cardiac function (derived from the same injection of radio-pharmaceutical), such as end systolic volume and filling rates (see below), can be converted to absolute units of volume and flow respectively. Another application is in the assessment of therapeutic embolization of systemic arterio–venous malformations, which can give rise to high output failure. Successful embolization results in a reduction of cardiac output.

7.2.2 Mean circulation time

Mean circulation time is the ratio of total blood volume to cardiac output and is the average time it takes for blood to undergo one circulation. The mean circulation times of plasma and red cells are slightly different; the haematocrit is different from organ to organ as a result of different regional transit times for plasma and red cells. Thus red cells take significantly longer to transit the spleen than plasma and the local haematocrit within the spleen is about 0.6. On the other hand, red cells transit the liver faster than plasma because local rheological factors promote axial streaming of the red cells. So a red cell, setting off from the aortic outflow tract, which finds itself going through the spleen may take two minutes to circulate back to the outflow tract whereas another traversing the liver (via the hepatic artery) may take only 30 seconds. The mean circulation time is the average of all the separate circulation times.

Circulation time can be measured from a single dose of an intravascular marker. Whether plasma or red cell transit time is measured depends on whether the tracer is human serum albumin or labelled red cells. Cardiac output is measured from equation 7.24 and total blood volume is measured from the dilution principle as described in Section 10. A simple approach, requiring no blood sampling, is to divide the area under the first pass curve over the lung (recirculation corrected) (units: counts) by the count rate in the same region of interest at about 10 minutes after injection (units: counts/second), when intravascular mixing is essentially completed. This yields mean circulation time (in seconds).

7.3 Intrinsic parameters of cardiac performance

The concepts of preload and afterload have already been referred to. Both are important in determining the oxygen requirements of the myocardium. Drawing an analogy with the isolated muscle preparation, stroke volume is the equivalent of the height a load is lifted, while aortic pressure is the equivalent of the weight of the load. The product of stroke volume and aortic pressure is therefore the work performed by the myocardium in each heart beat. The same work performed by the myocardium may result in differing oxygen costs. Thus a high stroke volume at low systolic pressure uses less oxygen than the same work performed at low stroke volume and high systolic pressure. Stroke volume is therefore an important intrinsic parameter of cardiac performance.

Within a single heart beat, and at a given inotropic state, more oxygen is required for the development of wall tension (i.e. to contract isometrically), than for the subsequent fibre shortening (isotonic contraction) after opening of the aortic valve. End diastolic volume, which determines preload, is therefore another important intrinsic parameter of cardiac performance. Combining stroke volume and end diastolic volume gives ejection fraction, which is the ratio of the two. Ejection fraction does not by itself determine oxygen requirement since both its numerator and denominator are directly proportional to oxygen costs. Nevertheless ejection fraction is a useful and relatively simply determined variable, a directional change in which, in response to various stresses including exercise, is of diagnostic value.

7.3.1 Ejection fraction

7.3.1.1 Multiple gated cardiac imaging

Ejection fraction is most readily measured from multiple gated (MUGA) cardiac studies. Dynamic images are acquired in the left anterior oblique view,

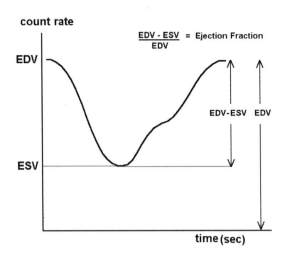

$$\frac{EDV - ESV}{EDV} = \text{Ejection Fraction}$$

▍ **Fig. 7.6** Basis for the calculation of ejection fraction, EF, from gated radionuclide ventriculography (MUGA). The curve represents a composite cardiac cycle, representing the average of many cycles, recorded by gated acquisition following intravenous injection of an agent which remains in the intravascular compartment. The highest count rate is recorded at the end of diastole when the left ventricular cavity is maximally filled with blood. The counts fall during systole to the end-systolic count rate and rise again as a result of re-entry of labelled blood. The difference between EDV and ESV represents the volume of blood ejected (stroke volume) while EDV represents maximal volume. [EDV − ESV]/EDV is therefore the ejection fraction. Additional information can be extracted from the overall slope of the curve (its first derivative — see below).

which allows the best separation of the two ventricles. A composite single cardiac cycle is constructed (Section 5.3.4). The computer on-line to the gamma camera automatically establishes an outline region of interest around the left ventricle in each frame of this composite cycle. The time–activity curve based on this region of interest (which of course is varying in size throughout the cardiac cycle) is then generated. It represents the time course of left ventricular blood volume, from which ejection fraction can be calculated (**Fig. 7.6**). The frame to frame left ventricular region of interest contains some pulmonary blood and so background subtraction is necessary. Various background subtraction techniques have been suggested.

Right ventricular ejection fraction is less reliably measured by this approach since on the left anterior oblique view there is considerable radioactivity in

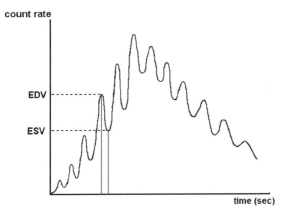

count rate

EDV

ESV

time (sec)

▌ **Fig. 7.7** Measurement of ejection fraction from a curve recorded by dynamic imaging during the first pass of tracer through a ventricular cavity seconds following intravenous bolus injection. The curve is saw toothed because of ejection followed by refilling of radioactivity in the left ventricle. The amplitude of each downslope is proportional to the stroke volume while the peak preceding each downslope is proportional to end-diastolic volume. Several cycles occur and can be averaged in the single pass. The technique is especially useful for measuring right ventricular ejection fraction because at equilibrium, as in a MUGA study, it is impossible to view the right ventricle from any angle without overlap from another chamber; this is not a problem during first pass since no tracer has yet reached the left side of the heart and the right ventricle can be 'captured' from the right anterior oblique projection.

the region of interest arising from blood behind the right ventricle (mainly from the right atrium) which is difficult to subtract. Conversely, in the right anterior oblique projection, the right ventricular signal is contaminated by signals from the left side of the heart. Right ventricular ejection fraction can however be measured with other techniques. One is based on first pass kinetics and the other on infusion of radiolabelled inert gases.

7.3.1.2 First pass

By acquiring dynamic data at a rapid frame rate in the right anterior oblique view (in which position the right ventricle is to the left of the right atrium and in front of the left ventricle), the bolus of radioactivity can be recorded as it passes through the right ventricle for the first time. The time–activity curve

so produced is 'saw toothed' each peak and trough representing end diastole and end systole of each cardiac cycle. The vertical distance from peak to next trough divided by the height of the peak is equal to ejection fraction (**Fig. 7.7**). Since for most of the period of this first-pass time–activity curve no activity enters the left ventricle, interference from this chamber is minimal. Using the same principle, left ventricular ejection fraction can also be measured from the first pass curve recorded by a detector or camera in the left anterior oblique position. The number of cardiac cycles available for measurement of ejection fraction by this approach is, of course, limited.

7.3.1.3 Inert gases

Following intravenous infusion, an inert gas is trapped in the lung as it rapidly enters the alveolar air spaces. Continuous infusion of krypton-81m, for instance, gives a steady state signal from the right side of the heart and lungs but almost none from the left ventricle. A MUGA acquisition can therefore be performed in the right anterior oblique position (without interference from the left ventricle) and analysed in the same way as the left ventricle in a conventional labelled red cell gated study (Sugrue *et al.* 1983).

Xenon-133 has also been used to measure right ventricular ejection fraction. Because of its long half-life, radioactivity builds up in the left ventricle as a result of the 5% or so that recirculates but, if the infusion is limited to a period of 20 seconds, long enough to acquire data over a reasonable number of cardiac cycles, it can be treated exactly like krypton-81m infusion and used to calculate right ventricular ejection fraction.

Simply by way of a theoretical comment, it can be pointed out that if technetium-99m macroaggregated albumin (MAA) is given as a tight bolus into the right side of the heart then the rate constant α of its removal from the right ventricle is a function of right ventricular ejection fraction and pulse rate, i.e.

$$\alpha = \text{ejection fraction} \times \text{pulse rate.} \qquad (7.27)$$

The rate constant of arrival in the lung, also k, can be recorded with a detector over the lung, and this therefore represents a simple method for measuring right ventricular ejection fraction (**Fig. 7.8**). The bolus has to be deposited instantaneously into and

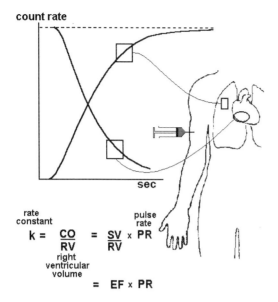

▌ Fig. 7.8 Simplified method for measuring right ventricular ejection fraction. With each cardiac cycle, the fraction of technetium-99m labelled macroaggregates (MAA) ejected from the right ventricle will be equal to right ventricular ejection fraction (RVEF). MAA will therefore leave the right ventricle with a rate constant k equal to RVEF × pulse rate and arrive in the lung with the same rate constant. Since it is not possible to deposit MAA instantaneously in the right ventricle, it is necessary to determine the input function to the right ventricle from a region of interest over the right atrium or superior vena cava. If RVEF is reduced the error resulting from the assumption of instantaneous bolus input to the RV will be small.

mix rapidly in the right ventricle. Nevertheless, k is relatively long in patients with impaired right ventricular function and reduced ejection fraction. With a region interest over the subclavian trunk for the input function, deconvolution analysis can be used to correct for bolus spreading.

7.3.2 End-systolic, end-diastolic and stroke volumes

Several cardiac volumes can be measured at the time of a MUGA study. If cardiac output is measured from the first-pass data, then stroke volume is obtainable from division of cardiac output by pulse rate. Ejection fraction, calculated separately as described above, is related to end systolic volume

(ESV) and end diastolic volume (EDV) as follows and can be used to calculate them:

$$EF = \frac{\text{stroke volume}}{\text{EDV}} \qquad (7.28)$$

$$= \frac{\text{EDV} - \text{ESV}}{\text{EDV}} \qquad (7.29)$$

The accuracy of this technique is limited by the geometric and background errors associated with measurement of ejection fraction and by the errors associated with measurement of cardiac output by first pass monitoring. It is of course possible to obtain these volumes exclusively from first-pass data.

Many other techniques have been described for measuring ventricular volumes from the equilibrium blood pool image. These are generally of two types:

(i) count-based (Links *et al.* 1982);
(ii) area–length measurements.

Area–length measurements are rather inaccurate because of the relatively poor resolution offered by scintigraphic imaging and by shaky geometric assumptions. Measurements based on gated SPECT should provide more accurate data, although this kind of approach is more suited to contrast angiography and, in future, magnetic resonance angiography (MRA). In the count-based methods, the count rate is recorded from a region of interest over the ventricle in an equilibrium image and is related to the blood volume contained within the chamber by counting a blood sample in a well counter, with allowances being made for photon attenuation based on the anatomic position of the chamber.

7.3.3 Rates of ventricular filling and emptying

As with the EDV, ESV and stroke volume, rates of ventricular filling and emptying can be calculated in absolute units of ml/min from an equilibrium MUGA study if cardiac output is known. Thus, from a knowledge of cardiac output, the y-axis units of the figure showing the cardiac cycle derived from multiple gated acquisition can be given units of volume (**Fig. 7.9a**). The maximum gradients of the downslope (i.e. systole) and up-slope (i.e. diastole) of the

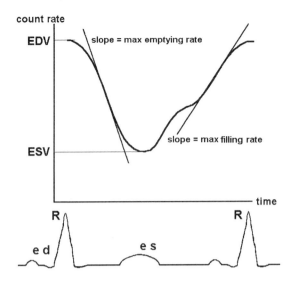

▌ **Fig. 7.9a** Cardiac emptying and filling volume curve.

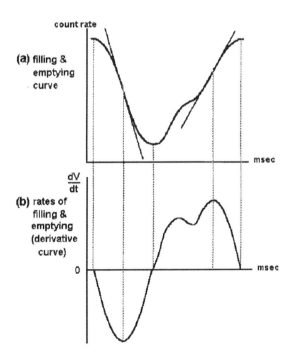

▌ **Fig. 7.9b** Actual rates of filling and emptying obtained from 7.9a by differentiating the volume curve. By differentiating the composite curve of left ventricular volume versus time, a curve (the first derivative) is obtained which depicts inflow and outflow rates. Such a curve may have diagnostic value, e.g. in showing times of peak emptying and filling.

cycle then represent the emptying and filling rates (**Fig. 7.9b**).

7.3.4 Intracardiac shunting

Intracardiac shunting may be the result of a congenital anomalous communication between the atria or ventricles, or between the pulmonary artery and aorta via a patent ductus arteriosus. Other, more complex, forms may exist. Initially the shunt is in the direction left to right because the systemic pressure exceeds the pulmonary. As a result of exposure to the high systemic pressure, irreversible changes occur in the pulmonary vascular bed, leading to progressive elevation of pulmonary arterial pressure, which eventually exceeds the systemic pressure. At this stage, described clinically as Eisenmenger's disease, the shunt may become bi-directional or reverse, resulting in hypoxaemia and cyanosis.

7.3.4.1 Left to right shunting

Left to right shunting may be intra-cardiac or through a persistent ductus arteriosus. Nevertheless the principle of measurement of the shunted flow applies to either (Treves 1980, Baker *et al.* 1985). A recirculating tracer is injected as an intravenous bolus and the first-pass time–activity curve over the lung is recorded. The principle of the measurement is to identify and measure a *second* time–activity curve over the lung that is the result of a fraction of the injected dose undergoing a second recirculation through the pulmonary vascular bed after it has undergone left to right shunting (**Fig. 7.10**). The *first* time–activity curve represents the entire dose on its first pass through the lungs (before any tracer has reached the pulmonary vein). The second curve, due to shunted activity, although partly superimposed on the first curve, can be separated from it in time because the shunted fraction is slightly delayed. The first curve is isolated by performing a gamma function fit from the take-off point to the point at which it is interrupted by the commencement of the second curve. This gamma function fit to the first curve is then subtracted from the recorded curve. The second curve can now be seen from its own take-off point up to the point of interruption by tracer recirculating from the systemic vascular bed. A gamma function fit up to this point of recirculation generates the second curve. If, say, half the total pulmonary venous blood flow shunted back into the right atrium, right ventricle or pulmonary outflow tract, then the second pulmonary time–activity curve

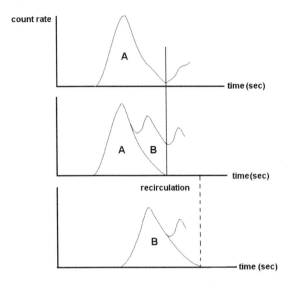

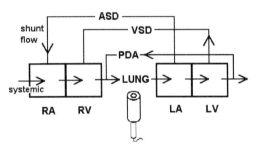

▊ **Fig. 7.10** Measurement of left-to-right vascular shunting by dynamic imaging of the lung following intravenous injection of a radioactive tracer. Normally the time–activity curve recorded over the lung is interrupted by recirculation when the curve is close to returning to baseline (top curve). If blood shunts from the left side of the heart, tracer appears in the lung before the normal time of recirculation and effectively produces a second curve (middle curve). These two curves can be resolved by gamma function fitting. Following its generation by fitting a gamma function, the first curve, A, is subtracted from the recorded curve to generate curve B which is then also fitted with a gamma function (bottom curve). The area under B is proportional to the flow of shunted blood, while the area under A is proportional to the total flow. The shunt is expressed as the quotient pulmonary flow (A) divided by systemic flow   [A – B] i.e. A / [A – B]. The site of the shunt may be deduced from the timing of curve B; it occurs earlier in an ASD than in a PDA.

would have an area half that of the first time–activity curve. If we denote the area under the first curve as A and the area under the second curve as B then

$$\frac{\text{pulmonary flow}}{\text{shunt flow}} = \frac{A}{B}. \qquad (7.30)$$

Systemic flow is the difference between pulmonary flow and shunt flow

$$\frac{\text{pulmonary flow}}{\text{pulmonary} - \text{shunt flow}} = \frac{A}{A - B} \qquad (7.31)$$

$$= \frac{\text{pulmonary flow } (P)}{\text{systematic flow } (S)}. \qquad (7.32)$$

The ratio of pulmonary to systemic flow is the conventional way to express the size of the shunt. The anatomical location of the shunt – atrial, ventricular or ductal – can be inferred from the timing of the second peak in relation to the first. Thus, if the shunt is inter-atrial, the first pulmonary curve (i.e. that representing the entire dose) is interrupted earlier than is the case for a ventricular shunt which, in turn, is interrupted earlier than is the case with a shunt through the ductus arterious.

7.3.4.2 Right to left shunting

Right to left shunting may follow a left to right shunt when pulmonary hypertension is established or may be the result of a pulmonary arterio–venous malformation. The measurement of right to left shunting using radionuclides is best accomplished with radiolabelled microspheres (Section 8.2.5). An intra-cardiac right to left shunt can also be measured from first-pass data using a technique analogous to that described above for left to right shunting. The region of interest is drawn over the left ventricle, so that shunted blood is now seen as an early curve preceding the curve given by radionuclide that has circulated through the normal route (i.e. the pulmonary vascular bed) (**Fig. 7.11**). Again the two curves can be resolved by gamma function fitting, first to the curve of shunted blood, then to the 'normal' (i.e. second) curve after subtraction of the first fitted curve from the composite curve. Then shunt flow is proportional to the area A under the first curve and the non-shunted flow proportional to the area B under the second curve; i.e.

$$\frac{\text{systemic flow}}{\text{pulmonary flow}} = \frac{A + B}{B}. \qquad (7.33)$$

This is usually expressed as the shunted fraction $A/(A + B)$.

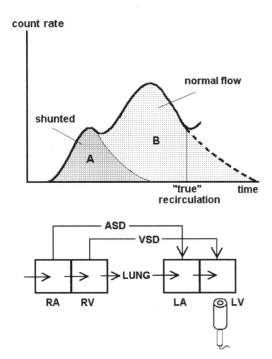

Fig. 7.11 Measurement of right-to-left shunting of dynamic imaging following intravenous injection of a radioactive tracer. In this case the first curve, A, recorded over the left ventricle represents shunted flow while B represents the non-shunted flow undergoing the longer route through the lungs. Systemic flow is proportional to [A + B] so the shunted fraction is equal to A / [A + B].

7.4 Myocardial substrate utilization

In the presence of oxygen, the myocardium preferentially utilizes fatty acids for energy production. Fatty acids are broken down within myocardial cytosol to 2-carbon fragments, acyl-CoA, which are then transferred to the mitochondria for entry into Kreb's cycle and subsequent generation of high-energy phosphate bonds. Transfer of these fragments into mitochondria is facilitated by the enzyme, acyl carnitine transferase. About 10–30% of normal myocardial energy production is through glucose which, following glycolysis, yields the 3-carbon fragment, pyruvate. This is also utilized in the mitochondria for oxygen-dependent energy production within Kreb's cycle. Under conditions of oxygen deprivation, fatty acid utilization is inhibited and the myocardium generates an increasing fraction of its energy requirement by glycolysis to the 3-carbon compound, lactate. Although this is often termed anaerobic glycolysis (in contrast to aerobic glycolysis), the term glycolysis specifically refers to the generation of 3-carbon fragments from glucose (a 6-carbon fragment) and is therefore anaerobic even in the presence of oxygen: i.e. all glycolysis is anaerobic. In the presence of oxygen, pyruvate is utilized in Kreb's cycle, whilst in the absence of oxygen, pyruvate is converted to lactate. Energy production by conversion of 6-carbon to 3-carbon fragments is relatively inefficient and requires increased glucose utilization. This, and the relative absence of oxygen, results in a decrease in the utilization of fatty acids.

7.4.1 Imaging fatty acid utilization

The normal myocardium can be imaged following the injection of a labelled fatty acid, which is rapidly taken up with an extraction efficiency of 50–60% as a result of the myocardium's normal preference for fatty acid as a source of energy. The single photon emitter iodine-123 has been complexed to fatty acid analogues (such as hexadecanoic acid), while for PET, carbon-11 labelled palmitic acid may be used (Schon *et al.* 1982). However only carbon-11 labelled fatty acids give a faithful representation of myocardial fatty acid kinetics since the radionuclide is an atom within the structure of the molecule, whereas when using iodine-123, which is a relatively large molecule, fatty acid analogues have to be constructed in which the inclusion of the iodine-123 is balanced by removal of a similarly sized side chain. This inevitably leads to alteration in the biokinetics of the agent. This points up a general advantage of PET over SPECT.

The signal from carbon-11 labelled palmitate in normal myocardium reaches a peak a few minutes after injection and then declines bi-exponentially (**Fig. 7.12**). The two exponentials have half-times of about 8 and 60 minutes respectively. The faster is thought to correspond to loss of carbon-11 from the myocardium as a result of immediate fatty acid oxidative metabolism because its time course corresponds to the time course of carbon-11 labelled carbon dioxide expiration. Furthermore, this exponential is greatly reduced by blockers of acyl carnitine transferase, the enzyme which facilitates uptake by the mitochondria of the 2-carbon fatty

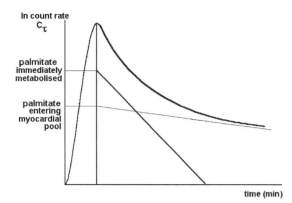

▋ **Fig. 7.12** Myocardial tissue concentration–time curve recorded by PET following intravenous injection of C-11 labelled palmitate. Following a peak representing the amount immediately deposited in the myocardium, there is a bi-exponential decline. The first exponential represents early loss of label as a result of immediate fatty acid oxidative metabolism with loss of C-11 as C-11 carbon dioxide. The second exponential represents slower turnover of the remaining C-11 labelled palmitate, most of which exchanges with circulating native fatty acid.

acid fragments utilized for energy production in Kreb's cycle. The second phase is thought to reflect the much slower rate of exchange of labelled fatty acid initially deposited in the neutral lipid pool of the myocardial cell with circulating native fatty acid. When the second exponential is extrapolated back to the time of peak of the total curve, it has a value approximately half that of the peak, indicating that half the labelled palmitate taken up is metabolised for immediate energy production and half deposited in lipid stores.

Several alterations are seen in these kinetics in the ischaemic myocardium. Firstly, the total amount of fatty acid taken up is reduced. This is not only a result of reduced perfusion *per se* but also a reflection of the reduced fatty acid utilization in ischaemic myocardium. Secondly, the fraction undergoing immediate energy utilization is reduced (because now glucose is the preferred substrate) resulting in an increase in the fraction deposited in the neutral lipid pool. Thirdly, there is increased back-diffusion into blood of unmetabolized fatty acid. The effect of increasing myocardial energy requirements by pacing, exercise or dipyridamole amplifies differences in these fatty acid kinetics, in comparison with the normal, and produces inhomogeneity in PET images at various times after injection.

Iodine-123 labelled fatty acid analogues, whilst giving information qualitatively similar to that of carbon-11 labelled palmitate, are more difficult to interpret with respect to fatty acid metabolism because of the effects of:

(a) the iodine-123 molecule on the biokinetics;
(b) the appearance of free iodine and its metabolic fate.

7.4.2 Glucose utilization

The myocardium increases its utilization of glucose (from about 20% of its requirements up to values approaching 100% of energy requirements) under two main conditions: increased availability (particularly if accompanied by insulin or a meal) and ischaemia. Fluorine-18 labelled deoxyglucose (FDG) competes with native glucose for uptake into the myocyte. Although it is phosphorylated by hexokinase to FDG-6-phosphate, it is not a substrate for any forward biochemical pathways. In common with other tissues like myocardium which lack glucose-6-phosphatase, especially brain and neoplastic cells, neither can FDG-6-phosphate be returned to blood. As deoxyglucose-6-phosphate, it is therefore metabolically trapped and provides an image of (or 'traces') glucose incorporation in myocardial tissue.

Following intravenous administration of fluorine-18 FDG to the fasting normal subject, there is a more or less homogeneous distribution of activity in the myocardium, reflecting the 20% or so of glucose utilisation by normal myocardium. Following a glucose load (usually 50 g by mouth) however normal myocardium increases its utilization of glucose and takes up more FDG under the stimulus of endogenous insulin which is secreted in response to hyperglycaemia and which also increases potassium uptake in skeletal muscle and myocardium. Ischaemic viable myocardium is already maximally vasodilated and preferentially using glucose and does not therefore increase its glucose utilization in response to a glucose load. Under fasting conditions, regions of ischaemic myocardium may take up more FDG than normal myocardium and be shown on contemporaneous perfusion imaging to correspond to defects of uptake of flow tracers such as rubidium-82 or nitrogen-13 labelled ammonia, producing so-called mismatched perfusion defects. After glucose

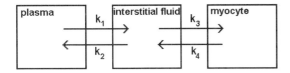

▌ **Fig. 7.13** Model representing glucose kinetics in the myocardium. This is 'traced' with F-18 FDG which is metabolically trapped in the myocyte because (a) it cannot be taken further metabolically after phosphorylation to FDG-6-phosphate by hexokinase and (b) cannot be dephosphorylated back to FDG since the myocardium lacks the enzyme glucose-6-phophatase. k_4 is therefore $\cong 0$. Steady-state FDG clearance is equal to $[k_1 \cdot k_3]/k_3 + k_2]$ or to the slope of a Patlak–Rutland plot based on myocardial and arterial FDG concentrations.

loading, however, a region of ischaemic myocardium may appear as a defect following FDG because now the normal myocardium is stimulated to increase its glucose uptake. The only tissues responsive to insulin are liver, myocardium and skeletal muscle. In contrast the, brain is entirely dependent on glucose for its energy requirements and does not increase its glucose utilization following glucose loading; instead it takes up less FDG as a result of increased competition with glucose. In order to standardize the insulin-dependent stimulus to myocardial glucose uptake, thereby allowing evaluation of myocardium purely on the basis of its glucose utilization rate (measurement of which is described a few lines below), it has recently been proposed and validated that FDG should be administered under conditions of hyperinsulinaemic euglycaemic clamping, achieved by continuous and simultaneous intravenous infusions of glucose and insulin (Knuuti *et al.* 1992).

A general model suitable for describing glucose uptake by the myocardium is described in Section 3.1.3.4. This consists of three compartments, corresponding to plasma, myocardial interstitial fluid and myocardial cell **(Fig. 7.13)**. Because FDG is metabolically trapped, k_4 can be assumed to be zero. The steady state FDG clearance Z_s is given by

$$\frac{Z_s}{V} = K_1 \cdot \frac{C_p}{C_a} \cdot \frac{k_3}{k_3 + k_2} \qquad (7.34)$$

where C_p and C_a are capillary and arterial concentrations respectively and K_1 is the PS product per ml of tissue for glucose transport from plasma to myocardial interstitial fluid.

If $C_p = C_a$,

$$\frac{Z_s}{V} = K_1 \cdot \frac{k_3}{k_3 + k_2}. \qquad (7.35)$$

More likely, $C_p < C_a$, in which case

$$\frac{Z_s}{V} = Z_{1,2} \cdot \frac{k_3}{k_3 + k_2} \qquad (7.36)$$

where $Z_{1,2}$ is FDG clearance per ml of tissue from compartment 1 to compartment 2.

As in the measurement of steady-state fluorine-18 clearance into bone, steady-state myocardial clearance of FDG can be measured from a Patlak–Rutland plot in which the ratio of FDG myocardial to arterial concentrations is plotted against the ratio of integrated arterial to arterial concentrations. The gradient of the plot is equal to $(Z_{1,2}.k_3)/(k_3 + k_2)$.

If the utilisation rates of FDG and native glucose were identical, the rate of regional myocardial utilization of native glucose ($_rM_{glu}$, mg/min/100 ml) would be equal to the product of plasma glucose concentration, C_{pglu}, and myocardial steady state FDG clearance: i.e.

$$_rM_{glu} = C_{pglu} \cdot \frac{Z_s}{V}. \qquad (7.37)$$

Clearance rates of the native substance and its tracer are not however identical: the clearance of glucose is about 50% greater than that of FDG. The proportionality constant relating the two clearance rates is known in the myocardial PET literature as the lumped constant, lumped because it incorporates differences in transport rates into the cell and in phosphorylation rates. Its value, 0.67, appears to be reasonably constant from patient to patient and from disease to disease, and can therefore be routinely used to derive glucose utilization rate from FDG clearance.

References

Araujo LI, Lammertsma AA, Rhodes CG, McFalls EO, Iida H, Rechavia E, Galassi A, De Silva R, Jones T and Maseri A. Noninvasive quantification of regional myocardial blood flow in coronary artery disease with oxygen-15-labeled carbon dioxide inhalation and positron emission tomography. *Circulation* 1991, **83**: 875–85.

Baker EJ, Ellam SV, Lorber A, Jones ODH, Tynan MJ and Maisey MN. Superiority of randionuclide over oximetric measurement of left to right shunts. *British Heart Journal* 1985, **53**: 535–40.

Bassingthwaite JB, Strandell T and Donald DE. Estimation of coronary blood flow by washout of diffusible indicators. *Circulation Research* 1968, **23**: 259–78.

Bergmann S, Herrero P, Markham J, Weinheimer CJ and Walsh MN. Noninvasive quantitation of myocardial blood flow in human subjects with oxygen-15 labeled water and PET. *Journal of the American College of Cardiology* 1989, **14**: 639–52.

Budinger TF. General thallium redistribution model explains false negatives, late redistribution, redistribution at rest, early and late redistribution after reinjection. *Journal of Nuclear Medicine* 1992, **33**: 915 (abstr).

Crone C and Levitt DG. Capillary permeability to small solutes. In: Renkin EM and Michel CC (eds) *Handbook of Physiology* section 2 : The cardiovascular system IV. American Physiological Society, Bethesda, Maryland: 1984, 375–409.

Dilsizian V, Roco TP, Freedman NM, Leon MB and Bonow RO. Enhanced detection of ischemic but viable myocardium by the reinjection of thallium after stress-redistribution imaging. *New England Journal of Medicine* 1990, **323**: 141–6.

Gambhir SS, Schwaiger M, Huang S-C, Krivokapich J, Schelbert HR, Nienaber CA and Phelps ME. Simple noninvasive quantification method for measuring myocardial glucose utilization in humans employing positron emission tomography and fluorine-18 deoxyglucose. *Journal of Nuclear Medicine* 1989, **30**: 359–66.

Goldstein RA, Gould KL, Marani SK, Fisher DJ, O'Brien HA and Loberg MD. Myocardial perfusion imaging with rubidium-82. I. Measurement of extraction and flow with external detectors. *Journal of Nuclear Medicine* 1983a, **24**: 898–906.

Goldstein RA, Mullani NA, Marani SK, Fisher DJ, Gould KL and O'Brien HA. Myocardial perfusion imaging with rubidium-82. II. Effects of metabolic and pharmacologic interventions. *Journal of Nuclear Medicine* 1983b, **24**: 907–15.

Knuuti MJ, Nuutila P, Ruotsalainen U, Saraste M, Harkonen R, Ahonen A, Teras M, Haaparanta M, Wegelius U, Haapanen A, Hartiala and Voipio-Pulkki L-M. Euglycemic hyperinsulinemic clamp and oral glucose load in stimulating myocardial glucose utilization during positron emission tomography. *Journal of Nuclear Medicine* 1992, **33**: 1255–62.

L'Abbate A and Maseri A. Xenon studies of myocardial blood flow: theoretical, technical and practical aspects. *Seminars in Nuclear Medicine* 1980, **10**: 2–15.

Links JM, Lewis BA, Becker C, Schindledecker JG, Guzman P, Burow RD, Nickoloff EL, Alderson PO and Wagner HN. Measurement of absolute left ventricular volume from gated blood pool studies. *Circulation* 1982,

Mullani NA and Gould KL. First-pass measurement of regional blood flow with external detectors. *Journal of Nuclear Medicine* 1983, **24**: 577–81.

Sapirstein LA. Regional blood flow by fractional distribution of indicators. *American Journal of Physiology*, 1958, **193**: 161–8.

Schelbert HR, Phelps ME, Huang S-C, MacDonald NS, Hansen H, Selin C and Kuhl DE. N-13 ammonia as an indicator of myocardial blood flow. *Circulation* 1981, **63**: 1259–72.

Schon, Schelbert HR, Najafi A, Huang S-C, Hansen H, Barrio J, Kuhl DE and Phelps ME. C-11 palmitic acid for the noninvasive evaluation of regional myocardial fatty acid metabolism with positron computed tomography. 1. Kinetics of C-11 palmitic acid in normal myocardium. *American Heart Journal* 1982, **103**: 532–47.

Selwyn A, Allan RM, L'Abbate A, Horlock P, Camici P, Clark J, O'Brien H and Grant PM. Relation between regional myocardial uptake of rubidium-82 and perfusion: absolute reduction of cation uptake in ischaemia. *American Journal of Cardiology* 1982, **50**: 112–121.

Selwyn A, Jones T, Pratt T and Lavender JP. Continuous assessment of regional myocardial perfusion in dogs using krypton-81 m. *Circularion Research* 1978, **42**: 771–9.

Sugrue DD, Kamal S, Deanfield JE, McKenna WJ, Myers MJ, Watson IA, Oakley CM and Lavender JP. Assessment of right ventricular function and anatomy using peripheral vein infusion of krypton-81 m. *British Journal of Radiology* 1983, **56**: 657–63.

Treves S. Detection and quantitation of cardiovascular shunts with commonly available radionuclides. *Seminars in Nuclear Medicine* 1980, **10**: 17–26.

Weisenberg G, Schelbert HR, Hoffman EJ, Phelps ME, Robinson GD, Selin CE, Child J, Skorton D and Kuhl DE. *In vivo* quantitation of regional myocardial blood flow by positron-emission computed tomography. *Circulation* 1981, **63**: 1248–58.

8 The lung

8.1 Mechanics of breathing

The functional unit of the lung as far as gas exchange is concerned is the alveolus. Within the alveolus, blood and air are separated by a thin barrier composed of three layers;

(1) the alveolar epithelium;
(2) a thin layer of interstitial tissue;
(3) the capillary endothelium.

During quiet breathing, the lung volume at functional residual capacity (FRC) is about 3000 ml of which 150 ml is in the anatomical dead space. Inspiration adds about 500 ml to this — the tidal volume. For a respiratory frequency of 15 per min, total ventilation (or minute volume) is 7500 ml/min of which about 5000 ml/min reaches the alveoli. Pulmonary blood flow is equal to cardiac output, about 5000 ml/min at rest, so the ventilation/perfusion ($\dot{V}/Q$) ratio is normally about unity.

As a result of branching, there are more than 20 generations of airway between the trachea and alveolar ducts. The respiratory zone (i.e. the zone within which gas exchange occurs) starts about generation 16. The total cross-sectional area of the airways, and therefore their airflow conductance, increases markedly and exponentially from about generation 10. In the proximal airways, therefore, the linear velocity of the airflow is rapid, whereas in the respiratory zone it becomes increasingly slow. Gas movement in terminal bronchioles and alveolar ducts is predominantly by diffusion. Because of their size, inhaled particles diffuse very slowly and therefore may not reach the alveoli. This is clearly of relevance to the use of aerosols for ventilation imaging and for the measurement of permeability of the blood gas barrier (see Section 8.4.2).

The essential force leading to lung expansion is the difference between atmospheric (or mouth) pressure and intrapleural pressure — the transpulmonary pressure. Because of the opposing elastic recoils of lung and chest wall, intrapleural pressure is negative at the end of quiet expiration. It then becomes increasingly negative during inspiration and returns towards its resting level during expiration. The change in lung volume per unit of applied pressure is the lung compliance; i.e. compliance $= \Delta V/\Delta P$. In the normal upright human, the weight of the lung and its contained blood causes the intrapleural pressure to be slightly more negative at the top of the lung than at the bottom. Also, because of this weight, the alveolar walls in the upper zones are more 'stretched' compared with the lower zones and ventilate slightly less than the lower zones (see Section 8.2). In addition to the resistance to expansion offered by the elastic recoil of the lung, the airways themselves offer resistance to air flow. Alveolar pressure must therefore fall below mouth pressure during inspiration in order to overcome airflow resistance. Conversely it rises above mouth pressure during expiration. Airway resistance is slightly less during inspiration than expiration because of the 'pull' on the airways during inspiration, and so the mean alveolar pressure over one respiratory cycle is slightly positive compared with mouth pressure (**Fig. 8.1**). (Note that alveolar pressure is equal to mouth pressure during breath holding with the glottis open.)

Airway resistance can be defined as the ratio of applied transpulmonary pressure to airflow. Distribution of ventilation between lung units depends inversely on the resistance to airflow to the unit and directly on the compliance of the unit. The product of resistance and compliance, discussed in Section 8.1.2, is called the time constant of the lung. The transpulmonary pressure (i.e. mouth minus intrapleural) is divided to overcome two forces in order to achieve lung expansion:

(a) mouth minus alveolar, to overcome airway resistance (including some viscous resistance which is the resistance offered by tissue planes sliding over each other);

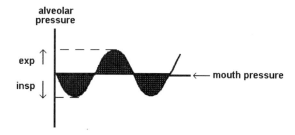

▮ Fig. 8.1 Trace of alveolar pressure with time. With the glottis open during breath holding, mouth pressure is equal to alveolar pressure. Alveolar pressure is negative during inspiration so air flows into the lungs. Alveolar pressure is positive during expiration, so air flows out. Resistance to air flow is slightly greater during expiration as a result of slightly lower airways diameter, requiring a higher pressure gradient to achieve the same flow. Mean alveolar pressure over one cycle is therefore slightly higher than mouth pressure.

(b) alveolar minus intrapleural, to overcome elastic recoil of the lung.

8.1.1 Regional ventilation

Measurement of the distribution of ventilation can be achieved with the single-photon-emitting radioactive inert gases, xenon-133 or krypton-81m. Although xenon-133 is a long-lived gas (with a half-life of 5 days) and krypton-81m an ultra short-lived gas (with a half-life of 13 seconds), the theory underlying their application to measurement of regional ventilation is the same.

Following a single inhalation of air containing xenon-133, the quantity M_{alv} of xenon-133 in a region of lung is given by the product of alveolar gas concentration C_{alv} and volume V_{alv}:

$$M_{alv} = C_{alv} \cdot V_{alv} \qquad (8.1)$$

and since

$$N = \frac{M_{alv}}{\gamma} \qquad (8.2)$$

where γ is a constant (with units, MBq/counts/min) relating the quantity of xenon-133 to the recorded count rate N,

$$N = C_{alv} \cdot \frac{V_{alv}}{\gamma}. \qquad (8.3)$$

That is, the count rate is proportional to the product of the alveolar concentration of gas and alveolar volume. It is intuitively obvious that the regional count rate is proportional to regional gas distribution from this single inhalation which in turn portrays regional ventilation.

If the xenon-133 is re-breathed from a closed circuit, equilibrium is soon reached in which the inflow rate of xenon-133 is equal to outflow rate in all lung regions; i.e.

$$V_i \cdot C_i = V_e \cdot C_{alv} \qquad (8.4)$$

where V_i and V_e are the inspiration and expiration flow rates, respectively. These are generally equal and represent minute ventilation $\dot{V}$ so that C_{alv} at equilibrium is equal to C_i. As C_i is constant, C_{alv} is also constant. Since

$$\begin{aligned} N &= C_{alv} \cdot V_{alv}/\gamma \\ &= C_i \cdot V_{alv}/\gamma \end{aligned} \qquad (8.5)$$

N must be proportional to regional volume. In summary, following a *single* inhalation of xenon-133, regional count rate represents *regional ventilation*, while following *re-breathing* to equilibrium, regional count rate represents *regional alveolar volume*.

Although the count rate over the chest following a single inhalation of krypton-81m is also proportional to regional ventilation, the half-life of krypton-81m is so short that a single inhalation is impractical. Instead, krypton-81m is continuously breathed to equilibrium which is reached very rapidly because of the short half-life of the isotope. Now, however, instead of representing regional volume, the steady state count rate N_{eq} represents regional ventilation (Fazio and Jones 1975). This was shown in Section 3.1.1 equations 3.14–3.18 but will be repeated for convenience.

Since there is a steady state, the inflow rate of krypton-81m is equal to the outflow rate. But since the half-life is short; i.e. the decay constant (δ) high, physical decay contributes significantly to the outflow rate. Thus

$$\frac{dM_{alv}}{dt} = \dot{V}C_i - (C_{alv} \cdot \dot{V} + C_{alv} \cdot V_{alv} \cdot \delta) \qquad (8.6)$$

which, at steady state, is equal to zero. So $\qquad (8.7)$

$$\dot{V}C_i = C_{alv} \cdot \dot{V} + C_{alv} \cdot V_{alv} \cdot \delta \qquad (8.8)$$
$$= C_{alv}(\dot{V} + V_{alv} \cdot \delta). \qquad (8.9)$$

Re-arranging,

$$\frac{C_{\text{alv}}}{C_{\text{i}}} = \frac{\dot{V}}{\dot{V} + V_{\text{alv}} \cdot \delta}. \qquad (8.10)$$

Dividing both sides by V_{alv},

$$\frac{C_{\text{alv}}}{C_{\text{i}}} = \frac{\dot{V}/V_{\text{alv}}}{\dfrac{\dot{V}}{V_{\text{alv}}} + \delta}. \qquad (8.11)$$

This equation is analogous to equation 3.16, which relates tissue concentration of radioactivity (in relation to the arterial input concentration) to tissue perfusion during continuous infusion of labelled water or krypton-81m (Section 3.1.1.2). Now the count rate N is proportional to the quantity of gas M_{alv} present within a region of lung (equation 8.4) which, itself, is given by equation 8.1:

$$M_{\text{alv}} = C_{\text{alv}} \cdot V_{\text{alv}}.$$

So multiplying both sides of equation 8.11 by V_{alv}, and re-arranging, we arrive at

$$M_{\text{alv}} = \frac{\dot{V} C_{\text{i}}}{\dfrac{\dot{V}}{V_{\text{alv}}} + \delta}. \qquad (8.12)$$

Since $\dot{V}/V_{\text{alv}}$ is, under most circumstances of normal quiet breathing, low compared with δ, equation 8.12 reduces to

$$M_{\text{alv}} = \frac{\dot{V} \cdot C_{\text{i}}}{\delta} \qquad (8.13)$$

Since C_{i} and δ are constant, regional count rate is proportional to regional ventilation.

Note that equation 8.12 is general and applicable to long-lived as well as short-lived gases. For a long-lived gas such as Xe-133, δ is essentially zero so $\dot{V}$ cancels out, leaving

$$M_{\text{alv}} = V_{\text{alv}} \cdot C_{\text{i}}$$

which, during re-breathing, is essentially the same as equation 8.5.

8.1.2 Ventilatory turnover and the lung time constant

If, after a period of re-breathing xenon-133, the air supply is switched to non-radioactive gas, the xenon-133 is expired from lung regions at a rate which is proportional to the ventilation rate of each region. However the lung does not completely empty itself

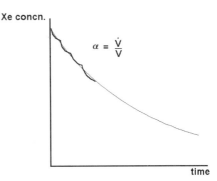

Fig. 8.2 Alveolar Xe-133 leaves from the lung as a result of expiration, each cycle of which removes a constant fraction of the xenon present. The disappearance curve is therefore exponential with a rate constant equal to air flow ($\dot{V}$) divided by lung volume (V) – ventilatory turnover. This applies whether the xenon is deposited in the alveolus as a result of inhalation or intravenous injection (after which pulmonary capillary xenon diffuses rapidly into alveolar gas as a result of its low aqueous solubility).

of air with each expiration, so a constant fraction of xenon-133 will be retained after each expiration. The xenon-133 is therefore cleared exponentially from the alveolus with a fractional rate constant; i.e. fractional turnover rate, equal to the ratio $\dot{V}/V$ (**Fig. 8.2**). This is the ventilatory turnover rate. If xenon-133 in saline is injected intravenously, it is also possible to measure $\dot{V}/V$, since the xenon-133 diffuses rapidly into the alveolar gas on first pass through the lung. It is then expired at a rate proportional to ventilation and inversely proportional to lung volume. However, in this case, the ventilatory turnover is measured only of *those alveoli that are perfused*.

Rather like the washout rate of intra-arterially injected xenon-133 from an organ for the measurement of organ perfusion, ventilatory turnover rate is actually the inverse of the mean transit time or residence time of xenon-133 in the lung. Also, like intra-arterial xenon-133, the washout rate from the lung is not truly mono-exponential, departing from a straight line on semilogarithmic replot at about 50% of the initial count rate. For the lung it can be shown that this is not necessarily due to non-homogeneous regional ventilatory turnover rates, since washout of inhaled (or intravenously injected) nitrogen-13, a positron-emitting gas less soluble in water than xenon-133, follows a mono-exponential time course down to about 10% of initial count rate. The explanation is, at least partly, due to recirculation of the more soluble xenon-133 and, in addition, some resulting uptake by the soft tissues of the chest wall.

Ventilatory turnover rate is a parameter of greater importance in clinical research than routine clinical diagnosis. It has the same units as, and is related to, the regional lung time constant, which is defined as the product of lung compliance and airways resistance:

$$\text{time constant} = \text{compliance} \times \text{resistance} \quad (8.14)$$

where

$$\text{compliance} = \frac{\text{change in lung volume}}{\text{applied pressure}} \quad (8.15)$$

and

$$\text{resistance} = \frac{\text{applied pressure}}{\text{air flow}}. \quad (8.16)$$

Although the applied pressures in equations 8.15 and 8.16 are different, their units cancel out, so

$$\text{time constant} = \frac{\text{change in lung volume}}{\text{air flow}} \quad (8.17)$$

with units

$$\frac{\text{ml}}{\text{ml} \cdot \text{min}^{-1}} = \text{min}.$$

Despite the reciprocal of the lung time constant having the same unit, min^{-1}, as ventilatory turnover, they are not the same variable. In the case of compliance, the applied pressure is the difference between intra-pleural and intra-alveolar pressures, while in the case of airway resistance it is the difference between intra-alveolar pressure and mouth pressure. Although these applied pressures are closely related, they are not identical. Nonetheless, the pressure units cancel out in the product, leaving the quotient volume to flow (i.e. time). In this sense, it is somewhat inappropriately named as it is the *reciprocal* of a fractional time constant. The lung time constant (or actual time to complete air filling) can be visualized to be short for non-compliant alveoli which initially fill rapidly and conversely, long for alveoli supplied by obstructed airways when, as a result of increased airways resistance, the alveoli continue to expand for a prolonged period of time (**Fig. 8.3**). The similarity between lung time constant and ventilatory turnover should be apparent from Fig. 8.3. Lung time constant is not usually measured by radionuclide

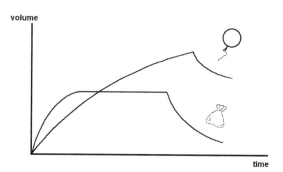

∎ **Fig. 8.3** The lung time constant is defined as the product of lung compliance (how easily the lung allows itself to expand) and airways resistance (the resistance to airflow). An asthmatic patient has increased airways resistance so the lung time constant is prolonged (like blowing up a balloon). In patients with low compliance (such as in interstitial lung disease with 'stiff' lungs) the time constant is reduced (like blowing up a paper bag). If the figure is turned upside down, the reader may appreciate that the lung with *short* time constant has *high* ventilatory turnover and *vice versa* for the lung with long time constant.

techniques but can be obtained by observing the time course of the count rate recorded over the lung during a single inhalation of xenon-133.

8.1.3 Lung gas volumes

8.1.3.1 Functional residual capacity and residual volume

Tidal volume is the difference between lung volume at the ends of inspiration and expiration during normal quiet breathing, the volume at the end of expiration being called functional residual capacity (FRC). Residual volume (RV) is the lung volume at the end of forced maximal expiration. Both FRC and RV can be measured from the dilution in the lung of rebreathed helium or from the measurement of nitrogen washout. They can also be measured, as a fraction of total lung capacity (TLC), with xenon-133 by comparing the count rate over the lung following a single inspiration of xenon-133 with that recorded after rebreathing xenon-133 to equilibrium. Imagine inspiring xenon-133 from residual volume (RV) to TLC and imagine that TLC is twice RV. The volume V_i of inspired gas containing xenon-133 will be diluted by an equal volume V_{alv} of alveolar gas in the lung containing no xenon-133, giving rise to a count rate N_0. If the xenon-133 is rebreathed to equilibrium, with the concentration of xenon-133 in the inspired gas remaining constant, the concentration of xenon-133 in alveolar gas will build up to an equilibrium concentration C_{eq} giving an equilibrium count rate of N_{eq}, twice that of the count rate N_0 recorded after a single breath. In general

$$N_0 = (\text{TLC} - \text{RV}) \cdot \frac{C_i}{\gamma} \quad (8.18)$$

or

$$N_0 = (\text{TLC} - \text{FRC}) \cdot \frac{C_i}{\gamma}$$

depending on whether the patient inhales from RV or from FRC and where γ is a constant converting MBq to counts.
Now

$$N_{eq} = \text{TLC} \cdot \frac{C_{eq}}{\gamma} \quad (8.19)$$

so

$$\frac{N_0}{N_{eq}} = (1 - \text{RV}/\text{TLC}) \cdot \frac{C_i}{C_{eq}}. \quad (8.20)$$

Thus the smaller the ratio RV/TLC the larger the value of 1-RV/TLC and the larger the ratio N_0/N_{eq}. However, at equilibrium,

$$C_{eq} = C_i$$

so

$$\frac{N_0}{N_{eq}} = 1 - \frac{\text{RV}}{\text{TLC}}. \quad (8.21)$$

If re-breathing is from a closed circuit then C_i will decrease and will need to be measured at equilibrium, so

$$\frac{N_0}{N_{eq}} = 1 - \frac{\text{RV}}{\text{TLC}} \cdot \frac{C_i(0)}{C_i(\text{eq})}. \quad (8.22)$$

The value of using xenon-133 for measuring RV and FRC is that regional values are obtainable. This is in contrast to the use of helium and nitrogen and to body plethysmography, which give total values.

8.1.3.2 Regional lung volume

Regional lung volume (V) can also be semi-quantified with xenon-133 in conjunction with krypton-81m. Following bolus intravenous xenon-133, the rate constant of disappearance of lung activity is recorded to give regional ventilatory turnover; i.e. $\dot{V}/V$. This is followed by a brief period of continuous krypton-81m inhalation, the regional count rate from which reflects regional $\dot{V}$. The ratio of these two measurements reflects regional lung volume. Because of differing energies and therefore counting geometries, this requires a homogeneous $\dot{V}/Q$ ratio. This may be a useful technique for determining whether an area of reduced ventilation is the result of lung compression (such as the left lower lobe by an enlarged heart) which is associated with low lung volume and a normal ventilatory turnover, or is the result of airway closure, which is associated with normal or increased regional volume and a reduced ventilatory turnover (Alexander *et al.* 1992). Xenon-133 clearance following intravenous injection gives the ventilatory turnover of perfused alveoli. Since continuous inhalation of krypton-81m measures total ventilation (including the ventilation of non-perfused alveoli), regional lung volume measured from simultaneous krypton-81m and xenon-133 should, at least from a theoretical standpoint, be based on xenon-133 lung washout following the *rebreathing* of xenon-133 to equilibrium rather than by intravenous injection.

Most nuclear medicine units that use xenon-133 routinely for ventilation imaging (by inhalation) perform a three phase study: wash-in, equilibrium and wash-out. The three phases reflect regional ventilation (Section 8.1.1), regional lung volume (Section 8.1.3) and regional ventilatory turnover (Section 8.1.2) respectively.

8.2 Pulmonary haemodynamics

The pulmonary vascular bed is in series with the systemic vascular bed, and has a blood volume about 10% of the total blood volume. However only a small proportion of this pulmonary blood volume, amounting to about 70 ml, is accommodated in the capillaries. Since mean pulmonary arterial pressure is low compared with systemic arterial pressure, and since the entire cardiac output passes through the lungs, it follows that the pulmonary vascular resistance is low. Furthermore, during exercise,

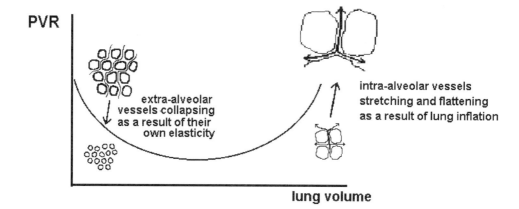

Fig. 8.4 Relationship between pulmonary vascular resistance, PVC, and lung volume. At low lung volume, vascular resistance is dominated by extra-alveolar vessels (larger than intra-alveolar capillaries) which have a natural tendency to collapse thereby raising PVR. At high lung volume however resistance is dominated by intra-alveolar capillaries which are compressed as a result of stretching of alveolar septa, thereby again raising PVR.

cardiac output may increase up to five fold without much increase in pulmonary arterial pressure, implying that under conditions of increased pulmonary blood flow, pulmonary vascular resistance becomes even lower. This is achieved by two mechanisms: distension of the vasculature and recruitment of previously closed capillaries.

Lung capillaries have the capacity to distend because of their intra-alveolar location, relatively unsupported in the alveolar septum. Medium-sized pulmonary arteries, as a result of their *extra-alveolar* location, tend to be held open by traction from the surrounding elastic structures of the lung, and they therefore tend to be opened by the elastic recoil of the lung. At low lung volumes, on the other hand, these extra-alveolar vessels tend to collapse as a result of their own elasticity and smooth muscle action. Their resistance therefore increases. The intra-alveolar capillaries, in contrast, increase their resistance at high lung volume because they become flattened as a result of the stretching of the alveolar septa. Lung volume therefore has two opposing effects on pulmonary vascular resistance with the result that the curve of vascular resistance (*y*-axis) against lung volume (*x*-axis) is concave upwards **(Fig. 8.4)**.

In the normal upright position, the distribution of neither ventilation nor perfusion is homogeneous, but favours the lower zones. In both cases this is predominantly due to gravity. Pulmonary vascular pressure is low and comparable to the vertical hydrostatic (gravitational) pressure resulting from

the column of blood in the lungs. Mean alveolar pressure is slightly greater than zero (relative to atmospheric — see Section 8.1) and, in the upper zones of the lung, may actually approach pulmonary arteriolar pressure (p_a), with the result that there is little blood flow. Further down the lung, as a result of gravity, alveolar pressure (p_{alv}) is exceeded by pulmonary arteriolar pressure but not by pulmonary venous pressure (p_v). Pulmonary blood flow is determined by the pressure difference between p_a and p_{alv}. In the lower zones, both p_a and p_v exceed p_{alv} and flow is determined, as in the systemic vascular bed, by the arterio–venous pressure gradient. These effects of gravity are seen whatever the position of the subject. Thus, after turning a subject upside down, the apices become better perfused than the bases, and similarly in the decubitus position the lower most lung is better perfused than the upper. A fourth zone has also been described in the lung bases where in the upright posture there is some degree of compression of extra-alveolar vessels with a resulting reduction in flow. Zone 4 can be abolished by deep inspiration which opens up these vessels.

Gravity also has an effect on the distribution of ventilation, and although the mechanisms are different compared with its effect on the distribution of perfusion, it results in preferential ventilation of the lower zones. Because of its elasticity, the lung behaves like a spring balance, being pulled down by its own weight and the weight of the blood contained within it. The alveoli in the upper zones of the lung

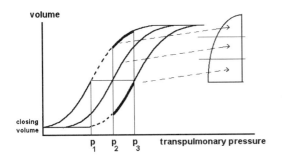

▌ Fig. 8.5 Pressure–volume relationship of normal lung. This is sigmoid in shape. Because of the weight of the perfused lung, the relationship is 'shifted' towards the right in lower lung regions. Thus, at the transpulmonary pressures p_2 to p_3, the regional lung volume is higher at the top as a result of lung stretching than at the bottom. Increasing transpulmonary pressure from p_2 to p_3 produces a larger increment in volume at the bottom than at the top (bold lines in the figure). Nevertheless this gradient can be altered by breathing between different points on the pressure axis such as from p_1 to p_2 (dotted lines on the figure).

are therefore more stretched than those in the lower zones. A decrease in intrapleural pressure, promoting lung expansion, therefore expands the upper zones less than the lower zones. Because of the weight of the lung, the curve of lung volume (*y*-axis) versus the transpulmonary pressure (mouth pressure–pleural pressure) is non-linear, being convex upwards (**Fig. 8.5**). At high lung volume (upper zone) the curve is not as steep as at low lung volume (lower zones) and so a given change in transpulmonary pressure expands the lower zones more. Intrapleural pressure is itself dependent on the weight of the lung and is more negative at the top of the lung compared with the bottom. As a result it is possible to alter the gravitational effect on the distribution of ventilation by breathing at different lung volumes. Imagine breathing at low lung volume. The upper alveoli are now less stretched and so ventilate better. Because the intrapleural pressure is less negative, they are now operating on a lower (steeper) part of the pressure volume curve. They may even ventilate better than the lower zones because of a phenomenon called closing volume. Thus when intrapleural pressure begins to exceed atmospheric pressure, as it may do at functional residual capacity, the lung starts to collapse. Because they are no longer pulled open, the airways also tend

to collapse, trapping air as a result. The effects of gravity on the distribution of ventilation can be elegantly demonstrated during continuous inhalation of krypton-81m while the subject lies in the decubitus position and consciously breaths at various lung volumes, i.e. towards functional residual capacity, at normal resting volumes, and towards total lung capacity. The vertical gravity-induced gradient is more marked for pulmonary blood flow than for ventilation. This results in a vertical gradient in the ratio of ventilation/perfusion ($\dot{V}/Q$ ratio), which is low at the base of the lung and increases exponentially towards the top.

Although the gravitational distribution of blood flow is similar in the infant as in the adult, the reverse is true for ventilation (Davies *et al.* 1985). Thus in a child lying in the decubitus position, the uppermost lung is better ventilated than the lowermost. The likeliest explanation is that because it has a more compliant chest wall, the infant normally functions at a lower pressure on the lung pressure volume curve (e.g. $p_1 \rightarrow p_2$ in Fig. 8.5). Furthermore, because the contents of the infant's abdomen weigh less, the lowermost diaphragm is relatively less 'splinted' than the uppermost compared with the adult. The distribution of ventilation in infants is of clinical importance because children with unilateral lung disease do better when they are nursed in the decubitus position in which their diseased lung is lowermost.

8.2.1 Pulmonary blood flow

Unless the patient has an intracardiac shunt, pulmonary blood flow is the same as cardiac output, the measurement of which is described in Section 7.2.1. In the presence of a right to left shunt (proximal to the lung) pulmonary blood flow is less than cardiac output by the amount of the shunt flow, and vice versa in the presence of a left to right shunt. The measurement of shunt flow in these directions is described in Sections 7.3.4 and 8.2.5.

8.2.2 Distribution of pulmonary blood flow

The distribution of pulmonary blood flow can be imaged with the gamma camera during the first pass through the pulmonary vascular bed of almost any intravenously injected tracer. The agents normally used to image the distribution of pulmonary blood flow, however, are macroaggregates of denatured human serum albumin (MAA) or microspheres of human serum albumin. These are particulate tracers which, on account of their size, are trapped in the first capillary bed they enter, as described in Section 3.3. Following intravenous injection therefore they microembolize in the lung. If the particles are completely mixed before leaving the right ventricle their distribution throughout the lungs is proportional to the distribution of pulmonary blood flow. Thus MAA gives no information on absolute values of pulmonary blood flow but only on its distribution.

MAA and microspheres are widely used with the gamma camera to image pulmonary vascular disease, in particular pulmonary embolism. A focal area of decreased or absent activity indicates a corresponding relative reduction in pulmonary blood flow to that area — a perfusion defect. Maintenance of an intact ventilation to the same area indicates that the architecture of the lung is intact (i.e. that the *systemic* [bronchial] supply is intact) and suggests the presence of focal *pulmonary* vascular disease. This is most often due to pulmonary embolism but may be due to other vascular diseases including vasculitis, veno-occlusive disease, vascular obliteration following radiotherapy or a congenital abnormality associated with an exclusive systemic supply (e.g. sequestrated segment). A common cause of a perfusion defect however is hypoxic vasoconstriction secondary to airways disease, especially bronchial asthma, and this gives rise to a ventilation defect in addition to the perfusion defect — a so-called matched defect. Here there is no vascular disease, as such, since hypoxic vasoconstriction represents a physiological response to alveolar hypoxia. A third type of perfusion defect is seen in destructive lung disease, including infarction, abscess and granulomatous disease, in which ventilation and perfusion are both reduced (although, in infarction, the area of reduced ventilation is not as large as the area of reduced perfusion). Some focal lung diseases are associated with more markedly reduced ventilation than perfusion, so called reversed mismatching. The main causes are alveolar consolidation, as in lobar pneumonia, lobar collapse and lung compression due to pleural effusions (in which the base is non-ventilated on the affected side) or cardiomegaly (in which, in the supine position, the left lower lobe is compressed). A reverse mismatch may also be seen in airways disease in the event of failure of hypoxic vasoconstriction. In the presence of lung compression, hypoxic vasoconstriction is less pronounced or absent.

Another group of agents for imaging the distribution of pulmonary blood flow are the inert gases. These are in principle similar to MAA and microspheres insofar as, following intravenous injection, they are trapped in the lungs on first pass as a result of their insolubility in water and rapid entry into the gaseous phase of the alveoli (see Section 3.1). For a short period after injection, or longer if the patient breath-holds, the distribution of the gas, and hence of pulmonary blood flow, can be imaged with the gamma camera or recorded with a scintillation probe. After breathing restarts, the gas is expired at a rate equal to the ratio of ventilation to lung volume (ventilatory turnover — see Section 8.1.3). Another difference between inert gas and microspheres is that, because the gas does not enter alveoli that are collapsed or consolidated (and where there is no air in them) but recirculates instead, the inert gas gives information on the distribution of pulmonary blood flow only within *aerated* lung.

Krypton-81m is an ultra short-lived inert gas with similar biophysical properties to xenon-133. Like xenon-133, it provides information on ventilation when given by inhalation and information on pulmonary blood flow when given intravenously. Because of its very short half-life, data are rather difficult to analyse when it is given as an intravenous bolus because the half-time of physical decay dominates the biological half-life. However, when given as a continuous intravenous infusion, it can provide elegant data on blood flow distribution (Section 3.1). A technical drawback with intravenous krypton-81m infusion used for this purpose is the very prominent image of the right side of the heart relative to the lungs which, again, is the result of the very short half-life.

8.2.3 Pulmonary blood volume and intravascular transit time

8.2.3.1 Pulmonary blood volume and haematocrit

A gamma camera image of the lungs following injection and complete intravascular mixing of an intravascular tracer, such as labelled red cells, portrays regional lung blood volume. Total pulmonary blood volume can be obtained from the transit time equation, $T = V/Q$ by measuring mean pulmonary vascular transit time of an intravascular tracer, such as labelled red cells (RBC), using residue detection and deconvolution analysis. The input function is obtained from a region of interest over the right ventricle, and the response (or output) function from regions of interest over both lungs. This generates the lung retention function curve; i.e. produces the curve that would have been obtained had the tracer had been deposited as a bolus in the lung without recirculation. If the area (which has x-axis multiplied by y-axis units) under this retention function curve is divided by the plateau height (which has y-axis units), mean transit time is obtained. Total lung blood volume can then be obtained by measuring cardiac output and inserting it for Q in the transit time equation. Since the tracer remains confined to the intravascular space, cardiac output can be obtained from the same first-pass curve recorded over any lung region (Section 7.2.1);

$$\text{cardiac output (CO)} = \frac{\text{injected activity}}{\Gamma \cdot \text{area under curve}} = Q \tag{8.23}$$

where Γ is a constant converting detector counts to $\text{MBq} \cdot \text{ml}^{-1} \cdot \text{min}$. By measuring the radioactivity in a blood sample taken when the tracer has completely mixed in the blood and recording the stable count rate over the same lung region of interest at the time the blood sample is taken, Γ can be determined and the first-pass curve calibrated in absolute units of tracer concentration, as explained in Section 7.2.1.

The need for deconvolution analysis in the above method for measuring mean pulmonary intravascular transit time can be eliminated by recording the count rate over the lung from technetium-99m labelled macroaggregated albumin (MAA) given before the intravascular agent. The MAA is completely retained on first pass and gives a count rate N_{MAA} which is constant and represents the plateau height of the deconvolved retention function curve that would be recorded with the same injected activity of the recirculating intravascular tracer; i.e. the MAA defines the height of the plateau that deconvolution analysis attempts to predict (**Fig. 8.6**).

The area under the first pass lung curve from RBC is independent of the input function, so mean

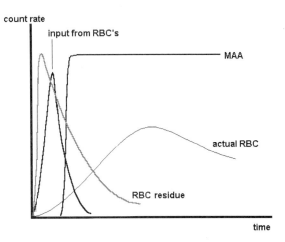

▌ Fig. 8.6 Use of labelled macroaggregated albumin to define the initial height of the red blood cell residue curve predicted by deconvolution analysis. The area under the RBC curve is independent of the shape of the input. Thus the height of the MAA signal curve (assuming equal initial activities of MAA and RBC) divided by the area under the recorded RBC curve (with correction for recirculation) gives mean pulmonary vascular transit time.

transit time is given by

$$T = \frac{\text{injected activity of MAA} \times \text{area under RBC curve}}{N_{MAA} \times \text{injected activity}_{RBC}}$$

$$\frac{\text{MBq} \times \text{counts} \cdot \text{min}^{-1} \cdot \text{min}}{\text{counts} \cdot \text{min}^{-1} \times \text{MBq}} = \text{min} . \tag{8.24}$$

After complete mixing of the labelled RBC in the circulation, the count rate over the lung (after subtraction of the signal from the preceding MAA) is proportional to lung blood volume. However, as the MAA is retained in the lung and therefore effectively calibrates the lung signal in units of MBq, total pulmonary blood volume (PBV), is given as a fraction of total blood volume (TBV) by

$$\frac{\text{PBV}}{\text{TBV}} = \frac{N_{MAA} \times \text{injected activity}_{RBC}}{N_{RBC} \times \text{injected activity}_{MAA}} . \tag{8.25}$$

Equation 8.24 can be further developed for *regional* mean intravascular pulmonary transit time $({}_rT)$ which multiplied by regional perfusion $({}_rQ)$ from equation 8.23 gives regional pulmonary blood volume $({}_rV)$.

Thus

$$_rQ = \frac{\gamma N_{MAA}}{\text{injected activity}_{MAA}} \times CO \qquad (8.26)$$

where γ relates regional count rate from MAA to MBq.

Combining equations 8.24 and 8.26,

$$_rV = \frac{\text{area under curve}_{RBC}}{\text{injected activity}_{RBC}} \times \gamma \cdot CO. \qquad (8.27)$$

Equation 8.27 states that $_rV$ is proportional to area (the other terms being constant) and therefore indicates that following the injection of any recirculating tracer, summation of the counts recorded during the first pass (with correction for recirculation) generates a parametric image of regional pulmonary blood volume and not, as might be imagined, regional pulmonary blood flow. With substitution for cardiac output, equation 8.27 reduces to $_rV = \gamma/\Gamma$, which simply indicates that after complete intravascular mixing of the red cells, the signal becomes constant and the distribution portrays regional lung blood volume.

Three-dimensional quantitative data on *regional* pulmonary blood volume and haematocrit can be obtained from PET using carbon-11 labelled albumin and carbon monoxide (labelled with oxygen-15 or carbon-11) to label red cells (Brudin *et al.* 1986). The concentration of radioactivity from labelled red cells in lung sections is compared with the concentration in peripheral blood to give the regional pulmonary blood volume in ml per ml of lung tissue. This is called the fractional lung blood volume, V_{iv}. It can be converted to lung blood volume in units of g blood per ml lung by multiplication with the density of blood ρ (taken as 1.05): i.e.

$$V_{iv} = \frac{C_{lung}}{C_{blood}} \times \frac{1}{\rho}. \qquad (8.28)$$

By this method, pulmonary blood volume is normally about 0.15 g/ml (Wollmer *et al.* 1984).

Regional pulmonary haematocrit can be measured using PET-labelled red cells and carbon-11-labelled human serum albumin. In lung sections this gives a haematocrit of 0.9 that of myocardial chamber blood. However, as less than 30% of pulmonary blood is present in small vessels, compared with 70% in large vessels with the same haematocrit as myocardial chamber blood, the haematocrit in small vessels is only about 0.67 that of myocardial chamber blood.

Thus, if h is small vessel haematocrit, then

$$(0.7 \times 1.0) + (0.3 \cdot h) = 0.9,$$
$$\text{so } h = 0.67 \qquad (8.29)$$

Since erythrocyte transit time shows a longitudinal gradient over the lung (see Section 8.2.3.2), there is probably also a corresponding gradient for *small vessel* haematocrit.

It is more difficult to obtain regional values for pulmonary blood volume using SPECT because of its quantitative limitations. SPECT performs more satisfactorily however for measurement of regional pulmonary haematocrit since two agents, labelled protein and labelled red cells, can be used. Quantitative SPECT under these circumstances is more reliable if both agents are labelled with the same radionuclide and imaging performed in sequence since only a count *ratio* is required.

8.2.3.2 Pulmonary intravascular transit time

Measurement of transit time for a whole lung region is described above as a means of deriving pulmonary blood volume. Regional pulmonary intravascular transit time is a variable of interest in its own right. In normal lung it displays a gravitational (longitudinal) gradient, decreasing down the lung (MacNee *et al.* 1989). In the experimental animal, regional erythrocyte transit time through pulmonary capillaries correlates with neutrophil transit time, although the latter is much longer.

Regional transit time can be measured using deconvolution analysis as described above with or without a preceding injection of technetium-99m MAA. Dividing an image of the labelled red cells continuously acquired over the duration of the first pass (i.e. the integrated first-pass RBC curve, representing regional volume) by the MAA image (representing regional perfusion), with appropriate scaling of the injected activities, generates a parametric image of regional pulmonary vascular transit time. A variant of this technique has been used in the experimental animal and in surgically resected human lung to measure red cell transit time by measuring radioactivity *ex vivo* in slices of frozen lung after intravenous injection of technetium-99m MAA (as a marker of regional perfusion) and chromium-51 RBC (as a marker of regional blood volume). This is clearly applicable to intact man using sequential SPECT (with technetium-99m labelling both MAA and red cells) or PET. A general limitation of the techniques for measuring regional pulmonary tranxsit time is that, like haematocrit, they are relatively insensitive to small vessel transit time.

8.2.4 Lung water

It is imperative for the lung to mobilize fluid crossing the vascular endothelium of the pulmonary capillary bed into the interstital space, since fluid accumulation in the alveoli effectively abolishes gas exchange. In clinical states promoting pulmonary oedema it may therefore be clinically useful to measure lung water and, in particular, extravascular lung water. This is performed using techniques which, in principle, are identical to those above for measurement of pulmonary blood volume, and based on the transit time equation, $T = V/Q$. Clearly the tracers must have a distribution volume which includes extravascular water and therefore be highly diffusible; V then refers to lung water volume, T to mean water transit time though the lung and Q to water inflow rate into the lung (i.e. pulmonary blood flow or cardiac output). The transit time T can be measured either by residue detection of a radioactive tracer or by outflow detection (Swinburne *et al.* 1982). From simultaneous measurement of flow, V can then be calculated. The tracer has to be sufficiently diffusible to equilibrate throughout lung water during a single transit through the pulmonary vascular bed and have a partition coefficient between water and blood that is either known or can be assumed to be close to unity. In order to measure *extravascular* lung water, which is the important component from a clinical point of view, as opposed to total lung water, then the labelled water (or its equivalent — see below) must be accompanied by an intravascular reference tracer, the transit time of which can be subtracted from the transit time of the labelled water.

Thus

$$V_{i+e} = Q \cdot T_{i+e} \qquad (8.30)$$

and

$$V_i = Q \cdot T_i \qquad (8.31)$$

where the subscripts i and e respectively refer to intravascular and extravascular.

So

$$V_e = V_{i+e} - V_i \qquad (8.32)$$

$$= Q(T_{i+e} - T_i). \qquad (8.33)$$

Using outflow detection, either the diffusible or reference tracer can be used to measure Q, although it is preferable to use the reference (i.e. intravascular marker), as in the measurement of cardiac output. For residue detection, the intravascular marker must be used.

Externally detectable extravascular markers which are also highly diffusible are few, and include the positron-emitting radionuclide, oxygen-15 labelled water and radio-iodinated antipyrine. Extravascular lung water is usually measured clinically by outflow detection rather than by residue detection. This requires rapid arterial sampling via an arterial line following the right atrial injection of appropriate tracers such as indocyanine green as the intravascular marker, and heat (e.g. cold saline) as the extravascular marker (used in a manner analogous to its use for cardiac output measurement). Transit time of a radiolabelled extravascular marker can be obtained from the ratio of the area under the residue curve to the initial height if the bolus is delivered directly into the pulmonary artery, or of the deconvolved retention function curve if the bolus is injected more distally. One of the major difficulties in measuring extravascular lung water is the presence of poorly perfused areas of lung which the extravascular marker is unable to penetrate. This is one reason why heat is a useful tracer because it diffuses 50 times faster than water itself. Another tracer which is externally detectable and has rapid diffusion is radioiodinated antipyrine.

Similarly to the expression of several other physiological variables as a quotient of a related variable, it may be useful to measure lung water as a quotient of pulmonary blood volume. Normally, the ratio extravascular lung water EVLW (which includes intracellular water) to pulmonary blood volume PBV is about unity (see below). Intravenous injection of two positron-emitting agents in sequence — labelled water followed by an intravascular marker — with external residue detection (which can be with scintillation probes) gives two time–activity curves. The ratio of their areas (following the appropriate corrections for respective doses and physical decay of the radionuclides) is equal to the ratio of their transit times and therefore to their distribution volumes; i.e. to (EVLW + PBV)/PBV.

The clinical value of lung water measurement is, at present, limited, largely because of its invasive nature. It may be useful if single photon emitting tracers could be developed that would provide rapid simple non-invasive measurements of lung water. A technique, developed by Snashall and his group (Briggs *et al.* 1987), involves non-invasive measurement of the compartmental distribution of fluid in the lung by combining transmission and emission scintigraphy. A transmission scan is analogous to a chest X-ray in that an image of the lung is obtained with the patient positioned between a flood source and the gamma camera. The fraction of emitted photons absorbed by the chest is a linear function of the water content of the chest. Therefore, using the transmission data to define the extent to which different regions of the lung attenuate gamma photons of the energy of technetium-99m, the regional 'thickness' of blood and extravascular fluid can be calculated from conventional emission scanning following an intravenous injection of technetium-99m labelled red cells and technetium-99m DTPA which respectively label the blood and extracellular fluid compartments of the lung.

Imagine radioactivity homogenously distributed in a cylinder of tissue, depth x cm, presenting an area of 1 cm^2 at the chest wall (**Fig. 8.7**): if there is no attenuation of the signal by tissue, let the count rate recorded at the chest surface from a plane of negligible thickness be $n(x)$. The total signal N_0 recorded would be the sum of all the $n(x)$ values

$$N_0 = n \cdot x. \qquad (8.34)$$

However, in reality, counts are lost from a plane depending on its depth. The total signal N recorded under the conditions of attenuation, is the area under the exponential which decreases to the count rate recorded from the most distant slice: i.e.

$$N = \int_0^x n(x) e^{-\mu x} dx \qquad (8.35)$$

where μ is the linear attenuation coefficient of the radionuclide in tissue relating depth to count rate. So

$$N = \frac{n}{\mu} - \frac{n \cdot e^{-\mu x}}{\mu} \qquad (8.36)$$

$$= \frac{n(1 - e^{-\mu x})}{\mu}. \qquad (8.37)$$

Dividing equation 8.34 by equation 8.37,

$$N_0 = \frac{N \cdot \mu x}{(1 - e^{-\mu x})}. \qquad (8.38)$$

The purpose of the transmission scan, obtained by placing the patient's chest between a flood source and the gamma camera, is to obtain μx; thus

$$N_{\text{trans}}/N_{\text{trans}}(o) = e^{-\mu x} \qquad (8.39)$$

where N_{trans} and $N_{\text{trans}}(o)$ are the count rates recorded from the flood source with the patient respectively between and not between source and camera. So, if the counting efficiency of the camera is known, then, by knowing N_0, the amount M of radioactivity in the tissue cylinder can be calculated. If the injected tracer is technetium-99m labelled red cells, then a blood sample taken at the same time as emission scanning can be used to relate the blood technetium-99m concentration to M, thereby obtaining the volume V of blood in the cylinder. The cylinder has already been defined as projecting an area of 1 cm^2, so V is numerically the same as the antero–posterior thickness in cm of blood in the thorax. Count rates recorded per pixel can be converted to count rates per cm^2 from a knowledge of pixel dimensions. The extracellular water in the thorax, i.e. interstitial thickness, can be similarly obtained after an injection of technetium-99m DTPA, allowing a little more time for this tracer to equilibrate between pulmonary intravascular and extravascular water. Briggs *et al.* (1987), measured chest wall thickness from a chest radiograph and then, in order to derive lung tissue thickness, subtracted it from total chest (transthoracic) thickness as measured from the transmission scan using equation 8.39 and an assumed value for μ. Nevertheless, the calculated blood and interstitial thickness include respective contributions from the chest wall, probably negligible for blood but not for interstitial fluid. Making the measurement within 5 min of DTPA injection, potentially before equilibration between plasma and interstitial fluid, minimizes the chest wall contribution without significantly underestimating the lung thickness because DTPA equilibrates more slowly in the chest wall than in the lung.

Normally about 50% of trans-thoracic tissue thickness is accounted for by blood and 25% by interstitial water, leaving about 25% for intracellular water. Values for the lung itself will be similar if not less for interstitial water. Blood thickness is reduced

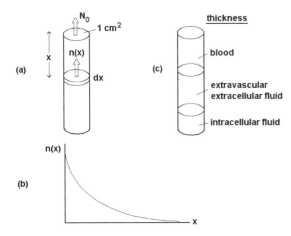

∎ **Fig. 8.7** Principle of measurement of regional fluid 'thickness' in the lung. The count rate N_0 projected at the body surface from a 'tissue' cylinder of cross-sectional area 1 cm² depends on the amount M of radioactivity in the cylinder, the depth of the radioactivity (x) and μ the linear attenuation coefficient of the tissue for that radionuclide energy (a), (b). From a knowledge of μ, M can be measured following injection of tracer that respectively remains in blood or distributes in the ECF. M can be converted into a volume V by measuring the concentration of tracer in a blood sample. Since the area of the cylinder is taken as 1 cm², V is numerically identical to thickness which, if the injected tracer was labelled red cells, would be the 'blood thickness' within the region (c). Similarly ECF thickness can be determined following injection and subsequent equilibrium of technetium-99m DTPA.

in emphysema, with a blood to interstitial water thickness ratio of about one. On the other hand, interstitial water thickness is increased in several diseases, including chronic interstitial pneumonitis, sarcoidosis, cryptogenic fibrosing alveolitis and pneumocystis carinii pneumonia.

A variant of this technique has been developed using PET (Wollmer *et al.* 1984). The sectional concentration of activity is measured following injection of carbon monoxide labelled red cells as for the measurement of regional pulmonary blood volume in units of g/ml, described above. This is compared with the sectional transmission scan obtained with an extended ring source, which gives lung tissue density, also in units of g/ml. The difference between intravascular density and lung density (i.e. between emission and transmission scans) gives regional *extravascular* lung density. In the

normal subject, the vascular lung density (about 0.15 ml/g) is close to extravascular lung density, a similarity which agrees well with the 'thickness' measurements described by Snashall's group. Furthermore, like interstitial water thickness, extravascular lung density is increased by interstitial lung disease.

8.2.5 Intrapulmonary vascular shunting

The causes of intrapulmonary arterio–venous shunting include congenital malformations (AVMs), trauma and cirrhosis of the liver. The shunt is from right to left and its measurement is, in principle, identical to measurement of right to left intra-cardiac shunting using labelled albumin microspheres (Section 7.3.4).

Following intravenous injection, a fraction of microspheres bypasses the pulmonary vascular bed via the shunt and micro-embolizes systemically. Quantification either of the activity remaining in the lung or the activity in the rest of the body relative to the injected dose gives the shunt as a fraction of cardiac output. Thus

$$1 - \frac{\text{shunt flow}}{\text{cardiac output}} = \frac{\text{lung activity}}{\text{injected activity}} \tag{8.40}$$

or

$$\frac{\text{shunt flow}}{\text{cardiac output}} = \frac{\text{whole body activity} - \text{lung activity}}{\text{injected activity}} \tag{8.41}$$

$$= \frac{\text{total systemic activity}}{\text{injected activity}} \tag{8.42}$$

Systemic micro-embolization is difficult to quantify because the activity is widely distributed. Furthermore equation 8.40 is rather sensitive to error because lung activity is not much less than the dose, unless the shunt is very large. The assumption can be made however that 10% of the cardiac output serves each kidney, so that by quantifying the activity in one kidney and multiplying it by 10, total systemic activity can be derived (Whyte *et al.* 1992). Activity in the right kidney is easier to quantify than in the left because of difficulty in separation of splenic activity from the left kidney. In contrast background activity is quite low on the right because the majority of hepatic blood flow is cleared of shunted microspheres by the splenic and mesenteric beds. Photon attenuation from the right kidney can be measured by taking a right lateral image and directly measuring the depth of the kidney or, alternatively, using a height and weight nomogram.

The injected dose should be measured carefully because microspheres easily stick to any surface with which they come into contact, so it is necessary to measure the residue in the syringe and in the intravenous line. Because of this difficulty, a more convenient way to measure the shunt is to assume the dose is effectively equal to the sum of total lung activity plus 10 times the right kidney activity. Then

$$\frac{\text{shunt flow}}{\text{cardiac output}} = \frac{10 \times \text{kidney counts}}{[10 \times \text{kidney counts}] + \text{lung counts}} \quad (8.43)$$

Attenuation corrections for both lung and kidney can be ignored as they are almost identical. This may seem surprising in view of the kidney's location towards the posterior of the abdomen. However their proximity to the gamma camera on the posterior view (giving rise to relatively less attenuation) is counterbalanced by the fact that the lungs contain air, which attenuates photons much less than does water. This approach is the simplest method of measuring shunt flow and appears to be accurate compared with the 'gold standard' 100% oxygen rebreathing method.

An interesting disparity between shunt flow measurement based on microspheres and based on oxygen measurement may be seen in patients with abnormal vessels of about 50 μm diameter in which some oxygen exchange takes place. Shunting measured with microspheres may therefore be larger than that recorded with oxygen, if the spheres are smaller than 50 μm. If they are bigger and embolize in the abnormal vessels, they may underestimate the shunt given by the oxygen method. If the size range of microspheres overlaps the diameter range of abnormal vessels, then the measured shunt will depend on the overlap. In theory it should be possible to determine the diameter of abnormal vessels from microspheres of defined and narrow size ranges. Unfortunately these are not available commercially at present.

Measurement of right to left shunt flow is of clinical value, particularly in the evaluation of therapeutic embolization. As it is non-invasive, it is also useful for assessing the effects of acute physiological interventions on shunt flow, such as exercise. Cardiac output is redistributed during exercise so the kidney can no longer be assumed to receive 10% of it. An alternative technique therefore is to place regions of interest around both lungs and to compare the counts (expressed in relation to the injected activity) before and after exercise. The regions must encompass both lungs because the distribution of lung blood flow between apex and base may change on exercise. If the baseline shunt fraction is S, then $(1 - S)$ of the activity will be retained in the lungs. If the lung counts per MBq of injected activity change on exercise by a factor f so that lung counts per MBq of injected dose are now equivalent to $[f(1 - S)]$, then the shunt will have changed to $1 - [f(1 - S)]$, from which a percentage change in shunt flow can be calculated: i.e.

$$\text{percent change} = \frac{1 - [f(1 - S)]}{S} \times 100. \quad (8.44)$$

8.3 Pulmonary granulocyte kinetics

The lung is an important organ with respect to granulocyte kinetics since it has been suggested, mainly by respirologists, that the lung is the major site in the body for granulocyte margination (Hogg 1987, MacNee and Selby 1990). It is also important because of the strong evidence in favour of a role for granulocytes in the pathogenesis of acute and chronic lung injury.

The physiological role of the lung in granulocyte kinetics is controversial. Some authors consider the pulmonary vascular bed to be the major site in the body for granulocyte margination. The lungs however are usually only faintly seen in clinical white cell scanning. Lung activity may be very prominent immediately after injection of labelled cells, but its intensity has been shown to correlate with labelling techniques (Savermuttu *et al.* 1983). Thus granulocytes isolated on Percoll-saline columns undergo prolonged lung transit following injection compared to cells isolated on Percoll-plasma columns, suggesting that no more than a modest amount activity in the lungs should be regarded as normal. When the lung activity is initially marked, it clears quite rapidly with irreversible diversion of the cells to the liver and spleen, and a very low recovery in circulating blood. Cells activated inappropriately *in vitro* appear to adhere to the first endothelial surface they encounter following intravenous injection. They are probably abnormally 'stiff' and swollen and, as a result, are mechanically trapped in the lung capillaries, the diameters of which are less than the diameter of a granulocyte. The sequestered granulocytes do not however migrate into the pulmonary interstitium: this presumably would require simultaneous endothelial activation.

Although the term margination can be applied to the lung, it should not be assumed that the same physiological process occurs as in the peripheral tissues, for which the term margination was originally applied. From a kinetic point of view, margination implies a prolonged mean transit time through a vascular bed in comparison with red cells or plasma and in this respect is identical to cell pooling (Chapter 10). In the classical view, margination in the peripheral tissues applies to a discrete population of cells, the marginating granulocyte pool (MGP), rolling along the endothelium and exchanging dynamically with a discrete population in the axial stream, the circulating granulocyte pool (CGP), the two populations together comprising the total blood granulocyte pool (TBGP). In the lung however the mean transit time of granulocytes reflects a continuous spectrum of transit times as granulocytes negotiate pulmonary capillaries with smaller diameters than their own. They do not obstruct red cells because the capillaries far outnumber the granulocytes in transit through the lung. The lung is unusual in comparison with the rest of the body in that granulocytes marginate within and migrate through pulmonary capillaries rather than post-capillary venules.

It is likely that in order to damage the lung, granulocytes must migrate through the pulmonary vascular endothelium into the interstitial space; they appear to cause little damage if contained within the pulmonary vascular space. It may therefore be important to separately quantify granulocyte margination and extravascular migration.

8.3.1 Pulmonary granulocyte pooling

Several methods are available for measuring the pulmonary vascular granulocyte pool following intravenous injection of radiolabelled granulocytes, including simple measurement of the $t_{1/2}$ of decrease of the lung signal over a period of about 30 min following injection, comparison with the signal from a preceding injection of labelled red cells (Section 10.3.2) and techniques based on the first pass.

The aim of the first pass technique is to quantify the pulmonary vascular granulocyte content (PGP) as a fraction of the whole body total blood granulocyte pool (TBGP). The principle of the technique is to 'capture' the entire dose of labelled granulocytes in the lungs as they transit the lungs on first pass (Ussov *et al.* 1995). The count rate $N(t)$ in a region of interest (ROI) over the lung at any subsequent time t expressed as a fraction of the first pass count rate in the same ROI N_1 will be equal to the ratio of the PGP expressed as a fraction of the whole body TBGP; i.e.

$$\text{PGP/TBGP} = N(t)/N_1. \qquad (8.45)$$

This assumes that no cells are irretrievably lost from the TBGP and that the cells have equilibrated throughout the marginating pools of the body at time t. This approach makes no distinction between granulocytes that are respectively in the circulating and marginating compartments, and is physiologically appropriate for the lung, given the continuum of transit times that probably exists. However, by expressing it in terms of the TBGP, the PGP would be dependent on margination elsewhere. For example, in a patient with splenomegaly and an increased splenic marginating pool, fewer cells would be available to the lung, and the ratio, PGP/TBGP, would be reduced. This can be accounted for by measuring labelled granulocyte recovery at time t, $R(t)$, which itself is a close approximation to the fraction of the labelled cells in the CGP. Provided equilibrium between the PGP and CGP is achieved when the lung ROI counts at time t are recorded, the first-pass count rate N_1 multiplied by $R(t)$ represents the cells available to the pulmonary vasculature, and so the count rate at time t in the lung ROI represents the PGP as a fraction of the whole body CGP; i.e.

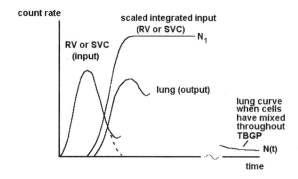

∎ **Fig. 8.8** Measurement of the pulmonary intravascular granulocyte pool (PGP). In principle, this compares the count rate $N(t)$ in a region of lung about 30 minutes after injection of labelled granulocytes with the count rate (N_1) in the same region that would have been recorded if all the intravenously injected cells had been *irrecoverably* trapped in the lung on the first pass. N_1 represents the dose of labelled granulocytes which will subsequently mix throughout the whole body total blood granulocyte pool (TBGP), while $N(t)$ represents the fraction of the dose present in the PGP. $N(t) / N_1$ is therefore equal to the PGP as a fraction of TBGP. N_1 is obtained using a technique identical in principle to measurement or organ blood flow as a fraction of cardiac output and relies on integration of an 'input' region (right atrium or SVC in this case) followed by scaling of the integrated curve to be parallel to the recorded lung curve.

$$\frac{\text{PGP}}{\text{CGP}} = \frac{N(t)}{N_1} \times \frac{1}{R}. \quad (8.46)$$

Equations 8.45 and 8.46 both assume that all the cells are temporarily trapped in the lung on first pass. This assumption is dealt with by a technique which is generally applicable to the measurement of blood flow from first-pass curves, such as renal blood flow (Section 11.1.1.3), and in principle predicts the plateau that the organ first-pass curve would reach if all the tracer arriving in the organ on first pass was retained. This requires an input curve, which for measurement of PGP uses the pulmonary arterial curve derived from ROIs over the superior vena cava, right ventricle, or pulmonary artery. After correction of one of these curves for recirculation, followed by integration, the integrated curve is scaled to be parallel to the lung curve, whereupon it gives an estimate of the required plateau, equal to N_1 (**Fig. 8.8**). Note that because they apply equally to N_1 and $N(t)$, no corrections are required for camera

sensitivity or counting geometry. However the further assumption is required that the fraction of the pulmonary arterial blood flow delivered to the lung ROI is equal to the fraction of the PGP in the ROI, an assumption that has been validated.

Pulmonary granulocyte pooling can be expressed in terms of the mean intravascular granulocyte transit time, either derived as such; i.e. with units of minutes, or as a quotient of red cell transit time. The latter technique is described in Section 10.3.2.2. Transit time can be derived in absolute units by deconvolution analysis based on the time–activity curve recorded over the lung and an input curve from an ROI over the right ventricle. This is described in Section 10.3.2.1 for non-pulmonary organs. It is of special interest in the lung because the technique reveals apparently two discrete populations of granulocytes with different transit times. The fraction of the total population with the longer transit time correlates with the fraction of cells seen on microscopy to be activated, suggesting that activation prolongs transit.

8.3.2 Pulmonary granulocyte migration

Granulocyte residence time in the circulation is about 10 hr, so the regional signal recorded from a tissue 24 hr after injection reflects granulocyte destruction in the reticuloendothelial system or extravascular migration. The 24 hr signal over the chest therefore represents a combination of granulocyte destruction in chest bone marrow and pulmonary extravascular migration. In normal subjects, there is a close linear relationship between the count rates respectively recorded from the chest and iliac bone (Ussov *et al.* 1994):

$$\text{chest} = [0.23 \times \text{iliac bone}] + 0.054 \text{ counts/}$$
$$\text{pixel/min/MBq} \quad (8.47)$$

By assuming no migration in normals, equation 8.47 can be used to subtract the chest bone marrow signal in patients with suspected migration. The resulting signal, with units of counts/pixel/min/MBq injected activity, gives a semi-quantitative index of granulocyte migration. In contrast to intravascular granulocyte pooling, the degree of migration correlates with indices of lung damage, specifically the $t_{1/2}$ clearance of inhaled technetium-99m DTPA (Section 8.4.2.).

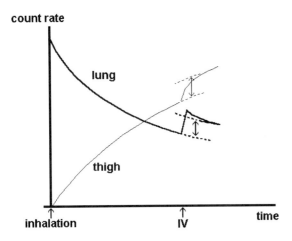

count rate

lung

thigh

↑ inhalation   ↑ IV   time

▌**Fig. 8.9** Subtraction of non-pulmonary background counts in a pulmonary technetium-99m DTPA aerosol clearance curve. When enough of the clearance curve has been recorded, DTPA is given intravenously producing sharp increments in lung and thigh (background) curves. By relating these increments to each other, the thigh curve can be appropriately scaled and subtracted from the recorded lung curve. The difficulty with the technique is that because the lung and thigh do not have the same proportion of plasma and interstitial fluid, the ratio of increments at, say, 20 minutes after inhalation does not accurately identify the scaling factor which may be appropriate for, say, the first 10 minutes of the lung clearance.

8.4 Capillary/alveolar transfer

8.4.1 Ventilation/perfusion ratio

Efficient gas exchange in the lung requires that, in any region, the delivery of air is appropriately matched by the delivery of blood. Ideally the $\dot{V}/Q$ ratio should be slightly less than unity. Various lung diseases can alter this ratio and lead to mismatching of ventilation and perfusion. A low $\dot{V}/Q$ ratio promotes hypoxaemia because pulmonary arterial blood with a low pO_2 is not oxygenated and is allowed to mix in the pulmonary venous blood with normally oxygenated blood from regions with normal $\dot{V}/Q$ ratios. Any cause of a reverse mismatch visible on a $\dot{V}/Q$ scan (i.e. a ventilation defect

greater than a perfusion defect or not matched by a perfusion defect) is therefore a potential cause for hypoxaemia. In lung units with a high $\dot{V}/Q$ ratio, on the other hand, ventilation is simply wasted with the result that the dead space (in this case alveolar dead space) is increased. This dead space adds to the anatomical dead space, the sum being known as the physiological dead space. Because of compensatory hyperventilation in alveoli with normal $\dot{V}/Q$ ratios, $\dot{V}/Q$ mismatching results in a greater abnormality of oxygen exchange than of carbon dioxide. A low $\dot{V}/Q$ ratio results in a physiological right to left shunt, in contrast to the anatomical right to left shunt in congenital heart disease or a pulmonary arterio-venous malformation.

Hypoxic vasoconstriction is a mechanism whereby the lung attempts to reverse a low regional $\dot{V}/Q$ ratio by reducing perfusion to a region of hypo-ventilated lung. This may be visualized on $\dot{V}/Q$ scanning in patients with obstructive airways disease, particularly bronchial asthma. Alveolar hypoxia is the principal stimulus for hypoxic vasoconstriction, which takes place in isolated lung segments as well as intact lung, indicating independence from neural mechanisms. Perfusion of alveoli with blood at low pO_2 does not induce the response. The precise biochemical mediator for hypoxic vasconstriction is obscure although the net effect is to redirect blood away from non-ventilated regions. Poor ventilation due to lung compression, such as by a pleural effusion or an enlarged heart, does not induce hypoxic vasoconstriction to the same extent as airway obstruction, perhaps because the alveolar air is not as hypoxic. The reverse of hypoxic vasoconstriction, namely redirection of ventilation away from units with reduced blood flow, following pulmonary embolism for example, is not seen on $\dot{V}/Q$ lung scanning, but there is evidence that an increase in alveolar dead space results in a reduction in compliance and an increase in airways resistance.

There are several non-radioactive methods for measuring $\dot{V}/Q$ ratio. The easiest conceptually is the simultaneous measurement of the physiological dead space (reflecting the presence of ventilated but non-perfused alveoli) and of right to left vascular shunting (reflecting the presence of perfused but non-ventilated alveoli). More complex techniques exist, one of which, described by Wagner *et al.* (1985) is based on the administration of six different gases of widely varying aqueous solubility and has given valuable data on global $\dot{V}/Q$ inequality.

Although regional $\dot{V}/Q$ mismatching can be imaged, it also occurs at a microscopic level and its existence may not be detectable scintigraphically because of inadequate image resolution. Thus separate $\dot{V}$ and Q images may show no apparent mismatch which, nevertheless, may be present to a significant degree. On the other hand, when there is obvious mismatching on imaging then there must be physiological right to left shunting which can be semi-quantified.

As will be apparent from above, regional $\dot{V}/Q$ mismatching may be identifiable from separate ventilation and perfusion images. Because neither $\dot{V}$ nor Q images are quantitative, it is not possible from the images to quantify $\dot{V}/Q$ mismatching in absolute terms (i.e. as a ratio of $\dot{V}$ in ml/min to Q in ml/min), but only to assess gross regional variations. SPECT of technetium-99m MAA and continuous krytpon-81m inhalation has been able to show gradients which are different for Q and $\dot{V}$, implying the existence of $\dot{V}/Q$ gradients (Weiner *et al.* 1990).

Regional variations in $\dot{V}/Q$ ratios can be imaged with xenon-133 given by continuous *intravenous* infusion (Anthonisen *et al.* 1966). After about 5 minutes of infusion, a steady state is almost reached in which the rate of xenon-133 expiration is equal to the difference between the rates of xenon-133 inflow in pulmonary arterial blood and xenon-133 outflow in pulmonary venous blood. Within a single alveolar unit, therefore, it can be stated that

$$Q \cdot C_a - Q \cdot C_v = C_{alv} \cdot \dot{V} \qquad (8.48)$$

where C is the concentration of xenon-133 in blood or alveolar air, with units of MBq/ml, and the subscripts a, v and alv refer respectively to arterial, venous and alveolar.

Since xenon-133 equilibrates between the end pulmonary capillary blood and the alveolar gas,

$$C_v = C_{alv} \cdot \lambda \qquad (8.49)$$

where λ is the partition coefficient of gas between blood and alveolus (considerably less than unity, i.e. in favour of alveolus).

Therefore

$$Q \cdot C_a - Q \cdot C_{alv} \cdot \lambda = C_{alv} \cdot \dot{V}. \qquad (8.50)$$

This can be rearranged to give

$$C_{alv} = \frac{C_a}{\dfrac{\dot{V}}{Q} + \lambda} \qquad (8.51)$$

and

$$\frac{\dot{V}}{Q} = \frac{C_a}{C_{alv}} - \lambda. \qquad (8.52)$$

[Note that $\dot{V}/Q$ and λ are both unitless.] The count rate N recorded in a region is proportional to the amount (M_{alv}) of xenon-133 present and therefore to the product of $C_{alv} \cdot V_{alv}$. By multiplying both sides of equation 8.51 by V_{alv} we can write

$$C_{alv} \cdot V_{alv} = \frac{C_a V_{alv}}{\dot{V}/Q + \lambda} = M_{alv}. \qquad (8.53)$$

Since C_a is constant, regional count rate is inversely proportional to the regional $\dot{V}/Q$ ratio for a given regional lung volume. Since λ is considerably smaller than a relatively normal $\dot{V}/Q$ ratio, this relationship is almost linear but becomes less so as $\dot{V}/Q$ decreases. It is also apparent that the regional count rate is also directly proportional to regional lung volume, which can be assessed by continuous inhalation of xenon-133 to equilibrium. As shown above (equation 8.3), this gives regional lung radioactivity,

$$M_{alv}(i) = C_{alv} \cdot V_{alv} \qquad \text{(same as equation 8.1)}$$

where $M_{alv}(i)$ is the alveolar radioactivity following *inhalation* to equilibrium and proportional to the count rate recorded at equilibrium N_i. Combining equations 8.1 and 8.53, and assuming λ is zero, we can now derive an absolute value for $\dot{V}/Q$:

$$\dot{V}/Q = \frac{N_i}{N_p} \times \frac{C_a}{C_i} \qquad (8.54)$$

where N_p is the recorded count rate following *infusion* to equilibrium.

Both C_a and C_i (the respective input concentrations) are constant for all lung regions, indicating that regional $\dot{V}/Q$ is reflected by the regional ratio N_i/N_p. The concentrations C_a and C_i can be measured from a mixed venous blood sample and a sample of inspired xenon-133 respectively, thereby allowing measurement of regional $\dot{V}/Q$ in absolute units.

Equation 8.52 can be developed for krypton-81m. We now have to take into account the removal rate of isotope due to physical decay, which is equal to

$V_{alv} \cdot C_{alv} \cdot \delta$. Incorporating this term into equation 8.50 we obtain

$$Q \cdot (C_a - C_{alv} \cdot \lambda) = C_{alv} \cdot \dot{V} + C_{alv} \cdot V_{alv} \cdot \delta$$

and rearranging

$$Q \cdot C_a = Q \cdot C_{alv} \cdot \lambda + C_{alv} \cdot \dot{V} + C_{alv} \cdot V_{alv} \cdot \delta. \tag{8.55}$$

Equation 8.55 can be further rearranged for C_{alv}. V_{alv}. Thus

$$C_{alv} \cdot V_{alv} = \frac{C_a \cdot V_{alv}}{\lambda + \dot{V}/Q + \delta \cdot \dot{V}_{alv}/Q} \tag{8.56}$$

$$= M_{alv}.$$

As λ is small compared with the other two terms in the denominator, equation 8.56 can be simplified to

$$M_{alv} = \frac{Q \cdot C_a}{\dot{V}/V_{alv} + \delta}. \tag{8.57}$$

This is identical to equation 8.12 for krypton-81m inhalation. As for krypton-81m by inhalation $\dot{V}/V_{alv}$ is small compared with δ so

$$M_{alv} \sim \frac{Q \cdot C_a}{\delta}. \tag{8.58}$$

For normal lungs, regional count rate is little influenced by regional $\dot{V}/Q$ and becomes, for krypton-81m, more dependent on regional Q and less dependent on $\dot{V}/Q$. This intuitively makes sense because, as for inhaled krypton, having been delivered by perfusion to a region of lung, the isotope decays before ventilation has the opportunity to clear it. By breath holding, the regional count rate can be made almost entirely dependent on regional perfusion, and krypton-81m infusion can be used as a means of monitoring regional perfusion as described in Sections 8.2.1 and 8.4.1.

Regional $\dot{V}/Q$ ratio has also been quantified by PET using nitrogen-13, an inert radioactive gas with a half-life of 10 minutes and which is even less soluble in water than xenon (giving an even lower value of λ, Rhodes *et al.* 1989). The value of δ for nitrogen-13 is about 1/50 of that of Kr-81m so the expression for V/Q is the same as that for xenon-133:

$$\frac{\dot{V}}{Q} = \frac{C_a}{C_{alv}} - \lambda \qquad \text{(same as 8.52)}$$

The concentration C_a can be measured from the blood in the chamber of the right ventricle. Since PET measures concentration as MBq per ml of total lung volume (air and tissue), it is necessary to determine the fraction of lung volume occupied by gas in order to determine C_{alv}. This fraction is then divided into the recorded pulmonary concentration to give the nitrogen-13 concentration of alveolar air. The volume of lung tissue is determined by a transmission scan, as for the measurement of extravascular lung density (Section 8.2.4), which gives tissue mass per unit volume of lung; i.e. g/ml. The density of gas-free tissue in the lung is taken as 1.04, so

$$\frac{V_{tissue}}{V_{total}} = \frac{\text{tissue density}}{1.04} \tag{8.59}$$

$$\text{with units} \quad \frac{g/ml}{g/ml} = \frac{ml}{ml}.$$

The air volume as a fraction of total volume is obtained from

$$\frac{V_{air}}{V_{total}} = 1 - \frac{V_{tissue}}{V_{total}} \tag{8.60}$$

and used to calculate C_{alv} from the recorded concentration.

A correction may also be made for the nitrogen-13 signal which arises from nitrogen dissolved in pulmonary blood by performing a subtraction based on a carbon-11-monoxide red cell scan. The count rate in the lung parenchyma is compared with that in the right ventricular chamber for both nitrogen-13 and carbon-11. Labelled red cells will occupy both pulmonary arterial and venous blood whereas nitrogen-13 only venous blood. A further correction can therefore be made based on the assumption that on average the blood nitrogen signal arises from 40% of pulmonary blood.

8.4.2 Alveolar epithelial permeability

Compared to the pulmonary vascular endothelium, the alveolar epithelium is about ten times less permeable to small hydrophilic solutes, the transfer rates of which from alveolar fluid into blood reflects, or are rate limited by, alveolar epithelial permeability. There has recently been great interest in the measurement of alveolar permeability using inhaled aerosols of small solutes, especially technetium-99m DTPA (O'Doherty and Peters 1996). The kinetics of solute transfer across the blood/gas barrier are similar to those of small solute transfer across microvascular endothelium in general. Thus the transfer rate is governed by the permeability coefficient, membrane surface area and concentration gradient across the barrier:

$$J = P \cdot S \cdot C_{alv} \qquad (8.61)$$
$$MBq/min = (ml/min) \cdot (MBq/ml)$$

where P is the permeability coefficient (cm/min), S is epithelial surface area (cm^2) and C_{alv} the concentration of tracer in alveolar fluid (MBq/ml).

Dividing both sides of equation 8.61 by M_{alv},

$$\frac{J}{M_{alv}} = \frac{P \cdot S \cdot C_{alv}}{M_{alv}} \qquad (8.62)$$

$$= \frac{PS}{V_{alv}} \qquad (8.63)$$

where V_{alv} is the volume of alveolar fluid (*not* air). The term J/M_{alv} is the fractional transfer rate (min^{-1}) of tracer from alveolus into pulmonary blood and recorded as the rate constant k of disappearance of tracer from the lung. It is directly proportional to alveolar permeability and surface area and inversely proportional to the volume of fluid in the alveoli.

If V_{alv} (cm^3) is divided by S(cm^2) an approximate value of alveolar fluid thickness d (cm) is obtained so

$$k = P/d \qquad (8.64)$$

(Widdicombe, 1997)

The techniques of generation and delivery of aerosol for permeability studies are the same as for routine ventilation imaging. The penetration of the lung by aerosol is dependent on particle size. Although the movement of gas in the airways beyond the sixteenth generation of bronchi is by diffusion rather than convection, there is evidence, based on particle technology, that these aerosols penetrate to the distal airways and alveoli. Thus, whilst the half-time of technetium-99m DTPA pulmonary clearance in normal dogs is about 20 min, it is increased by ligation of the pulmonary artery but not of the bronchial arteries. Occlusion of both pulmonary and bronchial flows greatly increases the half-time because collateral bronchial flow is responsible for the clearance after pulmonary arterial occlusion. The deep penetration into the lung of aerosol particles must depend to some extent on their kinetic energy.

The clearance rate of solutes from alveoli is dependent of several factors related both to the properties of the solute and of the lung. Lipophilic solutes are cleared extremely rapidly as a result of their ability to cross the epithelium by direct cellular penetration. Radio-iodinated antipyrine and technetium-99m HMPAO, for instance, enter the pulmonary circulation following inhalation almost as quickly as following intravenous injection. Their clearance from the lung is therefore blood flow dependent rather than diffusion dependent, and they have no value for the determination of epithelial integrity in the setting of radiolabelled solute clearance studies (but see Section 8.5). Hydrophilic solutes, in contrast, exchange across the alveolar epithelium much more slowly at a rate which is dependent on molecular charge and inversely proportional to molecular size. At normal levels of pulmonary blood flow, their transfer rate is diffusion dependent; i.e. unaffected by changes in blood flow. Nevertheless it should be realized that diffusion-dependent transfer will ultimately become blood flow dependent at very low levels of blood flow (such as after pulmonary embolism).

Hydrophilic solutes cross the epithelium by diffusing through the gaps in the inter-epithelial junctions. The gaps are electrically charged and this explains why transfer rates are dependent on solute charge as well as solute size. Thus neutral dextran has a shorter clearance half-time than similarly sized anionic or cationic dextran, a difference which can be abolished by injury to the blood gas barrier. The pulmonary factors of physiological importance in determining the rate of solute transfer include regional surface area available for exchange, regional lung volume, intra-alveolar pressure, the composition and volume of the fluid in the alveoli, surfactant, and solute back-diffusion from blood to lung interstitium. Surface area, lung volume and intra-alveolar pressure are closely inter-related in their effects on solute clearance rate. Surface area and lung volume have been compared by measuring the half-time of DTPA clearance at resting and elevated lung volumes, although lung volume itself and the increase in surface area that accompanies an increase in lung volume cannot be distinguished in their effects on clearance. Expansion of the lung might be expected to stretch epithelial cells and pull them apart, thereby enlarging the junction gaps. However, because of the arrangement of the alveolar

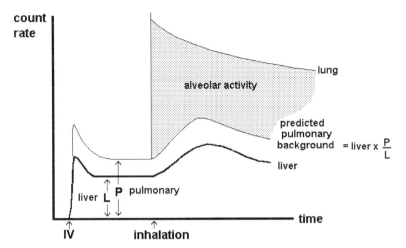

▌ **Fig. 8.10** An alternative method for background subtraction from a pulmonary DTPA aerosol clearance curve. In this technique the intravenous does is given first. Liver is used as the background tissue because it has a plasma / interstitial fluid ratio well matched to that of lung. Multiplication of the liver curve by *P/L* produces a curve which accurately predicts the non-alveolar, predominantly vascular, pulmonary DTPA. No correction is necessary for the intravenous activity itself since this is a component which is subtracted along with the DTPA that has moved from alveolus into plasma.

septa in pleats, expansion in lung volume may not necessarily be associated with stretching of the alveolar walls. Nevertheless positive end-expiratory pressure accelerates clearance, presumably by stretching epithelial cells and widening the junction gaps. Such stretching would also explain the finding that solute clearance is higher in the upper zones compared with the lower zones.

Surfactant seems to play a role in determining epithelial permeability to hydrophilic solutes, although the mechanism is unclear and the experimental evidence is based on rather unphysiological manoeuvres, such as the tracheal installation of detergents and the effects of surfactant depletion by bronchopulmonary lavage. As can be seen from equation 8.63, clearance should be inversely proportional to alveolar fluid volume. Nevertheless cardiogenic pulmonary oedema is not associated with reduced solute clearance implying that there is a counterbalancing increase in the permeability.

8.4.2.1 Measurement of alveolar epithelial permeability

Following inhalation, the radioactivity deposited in the lungs is monitored with a gamma camera or scintillation probe. The initial rate of disappearance of activity, over about the first 10 minutes, is mono-

exponential but, as tracer enters blood, recirculating pulmonary blood pool radioactivity makes an increasing contribution to the recorded signal, and the rate constant of disappearance decreases. This blood background signal requires correction by a subtraction procedure. This has usually been to monitor radioactivity over the thigh at the same time as recording over the lungs (**Fig. 8.9**). The appropriate factor by which to scale the thigh signal before subtracting it from the total lung signal is deduced by giving an intravenous injection of technetium-99m DTPA when the curve over the lung has fallen to about 50% of its initial value (Barrowcliffe *et al.* 1988). The factor is then calculated as the ratio of the respective sharp increments in the lung and thigh curves following intravenous injection (**Fig. 8.9**). This approach to blood background correction has a number of disadvantages. Firstly the signal from the thigh recorded after inhalation of the tracer becomes progressively weighted by extravascular activity as the DTPA moves from the intravascular compartment of the thigh into a much larger extravascular compartment. Secondly, relative to the intravascular compartment, the interstitial fluid compartment in the thigh is much larger compared with the lung. The thigh is therefore not an appropriate region on which to base background. More appropriate back-

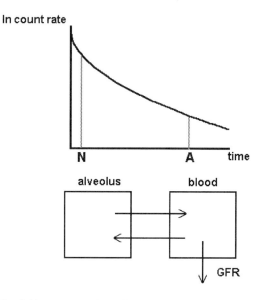

In count rate

N   A   time

alveolus   blood

GFR

▮ **Fig. 8.11** Hypothesis: Diffusion of DTPA from plasma back into alveolar fluid fully accounts for a bi-exponential pulmonary DTPA clearance curve. According to this model the gradient of the clearance should approach a rate constant which reflects GFR (or, more precisely, the ratio of GFR to extracellular fluid volume). This predicts that all clearance curves are bi-exponential. For a normal (i.e. slow) clearance, the relative recording time (effectively up to *N*) spans a small part of the clearance curve, is uninfluenced by GFR and appears linear. For a fast clearance (as in interstitial lung disease), the relative recording time includes a significant segment of the second exponential (up to *A*).

ground regions, in terms of relative volumes of intravascular and extravascular spaces, are the cranium and liver. DTPA does not penetrate the blood brain barrier, while the liver, like the lung, has a relatively small extravascular space. The extravascular tissues respectively in the scalp and in the anterior abdominal wall overlying the liver give radioactivity signals which match that from the extravascular tissues of the chest wall. In practice, the time–activity curve recorded over liver after intravenous injection of technetium-99m DTPA has a shape almost identical to that recorded over the lung, and is the background region of choice for alveolar permeability measurement (Peters *et al.* 1992). The cranium gives a somewhat more variable curve after intravenous injection but has the advantage compared with the liver that it can be

monitored with a scintillation probe. The liver is too close to the lung for probe counting, but is appropriate when the aerosol clearance is measured with a gamma camera.

Although the intravenous dose of DTPA is usually given after the aerosol, it is better to give it before, since subtraction is always more reliable when the signal for subtraction is smaller than the signal from which it is subtracted (Mason *et al.* 1995). Furthermore, when given first, the intravenous dose gives a signal over the lung which requires no subtraction itself from the subsequent lung curve recorded after tracer inhalation because inhaled tracer gaining access to the blood simply adds to the injected blood tracer, and the total is accounted for by the subtraction technique (**Fig. 8.10**).

In normal individuals, the clearance rate of technetium-99m DTPA is about 0.01 min^{-1}, or 1% per min, while in otherwise normal cigarette smokers, it is increased to about 4% per min. The half-time returns to normal if the subject abstains for about 10 days. This rapid clearance in smokers is a reflection of the sensitivity of the technique, but unfortunately also represents its major drawback in that the clearance rate resulting from severe interstitial lung disease is barely greater than in normal smokers. It is therefore difficult to apply the technique clinically to smokers, since the effect of the lung disease, on top of smoking, is not additive in terms of clearance rate. In an attempt to solve this problem, several authors have studied the comparative clearance rates of larger solutes with the aim of distinguishing between smokers and non-smokers. The rationale for this is based on the premise that smoking may increase clearance by increasing the size of the epithelial intercellular junction gaps so, with the use of a critically sized solute, the difference in clearance rates between smokers and non-smokers would be decreased. The inherent assumption is that interstitial lung disease either increases clearance by a different mechanism, perhaps involving an increase in pore numbers, or an increase in pore size by a greater degree than found in smokers. In any event, neither the mechanism responsible for the increased clearance in smokers nor the problems it creates with respect to the clinical use of the technique, have been resolved.

Interstitial lung disease generally results in an increased rate of clearance of DTPA from the lung.

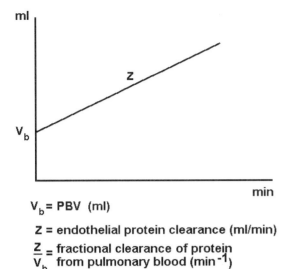

V_b = PBV (ml)

Z = endothelial protein clearance (ml/min)

$\dfrac{Z}{V_b}$ = fractional clearance of protein from pulmonary blood (min^{-1})

▌**Fig. 8.12** Measurement of endothelial protein transfer by Patlak–Rutland plot avoiding the use of labelled RBCs. The plot is virtually linear because of slow protein back-diffusion and represents the fraction of protein in pulmonary blood cleared through pulmonary endothelium per unit of time.

The diseases for which the technique has found the greatest clinical use are AIDS, ARDS and interstitial fibrosis associated with rheumatological conditions. In patients with AIDS, technetium-99m DTPA aerosol clearance is a sensitive marker for PCP and has been claimed to be the most useful non-invasive test for this complication, superior to chest radiography or gallium-67 scintigraphy. An interesting feature of the severely injured lung, in which permeability is markedly increased, is that the clearance curve is bi-exponential. It has been suggested that this is the result of two populations of lung units with different degrees of damage and correspondingly different clearance rates. The evidence for this is that in experimental lung damage, such as induced by intravenous oleic acid, the degree of injury is not homogeneous. However a biexponential curve is almost always seen when the clearance rate is increased from any cause and not necessarily under conditions in which heterogeneous lung damage might be expected, raising the possibility of other explanations for the bi-exponential shape. These include, firstly, deposition of aerosol more proximally in the airway, with slower clearance, and secondly, back-diffusion of tracer

from blood to interstitium. When the membrane becomes sufficiently damaged, and particularly when fluid accumulates within the distal lung, back-diffusion of solute from pulmonary blood may become detectable later in the clearance curve. Thus, from this argument, a bi-exponential clearance curve would be explained on the basis of the compartmental model (**Fig. 8.11**).

8.4.3 Pulmonary endothelial permeability

As with endothelium elsewhere, water, lipophilic solutes and small hydrophilic solutes have free access through the pulmonary vascular endothelium to the interstitial space. Water and lipophilic solutes penetrate the endothelium directly; i.e. through the endothelial cell, whereas hydrophilic solutes diffuse through the spaces between the endothelial cells at a rate inversely proportional to molecular size. Larger molecules, such as proteins, have restricted access to the pulmonary interstitial space.

Whereas alveolar epithelial permeability is quantified from the rate of clearance of tracer deposited in the alveolus, pulmonary vascular endothelial permeability is measured from the appearance rate in the pulmonary interstitium of tracer injected intravenously (Braude *et al.* 1986). Since the endothelium is considerably more permeable to hydrophilic solutes than the epithelium, a solute larger than technetium-99m DTPA is required for measurement of endothelial permeability, such as radiolabelled protein. DTPA, in contrast, is taken up into the lung interstitium at a rate which is dependent on blood flow rather than on diffusion. Another disadvantage of a small solute is that back-diffusion from interstitium to blood is early and rapid, especially as the interstitial fluid volume of the lung is relatively small. Radio-labelled proteins, to which the normal pulmonary vascular endothelium is essentially impermeable (Gorin *et al.* 1980), have therefore been used, either radio-iodinated albumin (molecular weight 68 000) or indium-111 labelled transferrin (molecular weight 75 000). Since the tracer is injected into the blood, the problem of blood background is greater when measuring endothelial permeability compared with epithelial permeability, and requires correction. This may be achieved with a simultaneous injection of radio-labelled red cells (see below) or by using a method of analysis, such as a Patlak–Rutland plot, which accounts for blood background.

The principle of measuring protein transfer across the pulmonary vascular endothelium is similar to the measurement of solute transfer across vascular endothelium elsewhere (Section 6.2.2.4.2). A scintillation detector or gamma camera region of interest is positioned over the chest, avoiding cardiac chambers and large blood vessels, and another over the heart for continuous recording of the blood level of radioactivity. Assuming that over a period of time t any radio-labelled protein diffusing into the interstitial space remains in the region of interest (i.e. does not move either back into the intravascular space or is carried away in pulmonary lymph) then

$$\frac{dM_e}{dt} = Z \cdot C_a \qquad (8.65)$$

where M_e is the quantity of protein in the interstitial space and Z is the clearance (ml/min) of protein from plasma into the interstitial space.

Therefore

$$M_e = Z \cdot \int C_a(t) \cdot dt. \qquad (8.66)$$

The total amount of radioactivity, which also includes intravascular protein M_i, is therefore

$$M_e + M_i = Z \int C_a(t) \cdot dt + V_b \cdot C_a \qquad (8.67)$$

where V_b is the volume of blood in the intravascular space within the lung region of interest. Dividing equation 8.67 by C_a

$$\frac{M_e + M_i}{C_a} = Z \frac{\int C_a(t) dt}{C_a} + V_b. \qquad (8.68)$$

If N_{lung} is the count rate recorded over the lung then

$$\gamma N_{lung} = M_e + M_i \qquad (8.69)$$

and similarly

$$\Gamma N_{heart} = C_a. \qquad (8.70)$$

Therefore,

$$\frac{\gamma N_{lung}}{\Gamma N_{heart}} = Z \cdot \frac{\int N_{heart}(t) \cdot dt}{N_{heart}} + V_b. \qquad (8.71)$$

Multiplying both sides of equation 8.71 by Γ/γ

$$\frac{N_{lung}}{N_{heart}} = \frac{\Gamma}{\gamma} \cdot Z \frac{\int N_{heart}(t) \cdot dt}{N_{heart}} + \frac{\Gamma}{\gamma} \cdot V_b. \qquad (8.72)$$

From equations 8.71, it is evident that a Patlak–Rutland plot of N_{lung}/N_{heart} against $\int N_{heart}(t) \cdot dt/N_{heart}$ gives a regression slope with a gradient α proportional to Z and an intercept c proportional to V_b. Hence α/c is equal to Z/V_b the fractional rate of clearance of protein from pulmonary blood to lung interstitium (**Fig. 8.12**).

In the case of a radio-labelled protein, equation 8.72 can be simplified because the blood level of radio-labelled protein should be relatively constant soon after injection. The term $\int N_{heart}(t) \cdot dt/N_{heart}$, which has units of time is, in this case, clock time. Compare this with equation 6.27 where the equivalent term, $\int C_a(t) \cdot dt/C_a$, although having units of time, is not clock time because C_a is not constant. It is sometimes called 'normalized' time. If C_a falls, normalized time numerically exceeds clock time. For a macromolecule such as labelled protein therefore equation 8.72 can therefore be re-written:

$$N_{lung}/N_{heart} = \propto t + c. \qquad (8.73)$$

In other words, to derive α, N_{lung}/N_{heart} is plotted as a function of time. As with measurement of extravascular clearance in peripheral soft tissues, α has the units of reciprocal of time; i.e. of a rate constant. In order to convert it to a variable with absolute units of ml/min (i.e. clearance rate of protein from intravascular into pulmonary interstitial space) a blood sample is required in order to determine Γ. If γ is known, equation 8.71 can be re-written in units

$$\frac{MBq}{MBq/ml} = \frac{ml.min}{min} + ml = ml$$

The parameter α then becomes Z, which is the rate at which the protein is cleared from the intravascular to extravascular space within the lung present in the field of view of the detector, or region of interest of the camera. It may come as a surprise to find that c is proportional to volume. Since it represents the y-axis intercept of the regression in equation 8.72, it must have the same units as those of the y-axis itself. When Z is expressed in terms of c, i.e. as α/c, it takes on units of min^{-1}. Blood sampling is not required, and detector sensitivity also cancels out. Clearance expressed in this way then represents the fractional rate at which intravascular labelled protein is cleared into the interstitial space.

The above approach represents another use for the Patlak–Rutland method of graphical analysis. How-

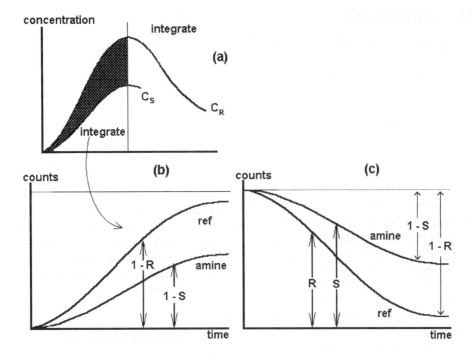

∎ **Fig. 8.13** Measurement of pulmonary amine extraction following intravenous amine injection. An intravascular non-diffusible, non-extractable reference tracer (red cells or albumin) given at the same time, defines the fraction of amine extracted. This is similar in principle to measurement of *PS* product by the indicator dilution technique (Fig. 6.6) except it is assumed that over the period of measurement, negligible extracted amine returns to the venous effluent. The similarity can be extended to include the use of residue detection to measure amine extraction fraction, as in the measurement of *PS* product illustrated in Fig. 6.7. Integration of pulmonary venous outflow curves (a) gives the cumulative venous outflow curves (b), which are mirror images of the pulmonary residue curves (c) recorded by the detector (*R* — reference signal, S — amine signal). Amine extraction *E* is then given by

$$E = \frac{\int C_R(t)\mathrm{d}t - \int C_S(t)\mathrm{d}t}{\int C_R(t)\mathrm{d}t} = \frac{(1-R)-(1-S)}{(1-R)}.$$

The certainty that *R* and *S* are impulse response curves can be increased by applying deconvolution analysis using a region over the superior vena cava or right ventricle as the input function (and lung as the output function).

ever most publications describing the measurement of pulmonary endothelial permeability have approached the correction of blood background by using two tracers, one a protein and the other a blood pool marker with restricted access to the pulmonary interstitial space, such as technetium-99m labelled red cells. Technetium-99m labelled red cells effectively serve to define *c*. They are however not necessary and in practice have the disadvantage of preventing the use of another tracer for studying a second biological entity alongside endothelial permeability, for example the simultaneous use of labelled neutrophils for cell kinetic studies or technetium-99m DTPA for measuring epithelial permeability.

Measurement of pulmonary vascular endothelial permeability generally has less clinical value than measurement of epithelial permeability. It is technically more difficult and the data obtained more 'noisy' compared with inhaled aerosol clearance. On the other hand, endothelial permeability, at least to protein, is not apparently increased in smokers. The technique has been used almost exclusively for the assessment of lung function in patients with ARDS, and it may have a role in predicting the onset of ARDS in patients at risk. Using radio-labelled protein, the test has proved rather insensitive, emphasizing the need to develop smaller molecules with more rapid rates of endothelial transit. A molecule intermediate in size between DTPA and transferrin, such as a peptide, may meet this requirement.

8.5 The metabolic functions of the lung

Imaging the metabolic functions of the lung has been centred on measurement of the extraction efficiency by the lung of intra-venously injected labelled amines and the subsequent rate at which they are cleared from the lung. The lung handles many important substances arriving in central venous blood. Firstly it filters particulate material, such as platelet aggregates, which are de-aggregated. This is probably why the arterial platelet count is marginally higher than the central venous count. It has also been suggested that megakaryocytes, after release from bone marrow and transportation in venous blood to the lungs, fragment into platelets by impaction on pulmonary arterial branching points; i.e. the lung may be the site of platelet production in the circulation. Secondly, it activates some physiological mediators. For example, by virtue of angiotensin converting enzyme in pulmonary endothelium, it converts angiotensin-1 into angiotensin-2. Thirdly, the lung inactivates several amines, including serotonin, bradykinin, some prostaglandins, and, to a lesser extent, noradrenaline and histamine. Bradykinin is inactivated by angiotensin converting enzyme. The extraction of amines by the lung is the metabolic function which has been most extensively studied by external radio-detection, and this has been facilitated by the availability of radio-iodinated amines and technetium-99m HMPAO.

8.5.1 Pulmonary amine extraction

Pulmonary uptake of iodine-123 labelled IMP following intravenous injection has been used as a non-invasive index of pulmonary metabolic function. Measurement of this uptake at a pre-determined time after injection, although simple, is only a semi-quantitative index of lung function. A physiologically better defined technique is measurement of the extraction fraction of an amine. This is based on quantification of unextracted amine leaving the lung in pulmonary arterial blood by comparing the residue curve of radio-labelled amine over the lung with that of an intravascular reference tracer such as labelled red cells or human serum albumin. The approach is, in principle, identical to the measurement of solute permeability in peripheral tissues by the indicator dilution technique, in which the venous effluent concentration of solute and reference tracers are compared immediately following upstream intra-arterial injection (Section 6.2.2.4.1). Under these circumstances

$$E_{\text{amine}} = \frac{C_{\text{ref}}(t) - C_{\text{amine}}(t)}{C_{\text{ref}}(t)} \quad (8.74)$$

where E and C are extraction fraction and concentration, respectively.

Equation 8.74 assumes that no extracted amine returns to the vascular space by time t. By the same token therefore E is obtainable from the cumulative venous effluent curves; i.e. the areas under the time/concentration curves of reference tracer and amine in venous blood (**Fig. 8.13a**).

External monitoring of pulmonary activity (i.e. by residue detection) makes it unnecessary to measure the pulmonary venous effluent solute concentration and reference concentration explicitly since the residue curves are mirror images of the cumulative venous effluent curves. If we assume that all the intravenously injected activity arrives in the lung instantaneously, and normalize the initial activity for both residue curves to unity, then the cumulative venous effluent curves can be described as $1 - R(t)$ and $1 - S(t)$ for reference tracer and amine respectively (**Fig. 8.13b**).
Therefore

$$E_{\text{solute}} = \frac{[1 - R(t)] - [1 - S(t)]}{1 - R(t)} \quad (8.75)$$

$$= \frac{S(t) - R(t)}{1 - R(t)}. \quad (8.76)$$

In order to strengthen the assumption of instantaneous arrival, E_{solute} can be derived from equation 8.74 using the impulse response curves over the lung. This requires deconvolution analysis using a region of interest placed over the superior vena cava or right ventricle.

Amines are retained in the lung as a result of binding to receptors on the pulmonary vascular endothelium, as can be demonstrated by showing saturable binding with increasing doses of amine. In this respect, therefore, amine extraction is different from solute uptake in the tissues, which is by diffusion into the extravascular space. Nevertheless, the theoretical approach is, as stated above, identical in principle to solute permeability measurement. As with the latter, it requires that bound amine does not return to the intravascular space in the interval up to t; i.e. does not dissociate from the receptor to which it becomes bound.

The receptors in the pulmonary vascular endothelium responsible for binding amines are saturable with high doses of amines. Extraction fraction for the amine can therefore be measured with increasing doses of amine and subjected to Scatchard analysis (Section 5.6). In this analysis, the ratio of bound to free ligand is plotted against free ligand. Extracted amine is taken to represent bound ligand whilst unextracted amine is taken to represent free ligand. Therefore, by measuring the extraction fraction of amine with increasing doses of amine, the dissociation constant between amine and its receptor can be calculated.

8.5.2 Lung clearance of receptor-bound amine

After injection, radio-labelled amines taken up by the lung are metabolized, and the rate at which the radioactivity is mobilized from the lung can be recorded and expressed as a clearance $t_{1/2}$ (Pistolesi *et al.* 1988). This is analogous to the clearance $t_{1/2}$ values expressed for labelled fatty acids following uptake by the myocardium. With respect to the lung, this approach gives a quantitative index which, although undefinable in simple physiological terms, may be useful for the monitoring of acute lung damage such as in the adult respiratory distress syndrome.

References

Alexander MSM, Peters AM, Cleland J and Lavender JP. Impaired left lower lobe ventilation in patients with cardiomegaly: an isotope study of mechanisms. *Chest* 1992, **101**: 1189–93.

Anthonisen NR, Dolowich MB and Bates DV. Steady state measurement of regional ventilation to perfusion ratios in normal man. *Journal of Clinical Investigation* 1966, **45**: 1349–56.

Barrowcliffe MP, Otto C and Jones JG. Pulmonary clearance of Tc-99m DTPA: influence of background activity. *Journal of Applied Physiology* 1988, **64**: 1045–9.

Braude S, Nolop KB, Hughes JMB, Barnes PJ and Royston D. Comparison of lung vascular and epithelial permeability indices in the adult respiratory distress syndrome. *American Revue of Respiratory Disease* 1986, **133**: 1002–5.

Briggs BA, Bradley TM, Vernon P, Cooke NT, Drinkwater C, Gillett MK and Snashall PD. Measurement of lung tissue mass, thoracic blood and interstitial volumes by transmission/emission scanning using [99m-Tc] pertechnetate. *Clinical Science* 1987, **73**: 319–27.

Brudin LH, Valind SO, Rhodes CG, Turton DR and Hughes JMB. Regional lung hematocrit in humans using positron emission tomography. *Journal of Applied Physiology* 1986, **60**: 1155–63.

Coates G and O'Brodovich H: Measurement of pulmonary epithelial permeability with Tc-99m DTPA aerosol. *Medicine 1986, 16, 275–84*

Davies H, Kitchman R, Gordon I and Helms P. Regional ventilation in infancy. *New England Journal of Medicine* 1985, **313**: 1626–8.

Fazio F and Jones T. Assessment of regional ventilation by continuous inhalation of krypton-81m. *British Medical Journal* 1975, **3**: 673–6.

Gorin AB, Kohler J and DeNardo G. Noninvasive measurement of pulmonary transvascular protein flux in normal man. *Journal of Clinical Investigation* 1980, **66**: 869–77.

Hogg JC. Neutrophil kinetics and lung injury. *Physiol Review* 1987, **67**: 1249–95.

MacNee W and Selby C. Neutrophil kinetics in the lungs, *Clinical Science* 1990; **79**: 97–107.

MacNee W, Martin BA, Wiggs BR, Belzberg AS, Hogg JC. Regional pulmonary transit times in humans. *Journal of Applied Physiology* 1989; **66** : 844–50.

Mason GR, Peters AM, Myers MJ, Ind PW and Hughes JMB. The effect of inhalation of platelet activating factor on the pulmonary clearance of Tc99m-DTPA aerosol. *American Journal of Respiratory and Critical Care Medicine* 1995, **151**: 1 621–4.

O'Doherty MJ and Peters AM. Pulmonary Tc-99m DTPA aerosol clearance as an index of lung injury. *European Journal of Nuclear Medicine* 1997, **24**: 81–7.

Peters AM, Mason GR and Hughes JMB. Appropriate background subtraction for pulmonary radioaerosol clearance. *Journal of Nuclear Medicine* 1992, **33**: 836.

Rahimian J, Glass EC, Touya JJ, Akber SF, Graham LS and Bennett LR. Measurement of metabolic extraction of tracers in the lung using a multiple indicator dilution technique. *Journal of Nuclear Medicine* 1984, **25**: 31–7

Pistolesi M, Miniati M, Petruzzelli S, Carrozzi L, Giani L, Bellina CR, Gerundini P, Fazio F and Giuntini C.

Pulmonary retention of iodobenzyl propanediamine in humans. Effect of cigarette smoking. *American Revue of Respiratory Disease* 1988, **138**: 1429–33.

Rhodes CG, Valind SO and Brudin LH Quantification of regional *VA/Q* ratios in humans by use of PET: 11 Procedure and normal values. *Journal of Applied Physiology* 1989, **66**: 1905–13.

Saverymuttu SH, Peters AM, Danpure HJ, Reavy HJ, Osman S and Lavender JP. Lung transit of 111-indiumlabelled granulocytes. Relationship to labelling techniques. *Scandinavian Journal of Haematology* 1983, **30**: 151–60.

Swinburne AJ, MacArthur CGC, Rhodes CG, Heather JD and Hughes JMB. Measurement of lung water in dog lobes using inhaled $C^{15}O_2$ and $H_2^{15}O$. *Journal of Applied Physiology* 1982, **52**: 1535–44.

Ussov W Yu, Peters AM, Hodgson HJ and Hughes JMB. Quantification of pulmonary uptake of indium-111 labelled granulocytes in inflammatory bowel disease. *European Journal of Nuclear Medicine* 1994, **21**: 6–11.

Ussov WY, Peters AM, Glass DM, Gunasekera RD and Hughes JMB. Measurement of the pulmonary vascular granuiocyte pool. *Journal of Applied Physiology* 1995, **78**: 1388–95.

Wagner PD, Smith CM, Davies NJH, McEvoy RD and Gale GE. Estimation of ventilation–perfusion inequality by inert gas elimination without arterial sampling. *Journal of Applied Physiology* 1985, **59**: 376.

Weiner C, McKenna WJ, Myers MJ, Lavender JP and Hughes JMB. Lung ventilation is reduced in patients with cardiomegaly in the supine but not in the prone position. *American Review of Respiratory Disease* 1990, **141**: 150H.

Whyte MKB, Peters AM, Hughes JMB, Henderson BL, Bellingan GJ, Jackson JE and Chilvers ER. Quantification of right to left shunt at rest and on exercise in patients with pulmonary arterio-venous malformations. *Thorax* 1992, **47**: 790–6.

Wollmer P, Rhodes CG and Hughes JMB. Regional extravascular density and fractional blood volume of the lung in interstitial disease. *Thorax* 1984, **39**: 286–93.

9 The gastro-intestinal tract and liver

9.1 Salivary glands

The salivary gland is one of the organs, along with gastric mucosa, thyroid gland and choroid plexus, that concentrates pertechnetate. The radionuclide is excreted in saliva at a rate that can be measured from dynamic imaging of the salivary glands. Obstruction of a salivary gland, as for instance by a stone in the salivary duct, produces a rising curve (sialogram), similar to the rising renogram of urinary obstruction. The similarity with renography can be extended by examining the effect on the sialogram of the administration of a sialogogue by mouth, such as lemon juice, 10 min after injection of pertechnetate. In the non-obstructed gland, radioactivity is briskly washed out, whereas no effect is seen in obstruction. Relative function of the glands on either side can also be assessed, analogously to differential renal function, either by imaging relative peak heights of the corresponding curves, or their maximum upslope gradients.

9.2 Motility in the gastro-intestinal (GI) tract

Identifying abnormal motility with radionuclides within the GI tract is usually based on transit time measurement. Thus, inert radiopharmaceuticals can be followed as they pass from the mouth to the stomach (oesophageal transit time), from stomach to duodenum (gastric emptying) and from small to large bowel (intestinal transit time studies).

9.2.1 Oesophageal transit time

Oesophageal transit can be investigated by scintigraphic monitoring of a bolus of a radio-labelled inert agent as it passes from mouth to stomach (Tolin *et al.* 1979). Multiple further swallows can be monitored. A region of interest is drawn around the

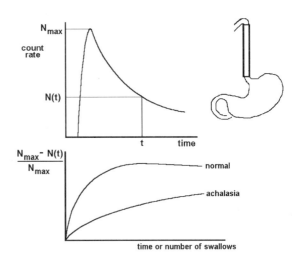

Fig. 9.1 Semi-quantification of oesophageal transit time.

entire oesophagus and a time–activity curve constructed. Transit time is usually expressed by graphically plotting $[N_{max} - N(t)]/N_{max}$ against time, where N_{max} is the maximum count rate recorded from the region of interest immediately after the bolus is initially swallowed, and $N(t)$ the activity remaining in the region at subsequent times t. With normal transit, this ratio rapidly reaches unity, whereas in conditions like achalasia and scleroderma, unity is reached more slowly (**Fig. 9.1**). As an alternative to expressing the ratio $[N_{max} - N(t)]/N_{max}$ as a function of time, it can be expressed as a function of the number of swallows.

Peristaltic activity can be investigated by a technique known as space–time matrix plotting, more fully described in Section 11.3 for application to the ureter, for which it has been used to study peristalsis ureteric and vesico-ureteric reflux. For the generation of a space–time matrix, several regions of interest are placed contiguously one above the other over the length of the oesophagus (**Fig. 9.2**) (Gibson and Bateson 1985). Time–activity information for each region is then generated and plotted on the matrix. The *y*-axis of the plot is the series of regions,

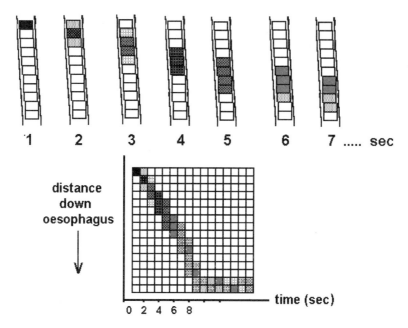

∎ Fig. 9.2 Space–time matrix to depict oesophogeal transit. The radiolabelled bolus passes down the oesophagus moving from one region of interest (ROI) to the next below. The counts recorded while the bolus is in the ROI determine the grey scale intensity in the display for that ROI. The counts will persist in a particular row on the grid (each row corresponding to one ROI) if the bolus fails to move to a lower ROI. Retrograde peristalsis can also be identified, if the bolus moves to the right and *upwards*.

i.e. representing distance down the oesophagus, and the x-axis is time. Each element in the grid matrix is colour or grey-scale coded for the counts collected in the corresponding region during a particular time frame. The peristaltic rate and velocity can then be visually assessed from the plot. As an alternative to several separate regions, one region of interest can be placed over the entire oesophagus and the computer programmed to generate contiguous one-pixel high regions with a width equal to that of the oesophagus. As before, the y-axis (space of the matrix) represents the distance down the oesophagus and the horizontal axis the time after administration. As the activity descends the oesophagus, blocks of colour representing the activity move down and to the right of the matrix display. This form of display is also known as a compressed image.

9.2.2 Gastric emptying

Stomach contents leave the stomach exponentially. A radioactive meal can be given to measure the $t_{1/2}$ of gastric emptying (Urbain and Charkes 1995).

There has been much argument as to what should be the precise physical state of the radioactive meal with respect to solid and liquid phases and to lipid and non-lipid phases. A labelled solid meal can be prepared by first injecting a live chicken with technetium-99m labelled colloid, which is taken up into the chicken's liver, and then cooking the liver for consumption by the patient. Less exotic meals involving, for example, labelled mashed potatoes and baked beans are usually used. A liquid component, such as orange juice, can be labelled with a second radionuclide for dual isotope studies. Furthermore, lipid and non-lipid phases can also be separately labelled. Measurement of gastric emptying is applied to patients with suspected pyloric stenosis and with post-gastrectomy syndromes.

9.2.3 Gastro–oesophageal reflux

Gastro–oesophageal reflux can be monitored and quantified using any of the labels described above for gastric emptying. The principles are the same as for measurement of vesico–ureteric reflux (Section

11.3.2). Thus a time–activity curve can be recorded from a region over the oesophagus and calibrated in volume units by:

(1) measuring the concentration of radioactivity in a sample of stomach contents;
(2) correcting for photon attenuation from the oesophageal region.

If it is assumed that the photon attenuations from tracer respectively in the stomach and in the oesophagus are the same, then reflux can be semi-quantified without sampling the stomach.

9.2.4 Duodeno–gastric reflux

This follows the same principles as above and is measured using an intravenous administration of technetium-99m labelled HIDA. Quantification is more cumbersome owing to the inaccessibility of the duodenum and unknown variations in attenuation but otherwise can be approached similarly to gastro–oesophageal reflux.

9.2.5 Intestinal transit time

Intestinal transit time can be measured by monitoring the progress of any inert, non-absorbed radiopharmaceutical through the gastro–intestinal tract, using a gamma camera. DTPA, labelled with technetium-99m or indium-111 is not significantly absorbed by the normal gut and can be used to measure intestinal transit time. It is however absorbed by diseased gut and, in conjunction with measurement of radioactivity in urine, can be used as a quantitative index of intestinal disease (see below, Section 9.5.3). Even in the presence of grossly abnormal absorption however the great majority of the activity remains in the gut lumen for measurement of transit time. This is the time it takes to reach various destinations in the gut, such as the terminal ileum, which marks the completion of small intestinal transit, and the various segments of the colon (Notghi *et al.* 1993). Transit time from duodenum to caecum normally ranges between 1.5 and 6 hr. In order to assess colonic transit time, indium-111 DTPA is preferable because of its longer physical half-life. Another agent for studying gastro–intestinal transit time is technetium-99m labelled sucralfate.

9.3 Hepatic organic ion transport

Bromosulphthalein (BSP), rose bengal (RB), indo-cyanine green (ICG) and iminodiacetic analogues (IDA) are examples of organic anions which share the same carrier-mediated transport system from plasma into the hepatocyte. They also share the same binding and carrier system for transfer from hepatocyte to bile canaliculus, as can be demonstrated by showing that the plasma concentration of a tracer dose of labelled anion can be increased transiently by the injection of a large amount of another, unlabelled, anion. The significance of this in clinical nuclear medicine is related to the fact that uptake of IDA analogues by the hepatocyte is decreased in jaundice. Urinary activity of IDA is also increased in jaundice, probably as a result of displacement of IDA from protein binding sites in plasma. The IDA analogues designed for use in jaundiced patients are less hydrophilic and cannot so easily be displaced from protein than the more hydrophilic analogues, such as diethyl IDA. On the other hand, they may have longer intrahepatic transit times than diethyl IDA, and might theoretically therefore at a slight disadvantage for imaging the biliary tree.

Following intravenous injection, organic anions such as BSP are normally cleared exclusively by the liver. From the hepatocyte, the substance is then actively transported into the bile canaliculus or diffuses back into plasma. So, whereas movement into bile is unidirectional, transport between plasma and hepatocyte is bi-directional. These kinetics can be represented by a closed-two-compartmental model with run-off (**Fig. 9.3**), and predict a bi-exponential plasma clearance curve (Clarkson *et al.* 1976). This is indeed the case, but because the extent of protein binding is unclear and because it is therefore not clear whether the distribution volume includes a significant extravascular component, bi-directional transfer of tracer between plasma and ECF could partly account for the bi-exponential nature of the disappearance curve from plasma. All of the organic anions, such as BSP, are probably handled in the same way, including IDA, although the extent of protein binding varies.

The fractional rate constants of organic anion transport along the pathways, k_1, k_2, and k are

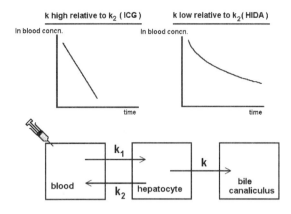

▮ **Fig. 9.3a** The two-compartmental model with run-off illustrating the kinetics of an organic anion such as IDA and predicting a bi-exponential blood disappearance curve following intravenous injection. If k is high relative to k_2 the plasma curve may appear to be a single exponential (as has been described for indocyanine green) since k_2 is given little chance to influence the curve. If k is relatively low (as is normally the case of IDA), then the blood disappearance curve appears clearly bi-exponential.

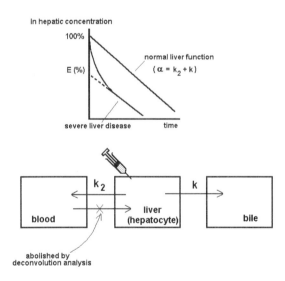

▮ **Fig. 9.3b** Deconvolution analysis of blood and hepatocyte curves in normal subjects or patients with biliary obstruction but otherwise normal hepatic function gives a mono-exponential IDA liver clearance curve with a rate constant $\alpha = k_2 + k$. An early fast exponential, seen in liver disease, is consistent with intravascular transit of unextracted tracer (probably through intrahepatic vascular shunts). The zero time intercept of the second exponential in this situation, relative to the total zero time signal, therefore reflects unidirectional hepatic extraction of IDA from blood to hepatocyte.

illustrated in Fig. 9.3. If the substance does not significantly enter the extra-hepatic extravascular space, the fractional rate constant k_1 is the fraction of the blood volume cleared per unit of time. These fractional rate constants can be measured from the parameters of the bi-exponential plasma disappearance curve using the techniques of compartmental analysis and curve stripping described in Sections 1.3 and 1.4 (see also the splenic handling of heat damaged red cells, Section 10.2.2.2). This curve is separated into two exponential curves with rate constants α_1 and α_2 and zero-time intercepts respectively A and B. The fractional rate constants of the model are related to the parameters of the exponential curves as follows:

$$k_1 = \frac{A\alpha_1 + B\alpha_2}{A + B} \tag{9.1}$$

$$k = \alpha_1 \cdot \alpha_2 / k_1 \tag{9.2}$$

$$k_2 = \frac{A\alpha_2 + B\alpha_1}{A + B} - k. \tag{9.3}$$

The values of these rate constants vary from one organic ion to another and may also vary between different IDA analogues (Chervu *et al.* 1982, Grainger *et al.* 1983, Burns *et al.* 1991). An important implication for this mechanism of handling is that, in the presence of unilateral biliary obstruction, IDA would not be expected to accumulate in, or show delayed drainage from, the obstructed lobe, because it will re-enter plasma and ultimately be cleared via the non-obstructed lobe. Although in practice it is impossible to image the parenchymal cell separately from the bile canaliculus, and because other factors may come into play following biliary obstruction, the authors have seen at least one instance of a well-documented case of unilateral obstruction of an hepatic duct in which the radionuclide hepatograms were reproducibly identical between obstructed and non-obstructed sides (**Fig. 9.4**).

9.4 Hepatic haemodynamics

The liver is unusual in that it has a dual blood supply. It receives arterial blood via the hepatic artery and a portal venous supply which comprises

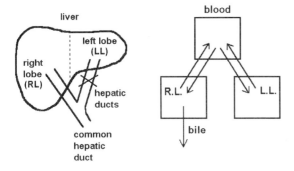

▌ **Fig. 9.4** The model shown in Fig. 9.3 explains why unilateral lobar obstruction may not become manifest on an IDA scan.

the splenic and the mesenteric venous outflows (i.e. from the entire gastro–intestinal tract). This means that total liver blood flow is substantial — about 1250 ml/min. The hepatic arterial flow is about 25% of this. Of the portal flow, about 250 ml/min serves the spleen. This blood flow arrangement is remarkable because not only are the two inflows at completely different pressures (the portal venous pressure is normally about 10 mm Hg), but their contents are different. For example, the portal flow carries to the liver all substances absorbed from the gastro–intestinal tract which therefore cannot gain access to the systemic arterial circulation until at least one pass through both the liver and the lung. The liver is also exposed first to the action of several gastro–intestinal hormones, including insulin, which are secreted into the mesenteric bed. Furthermore, the liver is the first vascular bed into which cytokines, bacterial products and occasionally malignant cells drain following release from pathological processes involving the gut.

The liver also has a substantial blood volume, which comprises about one quarter of total liver volume. The entire mesenteric vascular bed, including the liver, contains about one quarter of the total blood volume. It is easy to appreciate therefore that the liver and mesenteric bed are important in blood volume regulation and in the response to acute fluid shifts or depletion.

The intra-hepatic vascular functional anatomy has fascinated physiologists for decades. The nutrient vessel within the liver is the hepatic sinusoid which connects the terminal portal venules and hepatic arterioles to the central vein, a tributary of the hepatic vein. In contrast to the continuous endothe-lium of skin and muscle capillaries, the sinusoid has a fenestrated endothelium through which relatively large molecules can diffuse and which gives the sinusoid a high permeability. The interstitial space of liver is relatively small, and in this respect the liver resembles the lung and other solid organs like the spleen, pancreas and kidney. The hepatic arterioles and portal venules anastomose proximal to the sinusoid. On the basis of inert gas washout studies, it was thought for many years that they remained to some extent separated within the liver. Thus the washout rate of xenon-133 is apparently more rapid following injection into the portal vein than into the hepatic artery. However, various other explanations are available for this difference and it is currently thought that the two inflows completely mix proximal to the sinusoid (Mathie 1986).

Acute changes in portal venous flow result in reciprocal changes in hepatic arterial flow. Thus inflation of a balloon in the portal vein, with a resulting decrease in portal venous flow, causes an immediate increase in hepatic arterial flow. This is not the passive result of changes in intrahepatic vascular pressure but is a pre-sinusoidal active response, related possibly to local adenosine concentrations. Alterations in hepatic arterial flow have no effect on portal venous flow, of which there is no intrahepatic pre-sinusoidal control. Portal venous flow is not actively regulated by the liver and appears to be passively transmitted to the hepatic veins. Indeed portal venous resistance decreases with increasing portal flow as a result of passive vessel distension. The relationship between hepatic arterial and portal venous flows is important clinically, especially in cirrhosis and under circumstances such as portal venous thrombosis and therapeutic porto–caval shunting, which lead to changes in portal inflow to the liver.

9.4.1 Measurement of total liver blood flow

9.4.1.1 Indicator dilution

The classic method for measuring liver blood flow is based on hepatic organic anion uptake (Bradley *et al.* 1945). At steady state, the infusion rate (in mg/min) of an indicator, such as BSP, which is removed from the circulation only by the liver and excreted in bile, is equal to the output rate into bile (in mg/min).

From the Fick principle

$$\frac{dM_\tau}{dt} = Q(C_a - Cv) - Y \tag{9.4}$$

where M_τ is the amount of tracer in the liver, Q is liver blood flow, C_a and C_v are the arterial and hepatic venous concentrations of tracer respectively and Y is the biliary elimination rate (MBq/min).

At steady state,

$$dM_\tau/dt = 0 \tag{9.5}$$

so

$$Q(C_a - Cv) = Y$$

and

$$Q = \frac{Y}{C_a - C_v}. \tag{9.6}$$

If no other organ removes the indicator, then Y is equal to the infusion rate. The concentration C_v is measured from hepatic venous blood which requires catheterization of the hepatic vein. Although C_a should be measured from an arterial blood sample, a peripheral venous sample at steady state is an adequate reflection of the arterial concentration.

An alternative approach which does not require hepatic venous catheterization is to measure blood indicator clearance following bolus intravenous injection. Transfer between blood and the hepatocyte is bi-directional, while transfer from hepatocyte to bile canaliculus is uni-directional. The handling of the indicator by the liver can therefore be represented as a closed, two-compartmental model with run-off (**Fig. 9.3**). Since indicator returns to blood after entry into the hepatic cell, the *net* extraction efficiency and net clearance of organic anion are functions of time after injection, decreasing from a maximal value at zero time. It is important to grasp the concept of clearance and extraction efficiency at steady state and distinguish it from clearance and extraction efficiency at any other time after injection. Steady state clearance is the clearance existing during continuous infusion when the removal rate of indicator by the liver is equal to the infusion rate, and is obtainable as the ratio of infusion rate to arterial concentration ([mg.min^{-1}]/[mg.ml^{-1}] = ml.min^{-1}).

The steady-state clearance is also obtainable from the blood disappearance curve following intravenous bolus injection using the general equation for clearance Z:

$$Z = \frac{\text{injected administered activity}}{\text{total area under clearance curve}}. \tag{9.7}$$

Liver blood flow can be obtained from the steady-state clearance if steady-state extraction efficiency E_s is known. This is the extraction efficiency, defined as $(C_a - C_v)/C_a$, at steady state during continuous infusion when the hepatic concentration is constant. Liver blood flow can be measured from the blood disappearance curve following intravenous injection, *assuming that the extraction efficiency in the direction of plasma to hepatocyte is 100%* (see below). Thus following injection, an instant of time exists when the intra-hepatocyte content M_τ having risen from zero, is briefly constant before decreasing in parallel with the blood concentration. At this time,

$$dM_\tau/dt = 0. \tag{same as 9.5}$$

The instant at which M_τ is constant represents steady state, at which time

$$Q \cdot C_a = Y + Q \cdot C_v \tag{9.8}$$

But

$$E_s = \frac{Q \cdot C_a - Q \cdot C_v}{Q \cdot C_a} \tag{9.9}$$

so from equation 9.8

$$E_s = \frac{Y}{Y + Q \cdot C_v}. \tag{9.10}$$

Now at steady state, influx of tracer is equal to outflux, so provided that the extraction efficiency from plasma to hepatocyte is 100%, when clearance is equal to blood flow,

$$Q \cdot C_a = M_\tau \cdot k_2 + Y$$

and

$$Q \cdot C_v = M_\tau \cdot k_2 \tag{9.11}$$

where k_2 is the fractional rate constant (Fig. 9.3) determining transfer of indicator from hepatocyte to plasma. Furthermore

$$Y = M_\tau \cdot k \tag{9.12}$$

where k is the fractional rate constant (Fig. 9.3) determining transfer of indicator from hepatocyte to bile.

Substituting for Y and $Q \cdot C_v$ in equation 9.10,

$$E_s = \frac{M_\tau \cdot k}{M_\tau \cdot k + M_\tau k_2} = \frac{k}{k + k_2}. \tag{9.13}$$

(Note the similarity of this equation with equation 3.1.3.4 describing E_s in the 3-compartmental model for measurement of blood flow by PET.) Using equations 9.1 to 9.3 to calculate k and k_2, liver blood flow Q is obtainable from steady-state extraction fraction and plasma clearance Z (equation 9.7):

$$Q = Z/E_s. \qquad (9.14)$$

The right hand side of equation 9.13, $k/(k + k_2)$, is equal to E_s/E_0. Thus E_0 (the extraction efficiency at time zero) is effectively assumed to be equal to unity. This being so, liver blood flow can also be obtained from the rate constant k_1. Thus, if E_0 is 1, then assuming a negligible extravascular distribution volume,

$$k_1 = \frac{Q}{\text{total blood volume}}. \qquad (9.15)$$

Total blood volume (TBV) can be obtained by dilution from the zero time concentration and the injected activity:

$$\text{TBV} = \frac{\text{administered activity}}{(A + B)} \qquad (9.16)$$

where A and B are the zero time concentrations of the two exponentials, so

$$Q = k_1 \times \frac{\text{injected activity}}{(A + B)}. \qquad (9.17)$$

If some of the indicator diffuses from blood into the extravascular space, the distribution volume will be higher than blood volume. Nevertheless, equation 9.17 still gives liver blood flow because, provided extrahepatic equilibrium is reasonably rapid, it is also given by the product of k_1 and the distribution volume, the latter being equal to injected activity/$(A+B)$. Similarly, the use of equations 9.7, 9.13, and 9.14 will be unaffected. Thus, provided equilibration in the extravascular space is rapid, the clearance curve will still be recorded as bi-exponential from an early time after injection and equations 9.1–9.3 will be valid.

The rate constants depicted in Fig. 9.3 vary between organic anions. The blood clearance curve of indocyanine green, for example, is not obviously bi-exponential unless sampling is extended over several hours (Burns *et al.* 1991). This is consistent with a relatively high value for k compared with k_2 and explains why the initial gradient of blood clearance of this indicator has been used to measure liver blood flow without compartmental analysis.

The steady-state extraction fraction based on the kinetics of the clearance curve can be validated by measuring the ratio $(C_a - C_v)/C_a$ at the predicted time at which $dM_\tau/dt = 0$ (i.e. steady state) (Grainger *et al.* 1983). It can be appreciated from inspection of the model (Fig. 9.3a) that the time course of *hepatic* indicator M_τ is the difference between two exponentials **(Fig. 9.5)** (see Section 1.4) and is given by

$$M_\tau = -Ce^{-\alpha_1 t} + De^{-\alpha_2 t}. \qquad (9.18)$$

where C and D are the zero-time intercepts of the exponentials. The rate constants, α_1 and α_2, are the same as those in the blood clearance curve.

Since at time zero

$$M_\tau = 0,$$
$$C = D. \qquad (9.19)$$

Therefore, by differentiating,

$$dM_\tau/dt = -\alpha_1 Ce^{-\alpha_1 t} + \alpha_2 Ce^{-\alpha_2 t}. \qquad (9.20)$$

At steady state, since $dM_\tau/dt = 0$,

$$\alpha_1 Ce^{-\alpha_1 t} = \alpha_2 Ce^{-\alpha_2 t}. \qquad (9.21)$$

and after re-arrangement

$$t = \frac{\ln [\alpha_1/\alpha_2]}{\alpha_1 - \alpha_2}. \qquad (9.22)$$

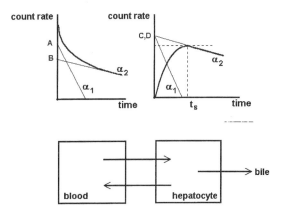

▮ **Fig. 9.5** The model shown in Fig. 9.3 predicts a *hepatocyte* time–activity curve which is the *difference* between two exponentials. Like the blood disappearance curve the hepatocyte curve approaches the slower of the two exponential curves. A steady state is transiently reached at which the rate of change of hepatocyte activity is zero. This time t_s can be determined from the rate constants of the two exponentials which are identical between blood and hepatocyte clearance curves.

So, the time after injection when hepatic concentration is maximal can be calculated from the blood disappearance curve, thereby providing validation of the compartmental technique for the measurement of liver blood flow. Thus it has been demonstrated for indocyanine green that the extraction fraction at the time of maximal liver concentration, calculated from equation 9.22, is very close to the extraction fraction measured at steady state by hepatic venous catheterization (Grainger *et al.* 1983). This also effectively validates the assumption that the initial extraction efficiency, i.e. the uni-directional extraction efficiency from blood to hepatocyte, is unity. Using IDA, the concordance between the predicted time of maximum liver activity and the recorded maximal value in the hepatic time activity curve can be demonstrated, supporting application of the model to IDA.

9.4.1.2 Liver blood flow and IDA extraction efficiency by deconvolution analysis

Another quantitative approach to the elimination of organic anions by the liver is hepatic IDA scintigraphy and deconvolution analysis, using an input function based on a cardiac region of interest. The resulting impulse response function is monoexponential (Brown *et al.* 1988) with a rate constant, α, which is the sum of k_2 and k (Fig. 9.3). In patients with impaired hepatocyte function, the impulse response function is bi-exponential with a fast initial exponential. The second exponential has a rate constant comparable to that seen in the normal mono-exponential clearance (**Fig. 9.3b**). The fast exponential has a time course compatible with hepatic vascular transit of unextracted tracer and so the y-axis intercept of the slow exponential relative to the total amplitude of the impulse response function at zero time has been interpreted to represent the hepatic extraction fraction of IDA. This is the extraction fraction from blood to hepatocyte and clearly not the steady state extraction fraction. There is little evidence of a preliminary exponential in normal subjects and in patients with biliary obstruction but otherwise normal parenchymal function, arguing in favour of an extraction efficiency from blood to hepatocyte which is normally almost 100%, as assumed by others (Clarkson *et al.* 1976, Grainger *et al.* 1983).

As described above, measurement of liver blood flow may be based on k_1, the fractional rate constant which expresses the fraction of total blood volume entering the liver in unit time or distribution volume if tracer enters the extravascular space.

An approach not influenced by extrahepatic distribution volume is to express the influx constant as hepatic clearance, i.e. (using the upper case symbol) as K_1. At steady state, when $dM_\tau/dt = 0$,

$$K_1 \cdot C_a = (k_2 + k) \cdot M_\tau. \tag{9.23}$$

But

$$k_2 + k = \alpha \tag{9.24}$$

where α is the rate constant of the impulse response curve determined by deconvolution analysis so

$$K_1 = \frac{M_\tau \cdot \alpha}{C_a}. \tag{9.25}$$

Dividing equation 9.25 by liver tissue volume V,

$$\frac{K_1}{V} = \frac{C_\tau \cdot \alpha}{C_a}. \tag{9.26}$$

If unidirectional extraction efficiency from plasma to hepatocyte is 100%, then K_1/V is hepatic perfusion which can be measured from the liver and arterial tracer concentrations at the time when the liver curve reaches its peak. Since this is no earlier than about 10 min after injection, arterial and venous tracer concentrations will have almost equalised, so C_a can be obtained from a venous sample. Using iodine-124 labelled rose bengal as the tracer, C_τ could be measured by PET using this approach, thereby enabling measurement of regional hepatic perfusion. Note that the hepatic activity needs to be corrected for the component due to the blood pool signal.

9.4.1.3 Hepatic clearance of gastro-intestinally absorbable agents

There are several compounds which are almost completely removed in one pass through the liver. These include galactose (Henderson *et al.* 1982) and D-propranolol (Feely *et al.* 1981). Unlike the organic anions described above, they do not re-enter plasma and are not excreted in bile. When given orally they are completely absorbed into the mesenteric blood and therefore provide a convenient technique for measuring liver blood flow. They generally have a high hepatic extraction efficiency but even when this is not the case the extraction efficiency can be accounted for by giving simultaneous oral and

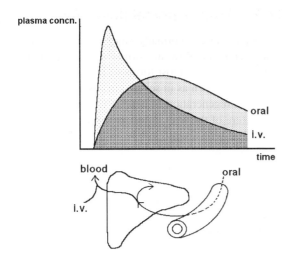

❚ **Fig. 9.6** Measurement of liver blood flow by oral and intravenous administration of a substance which is completely absorbed following oral administration and irreversibly extracted by the liver. The substance is labelled separately for oral and intravenous administration. If identical amounts are given, the difference between the respective areas under the time–plasma concentration curves from oral and intravenous administrations will depend on the fraction E of the substance extracted by the liver following oral administration. Having defined E, Q is then effectively obtained from the plasma disappearance curve since plasma clearance ($Q \cdot E$) is equal to injected activity divided by total area under the plasma clearance curve. The technique can be adapted to detect intrahepatic shunting, when E is reduced.

intravenous administered activities of the agent respectively labelled with different markers (or one labelled and the other unlabelled) (Feely *et al.* 1981).

The hepatic clearance Z of the intravenously administered activity is given by

$$Z = Q \cdot E = \frac{\text{injected activity}}{\text{AUC}_{\text{iv}}} \qquad (9.27)$$

where AUC_{iv} is the total area under the plasma time-concentration curve following the intravenous administration.

When the same amount of intravenous tracer is given orally, the area under the resulting plasma time concentration curve is less by an amount depending on how much is extracted during first pass through the liver after absorption from the gut (**Fig. 9.6**); in

fact this amount is equal to the oral administered activity multiplied by E.

Thus, combining equivalent equations for the intravenous (iv) and oral (o) administered activities,

$$\frac{\text{AUC}_{\text{o}}}{\text{AUC}_{\text{iv}}} = \frac{\text{activity}_{\text{o}} - (\text{activity})_{\text{o}} \cdot E)}{\text{activity}_{\text{iv}}} \qquad (9.28)$$

Re-arranging,

$$E = 1 - \left[\frac{\text{activity}_{\text{iv}}}{\text{activity}_{\text{o}}} \times \frac{\text{AUC}_{\text{o}}}{\text{AUC}_{\text{iv}}} \right] \qquad (9.29)$$

Substituting for E in equation 9.27, followed by re-arrangement,

$$Q = \frac{\text{activity}_{\text{iv}} \times \text{activity}_{\text{o}}}{\text{AUC}_{\text{iv}} \cdot \text{activity}_{\text{o}} - \text{AUC}_{\text{o}} \cdot \text{activity}_{\text{iv}}}. \qquad (9.30)$$

Using equation 9.30, E can be measured. It will be strongly influenced by any porto-systemic shunting that may be present, either intra- or extrahepatic (see Section 9.4.3). Obviously, the agent must not be excreted into the gut; i.e. undergo entero–hepatic circulation; this, for instance, invalidates the use of labelled bile acids or their analogues.

9.4.1.4 Colloid clearance

Colloidal particles are cleared by the liver with a high extraction efficiency and the plasma clearance is very nearly equal to liver blood flow (Shaldon *et al.* 1961). The clearance curve is mono-exponential, with a rate constant α equal to the fraction of total blood volume (TBV) cleared per minute.

Thus

$$Z = \alpha \cdot \text{TBV} \qquad (9.31)$$

and

$$\text{TBV} = \text{injected activity}/A \qquad (9.32)$$

where A is the zero time intercept of the mono-exponential time–concentration curve.

This technique has been extensively applied with various colloidal preparations. Currently available technetium-99m labelled colloids, such as sulphur colloid, tin colloid and antimony colloid, have hepatic extraction efficiencies ranging from 60–80% and do not give clearly mono-exponential curves. A source of error (promoting an over-estimation in liver blood flow) is bone marrow uptake, but this only becomes significant with liver failure. As splenic flow enters the liver, the effect of splenic uptake on colloid clearance is not immediately clear; the net effect is that a portion (approximately 250/1250 ~ 20%) of the hepatic circulation effectively has a higher extraction efficiency, since it is exposed to both hepatic and splenic phagocytes.

9.4.1.5 Inert-gas washout

The liver has been extensively studied by the technique of inert gas washout (Mathie 1986). Following injection into the liver, either via the hepatic artery or the portal vein, the clearance of inert gas is generally bi-exponential. Some studies have found a higher washout rate following portal compared with hepatic arterial injection, suggesting that the two inflows serve different vascular beds. This difference however can be accounted for by:

(1) 'contamination' of the hepatic arterial curve by portal recirculation of tracer injected into arterial branches serving the upper gastro–intestinal tract, such as the gastro–duodenal artery;

(2) accumulation of activity in gastro–intestinal gas following arterial injection.

Furthermore, like many other organ washout curves, hepatic xenon-133 washout curves may be multi-exponential. In contrast to, say, brain and kidney, there is no obvious anatomical basis for multi-exponential hepatic curves and it is likely that the slower exponentials are extra-hepatic artefacts. The sources of error mentioned above, along with a background signal from overlying pulmonary alveolar activity, can explain a multi-exponential curve. By counting krypton-85, which is a β-emitter, over the surface of the liver with a Geiger–Muller counter, thereby detecting only superficial local activity, it is possible to eliminate some of these errors. It is also possible to eliminate portal recirculation following hepatic arterial injection by tying off all non-hepatic branches of the hepatic artery. By so doing, it is possible to show identical monoexponential washout curves following both routes of injection, supporting the belief that the portal and arterial inflows mix completely upstream in the sinusoid.

9.4.2 Arterio–portal flow ratio

The hepatic artery normally supplies about 25% of total liver blood flow in normal man. The arterial supply increases in most forms of liver disease to as high as 90%, such as in severe cirrhosis. In the latter condition, regeneration of hepatic tissue disrupts the architecture of the liver, interfering more with portal inflow than with arterial inflow probably because the portal pressure is lower. Abnormal intra-hepatic shunts also develop between the portal and hepatic venous systems. The fraction of arterial blood serving the liver increases in metastatic disease because the tumours develop an exclusive arterial supply. Hepatic micro-metastases may significantly elevate the arterial fraction before otherwise becoming radiologically apparent.

9.4.2.1 Measurement of the arterio–portal ratio by first-pass kinetics

A simple technique for measuring the arterio–portal flow ratio is based on first-pass kinetics after intravenous bolus injection of a recirculating tracer. The technique rests on the principle that activity arriving via the portal vein is delayed by first passing through the splenic and mesenteric vascular beds, allowing the activity arriving via the hepatic artery to be first recorded and identified in a region of interest over the liver (Fleming *et al.* 1981). The smooth upslope gradient of the liver time–activity curve is interrupted by the arrival of isotope via the portal vein, and a new gradient is established **(Fig. 9.7)**. The arterio–portal index is taken as the ratio of the slopes before and after arrival of the portal isotope. From a quantitative point of view, the technique is fraught with difficulties and should therefore be regarded only as an index rather than a definable physiological entity. Thus:

(a) the hepatic arterial gradient is non-linear and it is uncertain if it reaches its maximum gradient before the arrival of portal activity;

(b) the gradient following arrival of portal activity reflects several processes, including residual arterial, mesenteric and splenic activities, and soon after, recirculating activity.

The gradients may be better defined from technetium-99m sulphur colloid compared with a recirculating tracer, since the ratio of the height at

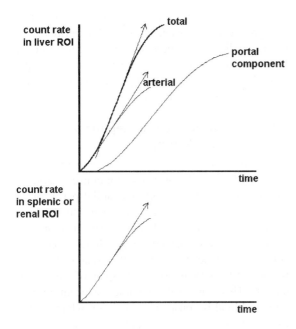

▮ **Fig. 9.7** Measurement of the arterio–portal ratio of liver blood flow from a first pass curve over the liver. Since arterial tracer arrives in the liver first, the initial gradient of the curve is proportional to arterial flow. The gradient then increases as portal tracer arrives, reaching a value proportional to total liver flow. Generating a simultaneous time–activity curve over the spleen or kidney may help to define the arterial component in the liver curve.

the inflection and the post-portal phase plateau can be used instead of the ratio of the gradients, but the sources of error are essentially the same.

By placing a region of interest over another structure such as the spleen or kidney, the time course of hepatic arterial activity can be better defined (Fleming *et al.* 1981). Thus the splenic curve can be scaled and superimposed on the hepatic arterial component so that it represents the curve that would be obtained over the liver if no portal blood was to arrive. This assumes that the transit of tracer through the spleen has an identical time course as that through the liver. The liver curve is then subtracted from the scaled splenic curve to yield the portal component of flow. Since the portal radio-activity is 'smeared' by passage through the mesenteric and splenic beds, the ratio of upslope gradients of arterial and portal components is weighted in favour of the arterial input. However this can be circumvented by comparing the areas

under the two curves by gamma function fitting since area is unaffected by bolus spreading. A variation of this approach is to apply deconvolution analysis to the first 2 or 3 minutes of the hepatic curve. This yields a bi-phasic impulse response curve which can be converted to a bi-phasic outflow curve by differentiation (see Section 2.1) and then resolved into arterial and portal components by gamma function fitting (Juni *et al.* 1986). The input curve is best obtained from the lung, since the left ventricular curve is contaminated by peaks from other structures, separated in time, as the bolus moves from venous to arterial sides of the circulation (see measurement of filtration fraction, Section 11.1.3). Although a portal venous curve would be the appropriate input function for the portal component of the hepatic curve, the lung curve, representing an arterial input, can be used for area-based measurement of the arterio–portal ratio (Juni *et al.* 1986). Thus the effect of the additional spreading of the bolus as it passes through the mesenteric and splenic beds is 'added' to the portal component curve, resulting in a flatter deconvolved curve, but not affecting the enclosed area.

9.4.2.2 Inert gas

A novel method for measuring arterial perfusion of liver, little used clinically, is to inject xenon-133 into the left ventricle or proximal aorta and then monitor the washout curve recorded over the liver (Holroyd and Peters 1980). Using the height/area approach for the calculation of mean perfusion (Section 3.1.1), it is possible to measure arterial perfusion, rather than total perfusion **(Fig. 9.8)**. The underlying theory is as follows.

If Q_a and Q_m are the hepatic arterial and portal venous blood flows respectively and V is liver volume, then

$$\frac{Q_a + Q_m}{V} = \frac{H}{A_a} \qquad (9.33)$$

where a and m refer to arterial and portal respectively, H is the initial height of the washout curve and A_a is the area under the washout curve resulting exclusively from isotope that has entered the liver via the hepatic artery. Because portal venous isotope arrives later, H is produced only by activity arriving via the hepatic artery. Note therefore that H/A_a is total liver perfusion and not arterial

▌ **Fig. 9.8** Measurement of arterial perfusion of the liver using xenon-133 injected into the left ventricle or aorta proximally to the liver arterial supply and assumed to mix before reaching it. The initial height of the curve represents arterial inflow. Dividing the initial height by the *total* area under the subsequent washout curve, which includes portal xenon, yields arterial blood flow per unit of liver tissue.

perfusion. According to the fractionation principle of blood flow measurement, assuming the tracer mixes completely above the coeliac axis; i.e. prior to its partitioning between hepatic arterial and portal circulations,

$$\frac{M_a}{M_a + M_m} = \frac{Q_a}{Q_a + Q_m} \qquad (9.34)$$

where M refers to quantity of radionuclide.

Now it is also true that

$$\frac{Q_a}{Q_a + Q_m} = \frac{A_a}{A_a + A_m} \qquad (9.35)$$

where A_m is the area under the washout curve contributed by portal isotope. By re-arrangement and substitution,

$$\frac{Q_a}{V} = \frac{H}{A_a + A_m}. \qquad (9.36)$$

In other words, the *arterial* perfusion of liver is equal to the initial height divided by the *total* area under the washout curve. The technique is invasive and has a rather high background because of the proximal injection of gas. Nevertheless as the liver

projects a large area, it is possible to avoid this background signal to a great extent. Furthermore, the theory applies to any perfusion-dependent tracer so, if recirculation could be corrected, the technique could be made non-invasive by using an intravenous bolus of oxygen-15 labelled water.

9.4.2.3 Measurement of hepatic arterial blood flow by PET

Continuous infusion of the short-lived tracers oxygen-15 labelled water and rubidium-82, as used for measuring cerebral and myocardial perfusion at steady state, are not readily applicable to the liver because of its dual blood supply. The fundamental principle of continuous infusion of these tracers is to compare residence time within the organ ($=V/Q$, see Section 2.1) with physical life-span of the radio-nuclide. This requires that the tracer concentration in afferent blood is constant, a condition which is met for organs with an arterial supply only. In the case of the liver however the portal supply will have a lower concentration than the hepatic artery as a result of physical decay during transit through the mesenteric and splenic vascular beds.

Hepatic arterial blood flow can be measured by PET using an intra-venous bolus injection of nitrogen-13 labelled ammonia (Chen *et al.* 1991). Since this tracer is largely cleared from portal blood or delayed during transit through the mesenteric or splenic beds, hepatic arterial perfusion is measured, rather than total perfusion. The technique is similar to the measurement of myocardial blood flow with labelled ammonia.

Thus, if E is the hepatic extraction fraction of ammonia and M_τ the quantity of radioactivity accumulated in the liver, through its arterial supply then

$$Q_a \cdot E = \frac{M_\tau(t)}{\int C_a(t) \cdot dt}. \qquad (9.37)$$

If the relationship between E and Q_a can be established then, as for myocardial blood flow, the hepatic permeability surface area product (PS) for ammonia[†] can be derived from

$$PS = -Q \cdot \ln(1 - E). \qquad (9.38)$$

Because of the liver's dual blood supply the

[†]Although the sinusoidal endothelium is fenestrated and must therefore be highly permeable to the ammonium ion, *PS* product is applied to the efficiency of uptake in the hepatocyte and not to the endothelial permeability.

sinusoidal tracer concentration falls as a result of dilution as well as tracer extraction and so PS, Q and E in equation 9.38 have to be redefined for tracers arriving only via the hepatic artery. Two possibilities can be considered: hepatic arterial and portal venous flows mixing (i) within, or (ii) proximal to the sinusoid.

(i) Assuming an exponential decrease in tracer concentration along the sinusoid (Section 6.2.2.1), (**Fig. 9.9**) then

$$PSC_p = Q_aC_a - (Q_aC_v + Q_mC_v) \quad (9.39)$$

where C_p is mean sinusoidal concentration as in Section 6.2.2.1. Therefore

$$PS = -Q_a\frac{(C_a - C_v)}{C_p} - Q_m\frac{C_v}{C_p}. \quad (9.40)$$

From equations 6.8 and 6.17 we can then say

$$PS = -Q_a \ln(1 - E) - Q_m\frac{C_v}{C_p} \quad (9.41)$$

(noting that because C_v is influenced by dilution with portal blood E measured as $(C_a - C_v)/C_a$ is greater than the fraction of incoming tracer actually extracted). From equations 6.8, 6.10 and 6.17 again, $PS/Q = \ln(1 - E) = (C_a - C_v)/C_p = E/C_p$ and $C_v = 1 - E$ then

$$PS = -Q_a \ln(1 - E) - Q_m\frac{(1 - E)}{E/\ln(1 - E)} \quad (9.42)$$

(ii) If the arterial tracer is diluted by portal blood *immediately* on entering the liver, followed by an exponential decrease along the sinusoid as a result of tracer uptake, then equation 9.38 is appropriate, except that Q is now total liver flow Q_{a+m} and E scaled down by Q_a/Q_{a+m} (**Fig. 9.10**):

$$PS = -Q_{a+m} \ln(1 - [E \cdot Q_a/Q_{a+m}]). \quad (9.43)$$

The purpose of these equations is to illustrate the effect of dual inflow on the derivation of PS with respect to the liver, especially relevant to PET. Nevertheless, if E is close to unity we can say

$$\frac{Q_a}{V} = \frac{C_\tau}{\int C_a(t) \cdot dt} \quad (9.44)$$

If tracer extraction in the vascular bed drained by the portal vein is significantly incomplete, the resulting

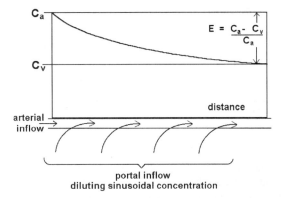

▌ **Fig. 9.9** The effect on the measurement of hepatic arterial perfusion, (for a substance which is delayed or extracted in the mesenteric / splenic beds) of progressive dilution of the arterial inflow along the sinusoid. Apparent E is then a function not only of tracer extraction but sinusoidal dilution from incoming portal blood.

error in equation 9.44 can be minimized by limiting the time (t) of acquisition.

The two-compartmental model used to measure myocardial blood flow using nitrogen-13 labelled ammonia has also been applied to the measurement of hepatic arterial flow. The mathematics are almost identical, except for the differential equation defining the rate of change of free activity, $M_f (= C_f \cdot V)$ (see Section 3.1.3.2 and 7.1.1.2). In the case of the liver, the hepatic arterial and portal inflows serve a common sinusoidal bed, so tracer freely distributed between plasma and interstitial fluid at concentration C_f, has an input $Q_a \cdot C_a$ but is washed out by total liver flow, Q_{a+m} (**Fig. 9.10**), so therefore,

$$\frac{dC_f}{dt} = \frac{Q_a}{V} \cdot C_a - (K_1 + Q_{a+m}/V)\frac{C_f}{V_1/V}. \quad (9.45)$$

In other words, there is a further unknown compared with myocardial flow and the complexity is beyond this text (cf. equation 3.39).

9.4.3 Porto-systemic shunting

Porto-systemic shunting results from portal hypertension. Normally the entire mesenteric and splenic outflows pass through the liver. Obstruction between the portal and hepatic venous systems results in

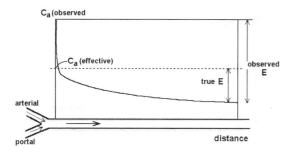

∎ **Fig. 9.10** The effect on the measurement of hepatic *PS* product (for a substance which is delayed or extracted in the mesenteric/splenic beds) of dilution of the arterial inflow proximal to the sinusoid. Effective or true *E* is equal to apparent or observed *E* multiplied by the arterial fraction of total hepatic inflow ($Q_a/[Q_a + Q_m]$), so

$$PS = -[Q_a + Q_m] \cdot \ln(1 - [E \cdot Q_a/[Q_a + Q_m]])$$

where subscripts 'a' and 'm' refer to arterial and portal respectively.

portal hypertension and the development of collaterals between the two systems. The sites of these collaterals include lower oesophagus, resulting in oesophageal varices, the anterior abdominal wall, where the collaterals may be visible, and the haemorrhoidal plexus. Porto-systemic shunting may also take place within the liver itself. Porto-systemic shunting is important not only because of the haemodynamic disturbances, which may result in serious bleeding, but also because bioactive substances, absorbed from the gastrointestinal tract and normally taken up by the liver, gain access to the systemic circulation and may cause hepatic encephalopathy.

Quantification of the fraction of portal venous blood bypassing the liver is difficult. Agents which undergo almost complete extraction, and retention, after one pass through the liver, and which are completely absorbed from the gut, have been mentioned above for measuring hepatic blood flow (Section 9.4.1.3) and, using equation 9.29, can be applied to shunt flow measurement assuming hepatic cellular extraction is not significantly reduced. *Intrahepatic* shunting can be quantified, using the same assumption, by deconvolution analysis of IDA scintigraphy which in severe liver disease generates an impulse response curve with an early rapid exponential thought to represent transit of unextracted intravascular tracer. Another approach is to

inject radio-labelled microspheres directly into the portal circulation and to count the radioactivity accumulating in the lung. The lung counts can be calibrated by an intravenous injection of a known administered activity of radio-labelled microspheres, which represents 100% shunting. Less invasive alternatives are to inject agents into the splenic pulp or to instil them in a segment of the gastro–intestinal tract from where they will be absorbed into a tributary of the portal circulation. Clearly it would be desirable for the agent to be completely extracted in both the hepatic nutrient capillary bed and the lungs. The porto-systemic shunt is then reflected by the amount of lung activity, which can be calibrated in terms of the fraction of the administered activity by a separate intravenous administered activity of the same agent. Radiopharmaceuticals that have been used include xenon-133 (which because of a delay in the hepatic vascular bed behaves to some extent like a microsphere), iodine-123 labelled iodoamphetamine and the potassium analogue, thallium-201. Since image resolution of the lungs is not a requirement for this approach, the use of nitrogen-13 labelled ammonia, in conjunction with scintillation probe counting over the lung, should be possible. A potential problem with this general approach is that *pulmonary* arterio–venous shunts may develop in association with cirrhosis of the liver.

9.5 Tests of gastro–intestinal permeability and absorption

Measurements of gastro–intestinal iron and calcium absorption are presented in the sections on haematology (Section 10.2.1.1) and bone (Section 13.2.3) respectively. In this section consideration will be given to techniques for quantifying absorption of sugars and bile acids, and diseases which result in the abnormal transfer of molecules from (a) gut to blood and (b) blood to gut.

9.5.1 Gastro–intestinal protein loss

Gastro–intestinal protein loss can be localized and/or measured using techniques analogous to those available for GI bleeding. Thus injection of chromium-51 labelled albumin followed by faecal chromium-51 counting can be used for measuring faecal protein loss, similarly to chromium-51 labelled red cells for measuring GI blood loss. As with GI bleeding, it may be more important to *localize* the site of protein loss within the GI tract when the underlying pathology, such as lymphoma, Whipple's disease or lymphangectasia, is focal. Protein then has to be labelled with a gamma-emitting radionuclide. Technetium-99m albumin gives images of high resolution, but the radionuclide binding is not sufficiently stable for imaging beyond a few hours after injection. Technetium-99m IgG is perhaps a preferable alternative. Another approach uses indium-111 labelled transferrin, which has about the same molecular size as albumin and a similar biological turnover. An advantage of indium-111 is that the imaging study can be combined with quantification of protein loss, either by faecal counting or, preferably, using the uncollimated gamma camera, as in the measurement of faecal indium-111 labelled granulocyte excretion (Carpani *et al.* 1996; Section 10.3.4). Indium-111 does not bind to transferrin as tightly as it does to cells. Since free indium-111 is taken up by the reticulo–endothelial system, rather than being excreted, this approach probably underestimates protein loss. Iodine-131 is a theoretical alternative for whole body quantification, although this radionuclide has the disadvantage, along with chromium-51, of undergoing urinary excretion after metabolism and dissociation from the protein, overestimating gut protein loss. Indium-111, in contrast, does not gain access to the urine.

9.5.2 Bile-acid absorption

The bile acids are synthesized in the liver from cholesterol, and, after conjugation to either glycine or taurine as bile salts, secreted in bile into the gut where they are involved in lipid absorption. The primary bile acids are cholic and chenodeoxycholic acids, the majority of which are re-absorbed in the terminal ileum by an active transport mechanism and are returned to the liver for re-conjugation and biliary secretion. The secondary bile acids are formed in the gut from the primary acids — deoxycholic from cholic and lithocholic from chenodeoxycholic — by dehydroxylation in the

presence of gut bacteria. This is physiological in the colon but pathological in the small bowel. The secondary bile acids are passively re-absorbed from the colon, re-conjugated in the liver and added to the bile acid pool. The cycle of secretion into and re-absorption from the gut is known as the entero–hepatic circulation. The high extraction efficiency of bile acids, by the liver from portal venous blood and by the enterocytes from gut, maintains the great majority of the bile acids within the enterohepatic circulation. Bile acids entering the systemic circulation are bound to albumin, which minimizes glomerular filtration and promotes their return to the liver. Any filtered acid is re-absorbed by the tubule, so the urine, like the feces, contains almost no bile acid.

Bile acids are lost from the body as a result of impaired absorption in the terminal ileum. A technique for the quantification of bile acid loss is the measurement of the whole body retention of a radiolabelled bile acid or analogue, given either intravenously or orally. Cholic acid can be labelled with carbon-14, but this requires faecal collection and measurement of the label by liquid scintillation counting. Alternatively, and more conveniently, bile acid retention may be quantified with an analogue of cholic acid, homocholic acid conjugated with taurine and labelled with selenium-75 (SeHCAT) (Merrick *et al.* 1982). Along with its metabolites SeHCAT is handled in humans similarly to the natural bile acids and their metabolites and, accordingly, is not excreted in urine. Whole body retention can be followed over time by whole body counting, either with a conventional whole body counter similarly to iron-59 absorption or an uncollimated gamma camera as with indium-111 granulocyte and protein loss measurement. Normally more than 20% of an administered activity of SeHCAT, given orally or intravenously, is retained at 7 days after administration. SeHCAT is more resistant to deconjugation and dehydroxylation than taurocholate, and may, by being less readily absorbed from the colon than the secondary bile acids, more sensitively and specifically reflect terminal ileal disease.

Because of a first pass hepatic extraction efficiency which is at least as high as that of other organic anions, bile acids, including SeHCAT, can be interchanged with bromosulphthalein and indocyanine green for the measurement of liver blood flow following intravenous injection (Gilmore and

Thompson 1981). Carbon-14 labelled cholic acid can also be used for this. The conjugated bile acids are extracted with a slightly greater efficiency by the liver than the unconjugated. Thus glycocholic acid has an extraction fraction in normal subjects of about 90% whereas for the secondary bile acid, deoxycholic acid, it is only about 70%.

9.5.3 Gastro–intestinal handling of sugars

The handling of small carbohydrates by the gut depends on molecular size. Small molecules such as mannitol (molecular weight, 182 Da) are passively absorbed through small pores in the lipid membrane of the enterocyte, whereas larger molecules, such as lactulose, a disaccharide of molecular weight 342 Da, and chromium-51 EDTA (molecular weight, 390 Da) are absorbed passively via the paracellular route. The gastro–intestinal epithelium, like the renal tubular epithelium, is very impermeable to solutes of this size, and normally less than 5% of an oral administered activity of chromium-51 EDTA can be recovered in the urine; absorption of solutes of this size is therefore *increased* in gastrointestinal disease. In contrast, physiological absorption in the monosaccharide size range is much greater and proportional to the surface area of the gut, so that, in disease, their absorption is *reduced*. This divergence in absorption characteristics has led to the combined oral administration of two solutes, one of each size, with measurement of their urinary concentration ratio. In theory, this circumvents problems associated with the ingestion of only one solute, namely variation in gastric emptying rate and renal function.

The use of dual markers to assess gut epithelial function relies on identical extravascular distributions, urinary handling and distribution of absorption sites throughout the gut. For example, if the latter is different for the two markers, their urinary concentration ratio will be dependent on the time after oral administration. Lactulose, mannitol and chromium-51 EDTA have all been shown to have identical renal handling after intravenous injection, all giving values for glomerular filtration rate within a few ml per min of each other (Elia *et al.* 1987). However, when given orally, the amounts of the substances accumulated between defined time intervals after ingestion vary between one another in a way that suggests that they are not absorbed from identical regions of the gut.

Many studies of intestinal integrity have relied on the use of one tracer only, usually chromium-51 EDTA, and have been based on the percentage of an oral administered activity accumulated in the urine up to 24 hr after ingestion. For EDTA, abnormal values up to 15% are recorded in patients with various enteropathies, such as Crohn's disease, chronic alcoholism and in chronic users of non-steroidal anti-inflammatory drugs. Typical normal values in spot urine samples for the *dual* marker approach are less than 0.01 (disaccharide/monosaccharide) normalized to administered activities, rising to as high as 0.15 in disease. An interesting finding in Crohn's disease is a correlation between an increase in intestinal permeability to ingested chromium-51 EDTA and an increase in pulmonary epithelial permeability to a similar molecule, technetium-99m DTPA, inhaled as an aerosol, suggesting a common mucosal abnormality.

References

Bradley SE, Inglefinger FJ, Bradley GP and Currey JJ. The estimation of hepatic blood flow in man. *Journal of Clinical Investigation* 1945, **24**: 890–7.

Brown PH, Juni JE, Lieberman DA and Krishnamurthy GT. Hepatocyte versus biliary disease; a distinction by deconvolutional analysis of technetium-99m IDA time-activity curves. *Journal of Nuclear Medicine* 1988, **29**: 623–30.

Burns E, Triger DR, Tucker GT and Bax DS. Indocyanine green elimination in patients with liver disease and in normal subjects. *Clinical Science* 1991, **80**: 155–60.

Carpani de Kaski M, Peters AM, Bradley D and Hodgson HJF. Detection and quantification of protein-losing enteropathy with indium-111 transferrin. *European Journal of Nuclear Medicine* 1996, **23**: 530–3.

Chen BC, Huang S-C, Germano G, Kuhle W, Hawkins RA, Buxton D, Brunken RC, Schelbert HR and Phelps ME. Non-invasive quantification of hepatic arterial blood flow with nitrogen-13 ammonia and dynamic positron emission tomography. *Journal of Nuclear Medicine* 1991, **32**: 2199–206.

Chervu LR, Nunn AD and Loberg MD. Radiopharmaceuticals for hepatobiliary imaging. *Seminars in Nuclear Medicine* 1982, **12**: 5–17.

Clarkson MJ, Hardy-Smith A and Richards TG. Measurement of liver blood flow by means of a single injection of bromosulphthalein without hepatic vein catheterization. *Clinical Science* 1976, **55**: 141–50.

Elia M, Behrens R, Northrop C, Wraight P and Neale G. Evaluation of mannitol, lactulose, and ^{51}Cr-labelled ethylenediaminetetra-acetate as markers of intestinal permeability. *Clinical Science* 1987, **73**: 197–204.

Fleming JS, Humphries NLM, Karran SJ, Goddard BA and Ackery DM. *In vivo* assessment of hepatic arterial and portal venous components of liver perfusion. *Journal of Nuclear Medicine* 1981, **22**: 18–21.

Feely J, Wilkinson GR and Wood AJJ. Reduction of liver blood flow and propranolol metabolism by cimetidine. *New England Journal of Medicine* 1981, **304**: 692–5.

Gibson CJ and Bateson MC. A parametric image technique for the assessment of oesophageal function. *Nuclear Medicine Communications* 1985, **6**: 83–9.

Gilmore IT and Thompson RPH. Direct measurement of hepatic extraction of bile acids in subjects with and without liver disease. *Clinical Science* 1981, **60**: 65–72.

Grainger SL, Keeling PWN, Brown IMH, Marigold JH and Thompson RPH. Clearance and non-invasive determination of the hepatic extraction of indocyanine green in baboons and man. *Clinical Science* 1983, **64**: 207–12.

Henderson MJ, Kutner M and Bain RP. First-order clearance of plasma galactose: the effect of liver disease. *Gastroenterology* 1982, **83**: 1090–6.

Holroyd AM and Peters AM. Measurement of arterial perfusion of the liver in man. *British Journal of Surgery* 1980, **67**: 179–81.

Juni JE, Rechle R, Pitt S and Meyers L. Quantitative measurement of hepatic artery and portal vein blood flow by deconvolution analysis. *Journal of Nuclear Medicine*, 1986, **27**: 957.

Mathie RT. Hepatic blood flow measurement with inert gas clearance. *Journal of Surgical Research* 1986, **41**: 92–110.

Merrick MV, Eastwood MA, Anderson JR and Ross HM. Enterohepatic circulation in man of a gamma-emitting bile acid conjugate 23-selena-25-homotaurocholic acid (SeHCAT). *Journal of Nuclear Medicine* 1982, **23**: 126–30.

Notghi A, Kumar D, Panagamuwa B, Tulley NJ, Hesslewood S and Harding LK. Measurement of colonic transit time using radionuclide imaging: analysis by condensed images. *Nuclear Medicine Communications* 1993, **14**: 204–11.

Shaldon S, Chiandussi L, Guevara L, Caesar J and Sherlock SJ. The estimation of hepatic blood flow intrahepatic blood flow by colloidal heat-denatured human serum albumin labeled with I-131. *Jounal of Clinical Investigation* 1961, **40**: 1346–54.

Tolin RD, Malmud LS and Reilley J. Esophageal scintigraphy to quantitate esophageal transit. *Gastroenterology* 1979, **76**: 1402–8.

Urbain J-LC and Charkes ND. Recent advances in gastric emptying scintigraphy. *Seminars in Nuclear Medicine* 1995, **25**: 318–25.

10 Haematology and the spleen

Introduction

Most of the subject matter relating to radionuclides and haematology covers blood cell kinetics. The most widely used techniques for the quantification of blood cell kinetics involve tagging the cells of interest with a radioactive marker for the quantification of cell traffic, either from blood sampling alone or, more usefully, in combination with external scintigraphic monitoring. In general, blood cells can be labelled either as a cohort (cohort labelling) or following isolation from peripheral blood, in which case they are sampled at random (random labelling). By cohort labelling is meant the simultaneous labelling, usually *in vivo*, of a cohort of cells all of the same age and at the same stage of development. It is generally achieved by the incorporation of a radiolabelled structural component of the cell, for example radio-iron for labelling red cells or selenium-75-labelled selenomethionine (an amino acid) for other cell types. Because it is based on a single peripheral blood sample, random labelling, which is more widely used than cohort labelling, involves the tagging of cells with a wide age range, including cells immediately released from bone marrow and senescent cells which are about to be removed from the circulation. It is helpful to divide blood cell kinetics into the kinetics of: (i) production; (ii) distribution; (iii) intravascular residence; (iv) destruction or extravascular kinetics after removal from the circulation.

10.1 Platelet kinetics

10.1.1 Platelet production

Under the stimulus of thrombopoeitin, platelets are produced in the bone marrow from megakaryocytes, which are large multinucleate cells. The marrow can increase platelet production in response to thrombocytopaenia but its limit, about four-fold the normal production rate, is less than the equivalent limits for red cell and granulocyte production, which are about ten-fold increases. The signal for increasing platelet production, mediated through thrombopoetin, is not well understood. The main afferent arm of the signal appears to be platelet biomass (i.e. the product of whole body mean platelet volume and whole body platelet count) rather than the peripheral circulating platelet count. Thus biomass may be relatively normal in the presence of thrombocytopaenia (for example in splenomegaly, see below), in which case the thrombocytopaenia remains uncorrected. An alternative view of platelet production has been proposed by Slater *et al.* (1983). Based on mathematical considerations of the distribution of platelet volume, which is log-normal, and the putative findings of intact megakaryocytes in right atrial but not arterial blood, they suggested that platelets are generated in the pulmonary circulation by impaction and subsequent fragmentation of megakaryocytes colliding with the 'buttress' vascular walls of the branching points of pulmonary arterioles.

The platelet production rate can be assessed from the rate of incorporation of selenium-75-selenomethionine into a cohort. This is seldom performed and it is easier to calculate the platelet production rate (PP) indirectly from the peripheral circulating platelet count (PC) and mean platelet life span in the circulation (MPLS) the measurement of which is described below (Section 10.1.3). Thus

$$PP = \frac{PC}{MPLS}.$$
(10.1)

This generates PP in units of cells produced per day per litre of blood. Because a considerable fraction SP_p of the circulating platelet population is pooled in the spleen (see Section 10.1.2) equation 10.1 has to be corrected for this as follows:

$$PP = \frac{PC}{MPLS} \times \frac{1}{1 - SP_P}.$$

10.1.2 Platelet distribution and the splenic platelet pool

A remarkable property of the spleen is its ability to pool blood cells; i.e. to impose a delay in their intravascular transit. Platelets and granulocytes, for example, take on average about 10 minutes to transit the spleen. Although not directly studied, because they are difficult to label, lymphocytes and monocytes probably also undergo a similar transit time of about 10 minutes (Allsop *et al.* 1992). Red cells are faster with a transit time of about one minute, though still significantly slower than in other organs. It seems therefore that the spleen delays all cells to about the same degree, except red cells. If red cells however are damaged, such as by heating, then they also undergo a transit of about 10 minutes. Plasma has a relatively fast transit time insofar as the intrasplenic haematocrit is considerably higher than the average for the whole body. The spleen can therefore be regarded as a 'cell sorter', with each component of inflowing blood being treated independently.

The route taken through the spleen by blood cells explains these times to some extent. After delivery to the splenic sinusoids via the arterial inflow, cells gain access to the splenic veins by passing through fenestrations in the sinusoidal endothelium (**Fig. 10.1**). As cell deformation is required for passage, rigid cells are delayed. Furthermore rigid intracellular inclusions, such as Heinz bodies, in otherwise non-rigid cells, are pinched off by the sinusoidal wall. This is how red cells are culled in the spleen and rigid inclusion bodies removed. This mechanism does not however entirely explain why platelets, which are much smaller, are retained.

It would clearly not be an advantage if red cells were subjected to the same transit time as other blood cells, as the 'queue' would lead to gross splenomegaly. Nevertheless, when the leucocyte count becomes markedly elevated, as in leukaemia, the spleen does become enlarged because leucocyte transit time remains at 10 minutes, with resulting severe 'passive' congestion. it remains physiologically unexplained why blood cells spend so much of their intravascular life span in the spleen, nor are the mechanisms understood.

10.1.2.1 Splenic blood flow

Measurement of splenic blood flow is considered here because one method of measuring it is based on

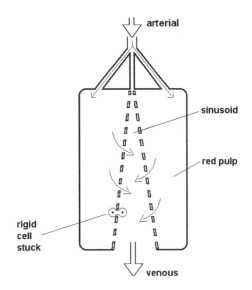

▮ **Fig. 10.1** Cartoon of splenic sinusoid. In the human spleen, 90% of the arterial inflow is delivered to the pulp from where it reaches the sinusoid by passing through gaps between the sinusoidal endothelial cells. The gaps are smaller than red cells and leucocytes which are therefore required to deform in order to negotiate the fenestrations. Rigid inclusion bodies within red cells, for example, such as Heinz bodies, are nipped off the trailing end of the red cell as it passes through, a process known as culling. The average transit time of normal red cells through the spleen is about one minute but this increases to 10–15 minutes if the cell is made rigid such as by heating (heat damaged red blood cells HDRBC). Leucocytes have a transit time of about 10 minutes. Plasma transits in about 30 seconds, so splenic haematocrit is high. In spite of a diameter comparable to that of the sinusoidal fenestration, a platelet also has a transit time of about 10 minutes. The spleen is therefore an excellent blood cell sorter and the term splenic blood volume has a rather special meaning as all the formed elements have different transit times.

the kinetics of platelet pooling within the spleen (Peters *et al.* 1980). Two other approaches have also been used: xenon-133 washout and first pass techniques. A further method, based on heat damaged red cell clearance, is in principle, similar to the method based on platelet pooling. Techniques based on positron emission tomography have not been applied to the spleen.

10.1.2.1.1 Splenic blood flow by measurement of platelet input

Following intravenous injection, radio-labelled platelets enter the splenic platelet pool. As a result of

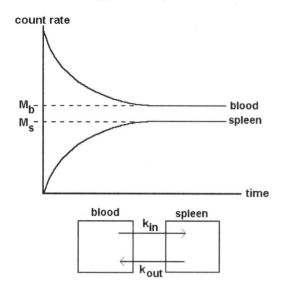

∎ Fig. 10.2 Measurement of splenic blood flow based on platelet pooling in the spleen. Platelet distribution can be represented by a closed two-compartmental model. The rate constant of transfer from blood to spleen k_{in} is equal to splenic blood flow SBF per unit of total blood volume. The reciprocal of k_{out} is the mean residence time of platelets in the spleen. At equilibrium, achieved about 20 minutes after injection, the partition of labelled platelets between blood and spleen, given by M_b/M_s, is equal to k_{out}/k_{in}. The rate constant of equilibration is equal to the sum of $k_{in} + k_{out}$. k_{in} can therefore be measured using these two equations.

platelet equilibration between circulating blood and the pool, the time activity curves of intravascular platelet-associated activity and intrasplenic activity are mirror images of each other, following the same exponential time course (**Fig. 10.2**). The rate constant of these exponential curves k is equal to the sum of the rate constants of input into and output from the spleen, k_{in} and k_{out} (see below). The input rate constant is the fraction of circulating platelets transferred from blood to spleen per unit of time and is therefore equal to splenic blood flow divided by total blood volume (TBV), while the output rate constant is the fraction of platelets in the splenic pool that re-enter the circulation per unit of time (Peters *et al.* 1980). The reciprocal of k_{out} is the mean residence (or transit) time of platelets in the spleen, while the reciprocal of k_{in} is the average time a platelet spends in the circulation before it returns to the splenic platelet pool. These kinetics can be formulated in two differential equations:

$$\frac{dM_s}{dt} = k_{in} M_b - k_{out} M_s \quad (10.2)$$

and

$$\frac{dM_b}{dt} = k_{out} M_s - k_{in} M_b \quad (10.3)$$

where M_s and M_b are the quantities of platelets respectively in the blood and spleen. If all the injected platelets were distributed and exchanging between the spleen and blood only (an assumption discussed below in this Section), then

$$M_0 = M_s + M_b \quad (10.4)$$

where M_0 is the injected dose.

Substituting for M_s in the differential equations and defining that at $t = 0$, $M_b = M_0$ and $M_s = 0$, the differential equations can be solved to give

$$M_b = M_0 \frac{k_{out}}{(k_{in} + k_{out})} + \\ M_0 \frac{k_{in}}{(k_{in} + k_{out})} (e^{-[k_{in} + k_{out}]t}) \quad (10.5)$$

and

$$M_s = M_0 \frac{k_{in}}{(k_{in} + k_{out})} (1 - e^{-[k_{in} + k_{out}]t}). \quad (10.6)$$

The derivation of these equations is shown in Section 1.4 as an example of the general situation of a closed two-compartmental model.

The reader needs only understand these two equations to the extent that they indicate that the time–activity curves for both spleen and blood pool have the same exponential term; in other words, the rate constant of equilibration (k_{eq}) recorded following injection of labelled platelets is equal to ($k_{in} + k_{out}$) and is the rate constant of both splenic uptake and blood disappearance towards their asymptotic values.

The rate k_{eq} can be measured from time–activity curves recorded either from a region of interest over the heart (reflecting the blood pool) or spleen. It is more accurately measured from the latter because:

(a) more counts are recorded from the spleen;
(b) it is less influenced by intravascular mixing and by early hepatic uptake (see below, this Section).

The ratio of k_{in} to k_{out} can then be measured from the partition of platelets between blood and spleen at equilibrium, when the rate of inflow of platelets into the spleen is equal to the rate of outflow. Thus since

$$M_b \times k_{in} = M_s \times k_{out} \qquad (10.7)$$

$$\frac{k_{in}}{k_{out}} = \frac{M_s}{M_b} \qquad (10.8)$$

where M_s/M_b is obtained from the blood pool curve as shown in Fig. 10.2. Platelets pooling in the liver equilibrate with blood platelets within about three minutes and damaged platelets are probably removed as quickly. The assumption that platelets distribute between only the spleen and blood therefore holds good from about four minutes after injection and this allows ample time to observe the splenic equilibration curve without interference from platelet uptake in the liver. In order to obtain M_s/M_b, the blood curve can be extrapolated back from four minutes either by conventional extrapolation on semilogarithmic replot (after subtraction of the asymptote) or by using the splenic curve (**Fig. 10.3**).

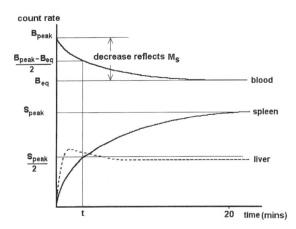

▌ **Fig. 10.3** Correction for hepatic uptake in the measurement of splenic blood flow from the kinetics of platelet equilibration. It is easier and less open to error to measure M_s from the blood curve rather than by quantitative splenic imaging. M_s is the difference between the equilibrium value and the zero time value in the curve recorded from a cardiac region of interest. Since the observed difference (based on the zero time value actually recorded) will be influenced by hepatic uptake, the zero time value is obtained indirectly, either by extrapolation of the cardiac curve to zero time from about 5 minutes or by using the splenic curve in which the increase in any segment is proportionally matched to the decrease in the cardiac curve between the same time points (0 and t).

Note that k_{in} is SBF/TBV. Because of minimal hepatic pooling, the measured TBV will include a liver blood volume which effectively includes the hepatic platelet pool; i.e. will be greater than 'true' TBV. In fact there are about 1.5 times as many platelets per ml in the hepatic vasculature as in central blood, so the apparent TBV is equal to (true TBV + [0.5 × LBV]). Assuming a liver blood volume of 10% of TBV, this will give an error in TBV of about 5%. Normal values for SBF/TBV are about 0.045, corresponding to an SBF of 250 ml/ minute (assuming a TBV of 5 litres).

10.1.2.1.2 Splenic blood flow measured by xenon washout

Xenon-133 washout has been used to measure splenic perfusion (Williams *et al.* 1968). The washout curve is essentially mono-exponential. The partition coefficient is normally taken to be 0.7. Normal values by this method are about 100 ml/ 100 ml/min.

10.1.2.1.3 Splenic blood flow measured by fractionation of cardiac output

Two first-pass approaches are possible, one using radio-labelled platelets (Peters *et al.* 1984a) or heat damaged red cells (Peters *et al.* 1982), the other using any recirculating radiopharmaceutical.

When radio-labelled platelets or heat damaged red cells are injected intravenously as a bolus, they enter the spleen, and are held up long enough for a brief plateau of activity to be seen from about 30 seconds after injection. Assuming that this plateau results from a transient cell extraction efficiency of 100% before pooled cells leave the spleen, then the principle of cardiac output (CO) fractionation can be adopted. Thus by measuring the dose and correcting for photon attenuation from the spleen, SBF/CO can be measured. Because of the shape of the spleen this attenuation correction is difficult. A modification of the technique, using platelets, which circumvents the need for attenuation correction and dose measurement, is to compare the splenic count rate N_s on first pass with the equilibrium count rate (i.e. after equilibration of platelets between spleen and blood). Thus

$$\gamma \cdot N_{s1} = M_{s1} \qquad (10.9)$$

where subscript 1 refers to first pass and the proportionality constant γ relates count rate to amount of activity M_s present. At equilibrium

$$\gamma N_s = M_s \qquad (10.10)$$

Now

$$\frac{SBF}{CO} = \frac{M_{s1}}{M_0} \qquad (10.11)$$

but

$$M_0 = M_s + M_b$$

so

$$\frac{SBF}{CO} = \gamma N_{s1} \times \frac{1}{M_s + M_b}. \qquad (10.12)$$

Substituting γ with M_s/N_s,

$$\frac{SBF}{CO} = \frac{N_{s1}}{N_s} \times \frac{M_s}{M_s + M_b} \qquad (10.13)$$

Note that M_s/M_b can be obtained from the blood pool curve, as described above (Fig. 10.3). Note also that this approach ignores the hepatic uptake; i.e. it assumes $M_s + M_b = M_0$, and therefore introduces an error of about 5%.

The fraction of cardiac output supplying the spleen can also be measured using the technique described in Section 11.1.1.3 for measurement of renal blood flow as a fraction of cardiac output. This approach has been used in measurement of splenic perfusion by dynamic CT, and has given results for perfusion similar to those published in the literature using radionuclide techniques (Miles *et al.* 1991). The attraction of dynamic CT is that, because the attenuation constant in soft tissue is such that one Hounsfield unit is equivalent to an iodine concentration of 25 mg/ml, it is, like PET, able to quantify tissue concentration of 'tracer' (i.e. elemental iodine) in absolute units. The theory of this technique is further discussed in Section 3.3.

10.1.2.1.4 Splenic blood flow measured from heat damaged red cell clearance

The kinetics of heat damaged red cell (HDRBC) distribution are qualitatively almost identical to those of platelet distribution. Following intravenous injection, HDRBC enter the splenic pool. On each pass in the normal subject, about half of the incoming HDRBC re-enter the circulation from this pool while the other half are trapped irreversibly (Peters *et al.* 1982). In other words, each HDRBC that enters the spleen has a probability of about 0.5 of irreversible entrapment. Eventually, all the HDRBC are irreversibly trapped and some hours after entrapment

undergo erythro-phagocytosis by splenic macrophages (Klausner *et al.* 1975). The HDRBC that are not irreversibly trapped on any one pass take on average, about 10 minutes to get out of the spleen (i.e. the mean intrasplenic transit time of HDRBC is about 10 minutes). In other words, reversibly trapped HDRBC undergo splenic pooling. The qualitative similarity with platelets may not immediately be obvious until it is considered that platelets are also destroyed in the spleen at the end of their normal life span and so a platelet entering the splenic pool also has a certain probability that it will remain irreversibly trapped. However, in this case, the probability (in the normal subject) is tiny compared with HDRBC, since normal mean platelet life span is 9 days, compared with an HDRBC mean life span in blood of about 1 hour.

Application of compartmental analysis to a model based on this distribution generates transfer rate constants for k_{in}, k_{out} and k (**Fig. 10.4**) in terms of the

In blood HDRBC counts

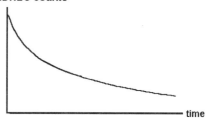

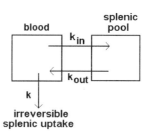

▌ **Fig. 10.4** Measurement of splenic blood flow using heat damaged red blood cells. HDRBC distribution can be represented by a two-compartmental model with run-off. $[k_{in} + k]$ is SBF/TBV, k_{out} is the rate constant of clearance from the spleen if HDRBC is not irreversibly removed and k is the transfer rate constant of irreversible removal of HDRBC from blood by the spleen. The reciprocal k_{out} is the mean residence time in the spleen of those HDRBC that return to the blood and is 10–15 minutes, similar to the residence time of platelets. The early part of the blood curve, up to about 8 minutes, is influenced by hepatic uptake of HDRBC.

two intercepts, A and B, and the two slopes α_1 and α_2 of the bi-exponential time activity curves obtained by monitoring the contents of the compartments:[†]

$$k + k_{in} = \frac{A\alpha_1 + B\alpha_2}{A + B} \qquad (10.14a)$$

$$k \cdot k_{out} = \alpha_1\alpha_2 \qquad (10.14b)$$

$$k_{out} = \frac{A\alpha_2 + B\alpha_1}{A + B}. \qquad (10.14c)$$

For HDRBC, there are two rate constants determining uptake in the spleen so SBF/TBV is given by $(k_{in} + k)$. As for platelets, there is some hepatic uptake of cells, which is completed by about 8 minutes. Analysis of the blood disappearance curve of HDRBC from 8 minutes onwards therefore allows calculation of SBF/TBV. Since hepatic uptake is largely irreversible, it does not distort TBV (cf. hepatic platelet uptake, above). It is important to appreciate that in its early phase (approximately 8–15 minutes) HDRBC disappearance from blood is largely a function of SBF and not a function of splenic reticulo–endothelial (phagocytic) activity.

10.1.2.2 Intrasplenic platelet transit time

Referring to Section 10.1.2.1.1,

$$k_{eq} = k_{in} + k_{out}. \qquad (10.15)$$

The measurement of SBF by the method based on platelet equilibration between blood and spleen simultaneously generates k_{out}, the reciprocal of the mean intrasplenic platelet transit time.

Mean intrasplenic platelet transit time can also be measured from deconvolution analysis applied to blood and splenic time–activity curves. Deconvolution analysis generates the splenic time–activity curve that would be obtained if the platelets were injected as a bolus into the splenic artery and did not recirculate. The technique generates, as would be expected, a mono-exponential splenic platelet washout curve, the rate constant of which is k_{out}, i.e. the reciprocal of intrasplenic platelet transit time. This has been shown to correlate well with splenic platelet transit time measured from compartmental analysis as described above (Peters *et al.* 1984a). An advantage of deconvolution analysis is its independence of extrasplenic kinetic events. In other words, this method is not influenced by extrasplenic platelet uptake, particularly in the liver, and can be used to calculate intrasplenic platelet transit time in conditions, like idiopathic thrombocytopaenic purpura, which are associated with extra-splenic platelet destruction and in which compartmental analysis is difficult. It is also useful when the spleen itself is involved in abnormal platelet destruction of a magnitude which leaves the platelet with a probability of irreversible removal, on each pass, approaching that of a heat damaged red cell and which therefore gives a splenic uptake curve which is no longer mono-exponential. The splenic disappearance curve generated by deconvolution analysis under these circumstances approaches an asymptote, which, relative to the initial height, represents the splenic extraction fraction of platelets on each pass (**Fig. 10.5**). Deconvolution analysis is also applic-

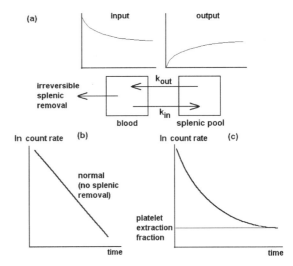

▮ **Fig. 10.5** Deconvolution analysis to generate a splenic impulse retention function using a cardiac region of interest for the input function, (a). In a normal subject, (b), the platelet retention function is exponential with a rate constant equal to k_{out}. In patients with severe thrombocytopenia resulting from premature destruction of platelets in the spleen, an asymptote may be seen (c). The amplitude of this asymptote, relative to the zero-time intercept of the retention function is the extraction fraction of platelets by the spleen. A similar retention function is obtained with HDRBC.

[†] Note that, in terms of the compartment into which the tracer is injected, this model is different from that used to describe HIDA kinetics and equations 14a-c are also different.

able to HDRBC blood disappearance and splenic uptake curves for the measurement of the corresponding variables (i.e. mean intrasplenic transit time and extraction fraction of HDRBC).

Intrasplenic platelet transit time has no obvious clinical value. This is largely the result of our ignorance of the factors that control platelet transit through the spleen. No conditions have been identified, empirically, to be associated with increased intrasplenic platelet transit time. Nevertheless it has clinical research potential and would be useful in studies aiming to throw light on the control of platelet traffic through the spleen. Furthermore it has led to a clearer understanding of the thrombocytopaenia associated with splenomegaly and, if the platelet transit time could be modified pharmacologically, might result in an elevation in the peripheral platelet count in patients with marked splenomegaly.

10.1.2.3 Splenic platelet pool

The intrasplenic platelet pool is important from a clinical standpoint since expansion in its volume takes place largely at the expense of the circulating platelet population. The association between splenomegaly, in which the splenic platelet pool is expanded, and peripheral thrombocytopaenia is well known.

The capacity of the splenic platelet pool is directly proportional to the variables, SBF and intrasplenic mean platelet transit time, since

$$\frac{M_s}{M_b} = \frac{k_{in}}{k_{out}} \qquad (10.16)$$

and

$$\frac{M_s}{M_b + M_s} = \frac{k_{in}}{k_{out} + k_{in}}. \qquad (10.17)$$

The splenic platelet pool can be measured, as a fraction of the total platelet population, from the blood disappearance curve of radio-labelled platelets since the fraction approximates to the ratio of $M_s/(M_b + M_s)$. The size of the splenic platelet pool quantifies the extent for which splenomegaly is responsible for peripheral thrombocytopaenia.

10.1.3 Mean platelet life-span

The mean platelet life-span (MPLS) is the average time between release of platelets from bone marrow

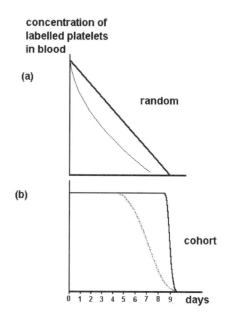

▮ **Fig. 10.6** Normal platelet survival profiles obtained with (a) random labelling and (b) cohort labelling. The profile with random labelling is essentially linear, cutting the time axis at the time of platelet life span. If the platelet life span is not one discrete value (i.e. there is a range of platelet life spans) then the profile would be curvilinear (dashed line). With cohort labelling, a cohort of platelets produced in the bone marrow at the same time is labelled simultaneously and so all appear in and disappear from the blood at the same time. Again, if the cohort had a range of life spans then the right side of the profile would 'tail off' (dashed line).

and their permanent removal from the circulation. Normally, platelets are destroyed when they become senescent, which is after about 9 days in the circulation. Although a cohort of platelets can be labelled with selenium-75 selenomethionine, platelets are usually labelled at random for the determination of MPLS and so comprise a complete spectrum of ages **(Fig. 10.6a)**. After reinjection therefore the platelets oldest at the time of labelling disappear from the blood first, while the youngest ones disappear last. Since the radiolabelled platelets are removed as soon as they become senescent, at 9 days of age, the radioactivity in blood disappears in a linear fashion with a profile of activity versus time which cuts the time axis at 9 days. A cohort of labelled platelets in contrast tend to disappear altogether after a period of about 9 days, producing a rectangular survival profile **(Fig. 10.6b)**.

MPLS may be reduced because of blood loss, platelet deposition in the peripheral circulation (as in thrombus) or premature destruction in the reticulo–endothelial system. All of these result in an element of random platelet loss. This has the effect on the cohort survival profile of introducing a gradual decline in circulating radioactivity because now platelets of all ages are disappearing from the circulation. The effect on the random survival profile is to introduce a degree of curvature; i.e. to make the profile curvilinear. Since cohort labelling is seldom performed, only MPLS determined by random labelling will be considered.

Whereas it is easy to calculate MPLS from a linear survival profile, it is difficult to calculate MPLS from a curvilinear profile, unless the degree of random destruction becomes so great, such as in severe idiopathic thrombocytopaenia, that the survival curve becomes mono-exponential. Under these circumstances MPLS is easy to measure because, as the disappearance is mono-exponential, MPLS is the reciprocal of the rate constant of disappearance. [It is worth noting that with a monoexponential disappearance, MPLS is identical to the mean residence time in blood from the time of labelling, in contrast to a curvilinear or linear disappearance in which MPLS (i.e. the time from platelet *release from bone marrow* to destruction) is longer than the time between labelling and disappearance.] Three approaches have been described for measurement of MPLS which is intermediate between normal and markedly reduced and which gives a curvilinear survival profile.

10.1.3.1 Weighted mean of linear and exponential fits

The profile is firstly considered to be linear and MPLS calculated as the time at which a linear profile, best fitting the data points, cuts the time axis. It is then assumed that the survival profile is exponential and MPLS calculated from the rate constant of the mono-exponential curve which best fits the data points. MPLS is then taken as the weighted mean of these linear and exponential fits, as follows

$$\text{MPLS} = \frac{[\text{MPLS(lin)} \times \text{SD(ln)}] + [\text{MPLS(ln)} \times \text{SD(lin)}]}{\text{SD(ln)} + \text{SD(lin)}}$$

(10.18)

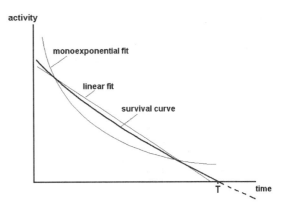

▌ **Fig. 10.7** Estimation of mean platelet life span based on a weighted mean of exponential and linear fits. The survival profile is 'curvilinear' cutting the time axis at the so-called 'deterministic' life span (*T*) i.e. the life expectancy. The exponential fit is asymptotic, theoretically never cutting the time axis. The linear fir cuts the time axis before the survival profile does. The linear fit always gives a higher estimate of mean life span than the exponential.

where SD refers to the sum of the squares of the deviations of the data points from the fitted lines and lin and ln to linear and exponential fits, respectively **(Fig. 10.7)**.

The other two approaches require computer facilities to calculate MPLS from the curvilinear survival profile.

10.1.3.2 Mills and Dornhorst equation

With this approach, originally developed for measurement of red cell life-span (Mills 1946, Dornhorst 1961), it is considered that platelets may reach senescence, and be removed in the normal way, at a time called the deterministic life-span, whilst at the same time facing a probability of premature random destruction. The deterministic life-span *T* is the time at which the profile cuts the time axis. The circulating platelet-bound activity *P(t)*, at any time *t* after injection, as a fraction of the level at zero time *P*(0), is given by

$$\frac{P(t)}{P(0)} = \frac{e^{-kt} - e^{-kT}}{1 - e^{-kt}}$$

(10.19)

where *k* is the fractional rate constant of random destruction and *T* the deterministic life-span. By measuring *k* and *T*, MPLS can be derived:

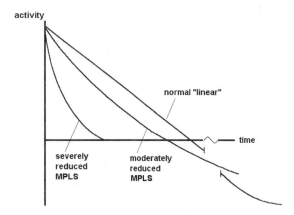

▮ **Fig. 10.8** Because there is always some random platelet destruction, even in the normal subject, all platelet survival profiles are theoretically potentially exponential. If the rate of random destruction is high then the curve approaches the time axis well before the deterministic life span and appears unequivocally exponential. The moderately reduced survival, which looks 'curvilinear', effectively approaches a negative asymptote which is never reached because of the deterministic life span. Similarly, the apparently linear profile has a negative asymptote which it approaches at infinite time.

$$\text{MPLS} = \frac{1 - e^{-kT}}{k}. \qquad (10.20)$$

When a curvilinear survival profile, generated from a moderately reduced platelet life-span, is extrapolated forwards on a linear plot it exponentially approaches an asymptote which has a *negative* value. A severely reduced MPLS gives the special case in which the y-axis asymptote is zero, in contrast to a negative value (**Fig. 10.8**). It should be appreciated that the asymptote is $-\infty$ for a survival curve which is linear. In fact it is likely that even in normal subjects a small number of platelets are destroyed at random and the survival profile is therefore exponential with a negative asymptote. In other words, all survival curves would approach negative asymptotes exponentially if they were not cut short by the limitation imposed by senescence (i.e. the deterministic life-span).

10.1.3.3 Multiple hit model

The other complex technique for measuring MPLS from a curvilinear survival profile is based on the so-called multiple hit model (Murphy and Francis 1971). In this model the platelet is considered to be ready for removal from the circulation after it has sustained a certain number of randomly occurring insults (or hits) during its life in the circulation. If one hit is sufficient to result in removal then the survival profile is mono-exponential. Such a hit, a big one, might be the attachment of an antiplatelet antibody, such as in ITP. On the other hand, if a platelet is removed only after sustaining an infinite number of infinitely small hits, as might be the case for a normal platelet circulating in a normal cardiovascular system, then the survival profile is linear. In intermediate circumstances, the number of hits (n) will be a finite number greater than one. Actually

$$\text{MPLS} = n \cdot a \qquad (10.21)$$

where a is the average time between uniform hits.

The attraction of the multiple hit model is that it generates values for the number of hits required, which gives information about the condition of the platelets, and the time interval between hits, which gives information about the state of the circulation. An example of the latter, for example, is seen in patients with prosthetic cardiac valves which are thought to cause mechanical damage to platelets.

Finally there is one simple method for calculating MPLS which is applicable to all shapes of survival profile between exponential and linear. This is to draw a tangent to the initial slope of the survival profile and extrapolate it to the time axis (**Fig. 10.9**). The MPLS is the time t at which the extrapolated line cuts the time axis. Although the tangent should be drawn to the earliest segment of the profile, it must not precede complete mixing of the labelled platelets between splenic pool and blood. It can be shown that MPLS derived by this approach is true for the extreme cases of linear and exponential survival profiles. Thus for a linear profile, the tangent will be superimposed on the profile right down to the time axis. For an exponential survival profile, on the other hand, the survival curve has the form $P(t) = P_0 e^{-kt}$ and the gradient of the curve is

$$dP/dt = -kP_0 e^{-kt} = -kP \qquad (10.22)$$

where P is the level of platelet-associated radioactivity which at zero time is P_0.

The tangent to the survival curve at $t = 0$ passes through P_0 and has a gradient $-kP_0$. It is a straight line with equation

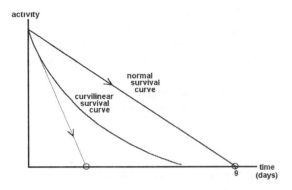

▮ **Fig. 10.9** Method for measuring mean platelet life span from early samples only. All survival profiles, whether they are exponential, curvilinear (obeying the maths of multiple hit or Mills–Dornhorst) or linear, have an initial gradient following equilibrium in the spleen (i.e. a tangent to the zero-time value) which when extrapolated forwards cuts the time axis at the MPLS. This technique has the potential to measure an MPLS of several days from a single patient visit (i.e. the first day). It does not work well, however (nor would it be necessary), for a patient with a severely reduced MPLS since it may be difficult to identify the completion of platelet equilibrium between blood and spleen.

$$P = P_0 - kP_0t \qquad (10.23)$$

and when $\quad P = 0, \quad t = 1/k \qquad (10.24)$

where t is the point on the time axis cut by the extrapolated line. So

$$t = \text{MPLS}. \qquad (10.25)$$

Since k is the rate constant of the survival curve, MPLS must be $1/k$.

It can be shown that for all curves intermediate between linear and exponential, this general approach holds true. It requires frequent early blood sampling to accurately establish the initial rate of loss. It also becomes difficult to use with a severely reduced MPLS since the initial falling blood radioactivity, due to mixing within the splenic pool, 'runs into' the phase due to platelet destruction. In any case, in such situations, it is relatively easy to calculate MPLS from the rate constant of disappearance, and there is no need to draw this tangent. The frequency of early sampling required is determined by the anticipated duration of MPLS.

Determination of MPLS is important with respect to both routine clinical haematology and clinical research. For routine clinical purposes, any of the simpler methods can be used, since an accurate determination of MPLS and associated parameters such as *n* and *a* (equation 10.21) are seldom required. However the more complex techniques are useful for clinical research where frequently the mechanisms underlying premature platelet destruction are addressed.

10.1.4   Platelet destruction

In normal subjects, platelets are removed from the circulation by the reticulo–endothelial system when they reach 9 days of age. In disease, additional loss may be in peripheral vessels or thrombus or through bleeding.

10.1.4.1   Measurement of intrasplenic platelet destruction

The progressive accumulation of radioactivity within the spleen following injection of indium-111 labelled platelets can be measured by day-to-day quantitation of activity in the spleen using quantitative scanning techniques (Section 10.4). In normal subjects, the splenic activity remains fairly constant, or may rise slightly, from a value of 30% of the injected dose at the time of equilibration of platelets in blood and splenic platelet pool at about 30 minutes after injection to about 35% of the injected dose at the time of disappearance of radio-labelled platelets from the circulation at 9 days. The total splenic activity does not increase by very much because the fraction of the total platelet population that pools in the spleen, and represents the activity seen at 30 minutes, is about equal to the fraction that is ultimately destroyed there, and represents the activity seen at 9 days, or whenever platelet disappearance is complete. It is simple to derive a value for splenic activity that represents the destroyed platelets as distinct from the pooled platelets at any time. The activity due to platelet pooling is, throughout platelet life-span, proportional to the circulating activity, so the platelet survival profile, determined from blood sampling, can be used to subtract the component in the splenic curve that is due to platelet pooling (**Fig. 10.10**).

It has been shown that the similarity between the fractions of the platelet population that are respectively pooled and destroyed in the spleen is retained over a wide range of pathologies in which the spleen

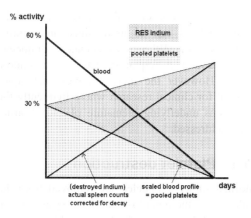

▌ **Fig. 10.10** Quantification of platelet destruction within the spleen. The initial splenic signal is the result of platelet pooling. Since the pool is in dynamic equilibrium between spleen and blood, it decreases over time in proportion to the blood activity. The splenic signal for platelet destruction increases over time faithfully reflecting destruction because the indium-111 is stably retained by macrophages following platelet engulfment. The recorded splenic signal which is the sum of pooled and destroyed platelet activity, remains fairly constant indicating a 'matching' of pooling and destruction. A steadily *rising* recorded signal indicates abnormally accelerated platelet destruction in the spleen, whilst a falling total signal indicates abnormal destruction (or consumption) elsewhere.

may be enlarged and/or MPLS reduced. It is as if, when the splenic platelet pool is enlarged (as in splenomegaly), a platelet is more likely to be in the spleen than in the other components of the reticuloendothelial system at the point in its life when destruction is imminent. Destruction is therefore appropriately shifted towards the spleen. A variable which recognizes this patho-physiological aspect of platelet destruction has therefore been proposed for measuring intrasplenic platelet destruction: the destruction/pooling (D/P) ratio (Peters *et al.* 1984b). This is the ratio of activities in the spleen:

(a) at the completion of platelet disappearance from blood;

(b) the completion of pooling equilibration in the spleen shortly after injection.

As shown above, the normal value is slightly more than unity. It is increased in ITP in which, as a result of immune mechanisms, platelet destruction is redirected towards the spleen, and the ratio may

reach 2 or more. It is reduced in abnormal intrahepatic platelet destruction, such as in severe ITP, and in peripheral platelet consumption or significant blood loss, and may fall to 0.5 or less.

10.1.4.2 Measurement of extrasplenic platelet destruction

Since there is no significant pooling of platelets in the liver, measurement of intrahepatic platelet destruction can be based directly on quantification of total hepatic activity following injection of indium-111 labelled platelets. Because of its diffuse distribution, radioactivity in the bone marrow cannot be quantified directly but can be measured indirectly by subtraction of the sum of activities in spleen, liver and blood from the total injected dose. This is not very satisfactory however since some activity is deposited diffusely in soft tissue, leading to an over-estimation of bone-marrow activity. It is also not possible to apply this technique in conditions associated with peripheral consumption, which may not be seen on imaging if it is diffusely distributed.

10.2 Erythrokinetics

Erythrocytes are produced from erythroid precursors in the bone marrow under the stimulation of erythro-poetin secreted by the kidney. As with other blood cells, the kinetics of red cells can be subdivided into four phases: production, distribution following release into the circulation, mean lifetime in the circulation and sites of removal from the circulation.

10.2.1 Erythrocyte production — ferrokinetics

Ferrokinetics are concerned with the kinetics of iron utilization in developing red cells. The models used are complex and only a summary of ferrokinetic measurements are given. Available radioactive forms of iron (Fe) are:

(1) Fe-59 that emits gamma radiation of energy 1.1 and 1.3 MeV and is therefore unsuitable for imaging with a gamma camera but may be counted *in vivo* with a large crystal surface counter or *in vitro* with most multisample well

counters. Its long half-life of 45 days is compatible with long term haematological studies.

(2) Fe-55 is a long ($t_{1/2} = 2.7$ year) low energy electron emitter and thus has very limited use in *in vitro* counting with a liquid scintillation counter.

(3) Fe-52 has a half-life of 8.3 hours and decays by gamma and positron emission to manganese-52m with a half-life of 21 minutes which in turn decays by high energy (1.4 MeV) gamma emission. Again the high-energy radiation makes this isotope unsuitable for gamma camera imaging though the positrons (and their associated annihilation gamma photons) are successfully imaged at low activities by PET. The short half-life (8.3 hr) allows only two days when measurements or imaging can be performed.

10.2.1.1 Gastro–intestinal iron absorption

Gastro–intestinal iron absorption is measured following an oral dose of iron-59. The iron which is not absorbed can be measured either by counting the radioactivity in faeces collected over several days or by whole-body counting in which absorption is expressed as the percentage difference between counts acquired immediately after injection and at 7 days. The variable is therefore unitless. The normal range is wide, with an average of about 30%. It approaches 100% in iron-deficiency anaemia.

10.2.1.2 Plasma iron clearance

Plasma iron clearance is the rate constant of clearance of intravenously injected iron-59 and therefore has units of fractional turnover; i.e. fraction cleared per unit of time. If the patient has a reduced transferrin binding capacity then iron-59 already bound to donor plasma should be used, otherwise the iron is taken up rapidly by the liver, to form ferritin. Clearance is normally 0.3–0.7 hr^{-1}. It is decreased in aplastic anaemia and increased in myeloproliferative disorders, haemolytic anaemia and iron-deficiency anaemia.

10.2.1.3 Plasma iron turnover

Plasma iron turnover is the product of plasma iron clearance and the plasma protein bound iron concentration. It therefore has units of mg/ml/min.

10.2.1.4 Red cell iron utilization

Red cell iron utilization (RCU) is the fraction of an injected dose of iron-59 that is incorporated into red cells. Daily blood samples are taken and the red cell volume (RCV) is multiplied by the red cell iron concentration in each sample:

$$RCU = \frac{RCV \times RBC \text{ iron concentration}}{\text{injected activity}} \quad (10.26)$$

with units

$$\frac{ml \times MBq/ml}{MBq}.$$

The highest daily fraction over a period of 2 weeks following injection of the iron is recorded as the RCU. It is normally 0.7–0.8. RCU is severely reduced (to less than 0.1) in aplastic anaemia, moderately reduced in myelofibrosis (0.1–0.5), and increased in iron-deficiency anaemia, haemolytic anaemia and polycythemia rubra vera (approximately unity).

10.2.1.5 Whole body iron utilization

An overall picture of ferrokinetics can be constructed by day-to-day surface counting with a scintillation probe over the liver, spleen, sacrum (for bone marrow) and heart (for blood pool) after intravenous injection of iron-59. Early counting gives information on sites of erythropoesis, which may be extramedullary, and later counting gives information on sites of red cell destruction. This investigation is rarely performed but does have some clinical value for determining the extent of extramedullary erythropoesis in the spleen prior to splenectomy.

Imaging of the distribution of iron utilization can be performed with iron-52, using a rectilinear scanner with high-energy collimators, a gamma camera with 511 keV collimators or a PET camera, which provides high-resolution images of the distribution of erythropoetic bone marrow within the skeleton. Other agents which gives high-resolution images of haematopoetic bone marrow are antigranulocyte monoclonal antibodies, which target cells of the myelogenous series, and nanocolloids which give images of the reticulo–endothelial component of bone marrow. Indium-111 chloride and labelled granulocytes give images which may reflect either the haematopoetic or reticulo–endothelial elements.

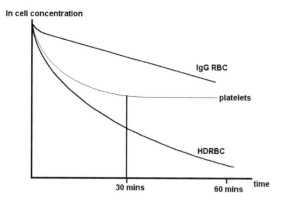

In cell concentration

IgG RBC

platelets

HDRBC

30 mins   60 mins   time

▮ **Fig. 10.11** Comparison of the shapes of the plasma disappearance curves of HDRBC, IgG-RBC and platelets over a period of about 60 minutes. Because they pool insignificantly, IgG-RBC disappear from plasma essentially mono-exponentially at a rate depending on the number of IgG molecules on the cell surface and the Fc receptors in the spleen which bind the IgG. HDRBC are simultaneously pooled and destroyed, thereby giving rise to a bi-exponential disappearance curve. Platelets show only pooling and therefore decrease to an asymptote the amplitude of which is inversely related to the size of the splenic pool. The initial gradients of the HDRBC and platelet curves are similar, both reflecting SBF / TBV.

10.2.2 Red cell distribution — intrasplenic kinetics

The mean transit time of red cells through the spleen is slightly less than one minute. Damaged red cells have a prolonged transit time and are consequently used as markers of splenic function. Damage may be by heating (heat damaged red cells; HDRBC) or by exposure to chemical damage. Red cells modified by coating with immunoglobulin (IgRBC) are also used to assess splenic function. IgRBC are not damaged however in the sense that they undergo prolonged transit (which is in fact normal) but are instead removed prematurely from the circulation as a result of immunodetection. Normal autologous red cells are also used to assess splenic function (Fig. 10.11).

10.2.2.1 Unmodified red cells

Unmodified red cells are used to determine the extent of red-cell pooling within the spleen, either in absolute units of local red cell volume or as the mean red cell transit time. Since this is a short-term study, a short-lived radionuclide, such as technetium-99m,

is an appropriate label. The capacity of the splenic red cell pool V_s can be measured by quantitative scanning following equilibration of labelled red cells between the splenic pool and circulating blood. We find that V_s is related to mean red cell transit time through the spleen T_{RBC} and SBF (expressed as the fraction of the whole body red cell volume [RCV] delivered to the spleen in unit time) as follows:

$$T_{RBC} = \frac{V_s}{SBF}$$

$$= \frac{V_s/RCV}{SBF/RCV}. \qquad (10.27)$$

Normally about 4% of the RCV is present in the spleen and splenic blood flow is 5% of total blood volume per minute so, from equation 10.27

$$T_{RBC} = 0.04/0.05 \text{ min}$$

$$= 48 \text{ sec}$$

Splenic red cell pooling is more difficult to measure from dynamic data, as used for the measurement of the splenic platelet pool, because the transit time of red cells through the spleen is fast compared with platelets and equilibrium is therefore completed rather rapidly — so rapidly as to make the time course of the splenic uptake curve critically dependent on other factors such as bolus width. It is possible however to measure splenic red cell transit time T_{RBC} from first-pass curves (Peters *et al.* 1987), analogous to the measurement of the extraction fraction for extracted tracers as described in Section 11.1.3 under measurement of filtration fraction. Following mixing of red cells in the circulation and equilibration in the splenic pool

$$\frac{N_s \gamma}{\text{injected activity}} = \frac{V_s}{RCV} \qquad (10.28)$$

where N_s is the splenic count rate and γ is the constant relating this to the amount of radioactivity in MBq. But

$$RCV = \frac{\text{injected activity}}{N_b \cdot \Gamma} \qquad (10.29)$$

where N_b is the count rate in a blood pool region of interest and Γ the constant relating this count rate to the *concentration* of activity in peripheral blood in MBq/ml of red cells. So, rearranging and substituting for whole body RCV,

$$V_s = \frac{N_s \gamma}{N_b \Gamma}. \qquad (10.30)$$

Now SBF can be related to the maximum gradient, dN_s/dt (counts per sec per sec), of the first-pass curve over the spleen, as described for renal blood flow measurement in Section 11.1.1.3. That is

$$\text{SBF} = \frac{(dN_s/dt)_{\max}}{N_{b\text{peak}}} \times \frac{\gamma}{\Gamma} \qquad (10.31)$$

where $N_{b\text{peak}}$ is the peak height of the first pass curve recorded over the blood pool region (see Section 11.1.1.3). Therefore, from equations 10.30 and 10.31.

$$\frac{V_s}{\text{SBF}} = T_{\text{RBC}} = \frac{N_{b\text{peak}}}{dN_s/dt} \times \frac{N_s}{N_b}. \qquad (10.32)$$

This approach gives a mean transit time for red cells through the spleen of about 40 seconds.

In splenomegaly the red cell pool is increased as is the platelet pool. Paradoxically, red cells take longer to equilibrate in the enlarged spleen compared with the normal sized spleen in contrast to platelets which equilibrate faster in the enlarged spleen compared with the normal. It has been suggested that the longer transit time of red cells is the result of a second compartment in the enlarged spleen, with a slower red cell turnover that is not present in the normal sized spleen. If this is true then platelets presumably do not enter it to any significant extent or have a fast transit through it.

Splenomegaly does not cause anaemia to the same relative extent as it causes thrombocytopaenia, and this is not surprising given the different intrasplenic transit times of red cells and platelets. The main clinical value for measuring the capacity of the splenic red cell pool is not so much for the assessment of anaemia, but rather for the assessment of polycythaemia. In secondary polycythaemia, the pool is normal whereas in primary polycythaemia it is expanded to greater than 5% of total red cell volume, up to 20%, and even higher with myelofibrosis typically reaching 30%.

10.2.2.2 Modified red cells

10.2.2.2.1 Heat damaged red cells

For many years heat damaged red cells (HDRBC) were used as a convenient marker for measuring splenic reticuloendothelial function. The rate of disappearance of radiolabelled HDRBC is in fact related to several functions of the spleen, including splenic HDRBC pooling and, in particular, splenic blood flow. The kinetics of HDRBC clearance can be represented by the model shown in Fig. 10.4 Splenic handling of HDRBC can be approximated to a two compartmental closed model with run off (see Section 1.4). This model is *identical* to that representing the kinetics of DTPA where the two compartments are the intravascular and extravascular extracellular spaces with run off into the kidney, and *similar* to that representing organic anion handling by the liver, where the two compartments are the blood and hepatocyte with run off into the biliary system. Such a model predicts a bi-exponential disappearance curve from blood (Section 1.4), and this is indeed observed for radiolabelled HDRBC **(Fig. 10.11)**. If hepatic uptake is ignored then, from the equations of this model, the rate constants k_{in}, k_{out} and k (Fig. 10.4) can be measured (Section 10.1.2.1.4). The term $[k_{\text{in}} + k]$ is equal to the ratio, spenic blood flow to total blood volume (SBF/TBV). The extraction fraction k of cells irreversibly removed on each pass (Peters *et al.* 1982) may reflect splenic reticulo–endothelial function. As damage is difficult to standardize, HDRBC are awkward to use for the measurement of SBF and splenic reticulo–endothelial function (Klausner *et al.* 1975). Another clinical use of radiolabelled HDRBC, more important than those above, is the selective imaging of functional splenic tissue, such as for the detection of splenunculi in a previously splenectomised patient.

10.2.2.2.2 Immune-coated red cells

Immune-coated RBC are occasionally used for quantifying splenic reticuloendothelial function and, since they are recognised by splenic macrophages via the macrophage Fc receptor, are probably a more specific probe for splenic reticuloendothelial function than HDRBC. Red cells coated with an IgG immunoglobulin are taken up exclusively by the spleen. The disappearance curve is mono-exponential, at least from about 3–5 minutes after injection, with a rate constant that is the product of (SBF/TBV) and splenic extraction fraction **(Fig 10.11)** (Peters *et al.* 1984c). A mono-exponential curve implies that IgGRBC not extracted on a single pass through the spleen have a relatively short mean intrasplenic transit time, very likely the same as normal red cells.

This is not surprising since the immune-coated cell, unlike the rigid HDRBC, retains deformability of its cell membrane and is therefore not delayed in the splenic sinusoids. The blood disappearance rate of IgGRBC has been shown to be proportional to the amount of IgG coating the cell. Again this is not surprising as the probability of interaction with a splenic macrophage Fc receptor is proportional to the number of available Fc terminals on the red cell. The extraction fraction of IgGRBC can be measured if SBF/TBV is separately measured with HDRBC or indium-labelled platelets (Walport *et al.* 1985). Extraction fraction measured by this means is then a quantitative index of splenic macrophage function (specifically, the Fc receptor population) and has clinical research potential for the investigation of immune complex disease, in which reticuloendothelial blockade is thought to play an important etiological role.

10.3 Granulocyte kinetics

The physiology of inflammation involves essentially three components, endothelial activation, leucocyte migration and resolution. Leucocytes and endothelium may be separately activated, and leucocyte migration initiated, by several pro-inflammatory mediators, including interleukin-1, tumour necrosis factor and phytohaemagglutinin.

In general activation of the endothelium is the first stage of inflammation. Endothelium is not a simple barrier separating the interstitial space and plasma but is a highly active, specialized tissue responsible for orchestrating cell migration in inflammation. It achieves this by synthesizing several substances called adhesion molecules, which are antigenic substances expressed on the endothelial luminal surface and which display functional selectivity for interaction with circulating leucocytes. They are activated in response to pro-inflammatory mediators (cytokines) liberated at the site of inflammation. Some adhesion molecules are constitutively expressed; i.e. expressed all the time, while others are only expressed in response to a specific stimulus. In the case of the latter, the time course of expression varies according to the stimulus. Because the adhesion molecules are antigenic, they potentially provide a means for imaging by targeting with

specific radiolabelled monoclonal antibodies. Inducible adhesion molecules, rather than those that are constitutively expressed, offer the best chance of success with this approach.

The following sequence of events occurs in an inflammatory process. Firstly, granulocytes arriving at the site of infection, marginate on the endothelial surface of small blood vessels, mostly post-capillary venules, by interacting with the endothelial adhesion molecule, E-selectin, which is synthesized in response to cytokines, also known as chemoattractants, released at the site of inflammation. Margination, which is reversible, is followed by endothelial adherence which is irreversible and mediated by endothelial adhesion molecules called integrins. These are widely distributed in nature and share the general property of holding cells together. Following adhesion, granulocytes undergo transmigration by negotiating the interendothelial junctions, which widen in response to the inflammatory stimulus. The separation of endothelial cells from each other forms the basis for the accumulation of macromolecules at sites of inflammation. Unless terminated, the inflammatory process may result in local tissue damage, and so the mechanisms which switch off inflammation are as important as those initiating it. However these are not as well understood.

10.3.1 Granulocyte production

Granulocytes are produced in the bone marrow from myeloid precursors over a maturation period of about 15 days. They than spend, on average, only about 10 hours in the circulation (see below), followed by a further 2–4 days in the tissues, if they migrate in response to an inflammatory stimulus. In other words, a granulocyte, unlike a red cell or platelet, spends a very small fraction of its life span in the circulation, which is not surprising since this is not where it performs its function. Radiolabelled anti-granulocyte monoclonal anti-bodies, recently introduced with the aim of imaging inflammation, give very good images of bone marrow, which is consistent with the notion that the majority of antigen is present in marrow and points up a fundamental problem that is likely to be faced by such agents. As with platelets, information on granulocyte production is potentially available from the peripheral count and intravascular life span, although the latter is seldom of clinical interest. Much of the experimental literature on granulocyte kinetics is based on cohort labelling *in vivo* with tritiated thymidine, but this has not been used in man.

10.3.2 Granulocyte distribution — intravascular margination

After intravenous administration only about 50% of radiolabelled granulocytes can be accounted for in the circulation. This is the result of reversible entry of cells into intravascular granulocyte 'pools' which collectively make up the so-called *marginating granulocyte pool* (MGP). The MGP, together with the *circulating granulocyte pool* (CGP), make up the *total blood granulocyte pool* (TBGP).

Because of the inefficient gamma emission of the radionuclides on which early observations were made, it was difficult to quantify the distribution of the whole body MGP, although, on the basis of organ arterio–venous differences in granulocyte count and surface counting studies, it was suspected that the lungs and spleen were important sites of granulocyte margination. Although the subject remains controversial, more recent studies with indium-111 labelled granulocytes and gamma camera imaging suggest that the spleen is the location of a significant granulocyte pool, as it is for platelets. The bone marrow is also an important site of pooling. Between them, the spleen, liver and bone marrow account for at least 75% of the whole body MGP. Granulocytes are delayed in their transit through the lung, but not so much as in the spleen and bone marrow. Furthermore, since the diameter of a granulocyte is larger than the pulmonary capillary, the slow transit through the lung is partly mechanical, so the term margination is inappropriate.

Although the pulmonary vascular granulocyte pool is only about the same as the average for the whole body, it increases in several diseases not only of the lung itself but also of other organs, including inflammatory bowel disease, systemic vasculitis and graft versus host disease. The mechanisms are probably related to granulocyte deformability but are not well understood and so measurement of pulmonary granulocyte pooling has important clinical research potential. It is also possible to quantify granulocyte migration in the lung (Section 8.3.2),

and this is also important because of evidence which suggests that increased margination does not by itself damage the lungs.

Although the description of granulocyte rolling, as a basis for margination, has been based primarily on observations made on peripheral vessels with continuous endothelium, the mechanisms responsible for granulocyte pooling within the sinusoids of the reticulo–endothelial system are uncertain. As with platelets, granulocytes pool in the spleen to an extent that splenomegaly may cause a significant granulocytopaenia. Indeed, using the techniques described below, granulocytes have been shown to have a very similar mean intrasplenic transit time to platelets — about 10 minutes. Furthermore granulocyte transit time through the bone marrow appears to be similar (Ussov *et al.* 1995).

The term margination has come into general use for describing granulocytes that are physiologically pooled, but should perhaps be reserved for the process of granulocyte rolling, mediated by E-selectin, prior to emigration from the vasculature in inflammation. In other words, margination is a pathological rather than physiological event. Nevertheless, the term will be used in its wider sense in this section.

10.3.2.1 Measurement of regional marginating granulocyte pooling from transit time

Assuming that there were no losses of granulocytes as a result of damage sustained during labelling, then the recovery R of a dose of infused radiolabelled granulocytes would be equal to the circulating granulocyte pool (CGP) as a fraction of the total blood granulocyte pool (TBGP), and the marginating pool (MGP) equal to $1 - R$. Granulocytes labelled *in vivo* with tritiated thymidine meet this assumption and can be regarded as equivalent to native granulocytes (Dancey *et al.* 1976). Granulocytes labelled *in vitro* with DFP-32 (Athens *et al.* 1961) also come close to reflecting the behaviour of native granulocytes. The advantage of indium-111 labelled granulocytes is that they provide information on the regional distribution of the MGP, although their disadvantage is the necessity for *in vitro* separation of granulocytes., which results in some activation and loss of viability, however carefully labelled.

The fraction of the whole body MGP M_G present within a particular organ can be determined by measuring the mean transit time T_G of radiolabelled granulocytes through the organ (Peters *et al.* 1985). A high degree of margination will be reflected by a long transit time, and conversely, a low degree will be reflected by a transit time which is close to that of red cells. Making use of the transit time equation,

$$V_G = T_G \times Q_G \qquad (10.33)$$

with units

$$MBq = min \times MBq \cdot min^{-1}$$

where V_G is the activity representing the total number of labelled granulocytes (or volume, analogous to splenic red cell volume; see above) in the organ (circulating plus marginating) and Q_G the rate of inflow of labelled granulocytes into the organ.

Expressing V_G as a fraction of the whole body CGP,

$$\frac{V_G}{CGP} = T_G \times \frac{Q_G}{CGP}. \qquad (10.34)$$

Now Q_G/CGP is equal to the organ blood flow (Q) expressed as a fraction of total blood volume (TBV), i.e.

$$\frac{V_G}{CGP} = T_G \times \frac{Q}{TBV} \qquad (10.35)$$

Rearranging and dividing both sides of equation 10.35 by whole body TBGP,

$$\frac{V_G}{TBGP} = T_G \times \frac{CGP}{TBGP} \times \frac{Q}{TBV}. \qquad (10.36)$$

Whole body CGP/TBGP can be measured as the recovery at the earliest time after complete equilibration between labelled and native cells. Since granulocyte survival in blood is relatively short, a correction to this ratio can be applied which takes into account those radiolabelled granulocytes that have been physiologically destroyed up to the time of measurement of recovery.

Division of V_G between circulating and marginating compartments of an organ requires a knowledge of the red cell volume (V_{RBC}) within the organ. The circulating C_G, in contrast to marginating M_G, granulocytes can be regarded as equivalent to red cells, which do not marginate, i.e.

$$\frac{C_G}{CGP} = \frac{V_{RBC}}{RCV} \qquad (10.37)$$

where RCV is whole body red cell volume; so

$$C_G = CGP \times \frac{V_{RBC}}{RCV} \qquad (10.38)$$

dividing both sides of equation 10.38 by TBGP,

$$\frac{C_G}{TBGP} = \frac{CGP}{TBGP} \times \frac{V_{RBC}}{RCV}. \qquad (10.39)$$

Although T_G can be measured, it is necessary to use assumed values for organ blood flow (Q) and red cell volume (V_{RBC}) in order to calculate $M_G/TBGP$.

As $C_G + M_G = V_G$

$$\frac{M_G}{TBGP} = \frac{V_G}{TBGP} - \frac{C_G}{TBGP}$$

and $M_G/TBGP$ can be calculated as the difference between equations 10.36 and 10.39. Transit time can be measured from the impulse response function (IRF) generated by deconvolution analysis using sampled blood or a region of interest well focused over the left ventricular blood pool as the input function. This gives transit time values for the spleen and liver of about 10 min and 2 min respectively (Peters *et al.* 1985). The IRF over the lung, using an input region over the right ventricle, consists of two exponentials, the relative amplitudes of which correlate with the fraction of granulocytes showing evidence of activation *in vivo* (unpublished).

10.3.2.2 Measurement of regional MGP from comparison with red cells

Another approach to expressing granulocyte margination is to compare the granulocyte mean transit time through the organ with that of the mean transit time of radiolabelled red cells (Peters *et al.* 1992). If the blood activity levels of the two cells were the same, the ratio of their transit times would be equal to the ratio of their respective signals recorded by a detector over the organ; i.e.

$$\frac{T_G}{T_{RBC}} = \frac{N_G}{N_{RBC}} \times \frac{B_G}{B_{RBC}} \qquad (10.40)$$

where T refers to transit times, N to detected count rates, and B to blood radioactivity levels. If both cell types are labelled with indium-111, photon attenuation can be ignored. The red cells, in a relatively small dose, are injected first and since they soon equilibrate without significant loss from the circulation, their signal can be regarded as a background signal prior to the injection of the labelled granulocytes (**Fig. 10.12**). Values for the ratio of

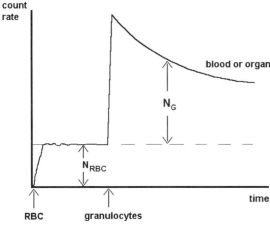

$$\frac{T_G}{T_{RBC}} = \frac{N_G \, (\text{organ})}{N_{RBC} \, (\text{organ})} \times \frac{N_{RBC} \, (\text{blood})}{N_G \, (\text{blood})}$$

▌ **Fig. 10.12** Measurement of mean granulocyte transit time (T_G) relative to red cell transit time (T_{RBC}). Indium-111 labelled red cells (RBC) are injected, and, after mixing, give stable signals in blood and over the organ of interest. Both signals increase after subsequent injection of indium-111 granulocytes. By normalizing the curves for organ and blood to the red cell signal, the size of the organ granulocyte signal gives a direct measurement of granulocyte margination which can be expressed either as the organ transit time in relation to (i.e. as a quotient of) red cell transit time or as a ratio of the organ MGP to organ CGP.

granulocyte to red cell transit time are about 7 for the liver and 14 for the spleen.[†] In the lung it decreases with time after injection from about 5, at 5 minutes after injection, to about 2.5 at 40 minutes after injection. This fall presumably reflects some granulocyte 'de-activation' when the cells are returned to their normal *in vivo* environment.

Using indium-111 granulocytes and these kinetics, the distribution of the MGP has been 'mapped out', showing that about one third is in the spleen, about the same in bone marrow and about 10% in the lung. The liver is difficult to interpret since activated and/or damaged granulocytes are sequestered (reversibly or irreversibly) within the liver. Only a small fraction exists in other tissues.

An assumption implicit in these techniqes, based on sampling of peripheral venous blood, is that the arterial granulocyte level is the same as in peripheral venous blood; i.e. that there is no arterio–venous granulocyte difference in the forearm (from which venous samples are usually taken). This may not be the case, especially early after injection, if the forearm contains a significant MGP. However this is unlikely. In any event, the time required for equilibration of cells between the MGP and CGP of the forearm is probably short compared with equilibration time in the spleen, because the transit time of the granulocytes in the forearm vascular bed is likely to be much shorter.

No clinical value has been demonstrated for measurements of regional granulocyte margination. However granulocyte margination within the pulmonary vasculature is increased in the adult respiratory distress syndrome and certain other diseases, including systemic vasculitis, graft-versus-host disease and inflammatory bowel disease. Measurement of mean granulocyte transit time in the lung has obvious clinical research potential, especially when combined with measurements of lung endothelial permeability (with radiolabelled protein) and alveolar epithelial permeability (with inhaled technetium-99m DTPA) and may have routine clinical value when measured in the intensive care unit with a mobile gamma camera.

10.3.3 Mean granulocyte life-span in blood

Granulocytes undergo a relatively long period of maturation in the bone marrow before being released into the circulation — about 15 days. There is no technique which is readily available for measurement of this period in man. Nevertheless, with the increasing use of anti-granulocyte monoclonal antibodies for imaging inflammation, the fact that most of the population of myeloid cells is in the bone marrow is of some practical importance since it explains why these antibodies give such impressive images of the bone marrow and why only a small percentage of the circulating activity (<10%) is bound to granulocytes.

Because the blood clearance curve of radiolabelled granulocytes is exponential, it can be said that

---

[†]It should be recalled that although a ratio of 7 seems high, red cells transit the liver faster than the spleen; thus intrahepatic haematocrit is lower while intrasplenic haematocrit is higher than central haematocrit.

granulocytes are removed from the blood at random. The mean residence time of granulocytes in blood is about 10 hours, rather short in comparison to red cells and platelets. In the absence of inflammatory disease, almost all circulating granulocytes are destroyed in the reticulo–endothelial system. Granulocytes which migrate into the tissues in response to a chemoattractant stimulus survive for up to a further 2–4 days.

Mean granulocyte life-span (in the blood) (MGLS) was initially measured with several non-imaging radiopharmaceuticals, including chromium-51 (Dresch *et al.* 1975), phosphorus-32 labelled di-isopropylfluorophosphonate (DFP-32) (Athens *et al.* 1961) and tritiated thymidine (Dancey *et al.* 1976). It is not necessary to isolate pure populations of granulocytes for labelling with these agents because the survival curves are based on measurement of the granulocyte-associated activity, determined by density gradient separation, in blood samples obtained following injection of the labelled blood. MGLS can also be measured with indium-111 labelled granulocytes, which give similar values to the classical techniques (Saverymuttu *et al.* 1985). Because of the presence of more than one exponential in the survival curves, and uncertainties in their interpretation, the best approach to measurement of MGLS is by forward extrapolation of the initial part of the survival curve to the time axis, as described above for mean platelet life-span (MPLS).

Although the measurement of MPLS has an established value for investigating patients with thrombocytopaenia, measurement of MGLS has no established value in patients with granulocytopaenia. There are several reasons for this: for example, granulocytopaenia usually has a fairly obvious cause; furthermore, the response of the bone marrow to granulocytopenia is greater in comparison with platelets, so granulocytopenia is not as difficult to interpret and usually due to marrow failure. Splenomegaly is a recognized cause of granulocytopenia.

10.3.4 Granulocyte destruction and whole body losses

Although it is possible to measure the relative quantities of granulocytes deposited in the liver, spleen and bone marrow using the same approach as for platelets, it is not routinely performed for

clinical use; we are rarely presented with the clinical problem of whether or not the spleen is responsible for abnormal destruction of granulocytes in a patient with granulocytopaenia and reduced MGLS. On the other hand, the measurement of granulocyte losses from the body is a technique with clinical potential, not in patients with abnormalities of granulocyte kinetics, but as a means of quantifying granulocyte migration as an index of the severity of inflammatory disease. The two diseases to which this has been applied are inflammatory bowel disease (IBD) (Carpani *et al.* 1992) and bronchiectasis (Currie *et al.* 1987), because in both of these conditions, granulocytes migrate into a lumen (gut or bronchus) and are then excreted. In fact, gamma camera images show complete mobilisation and excretion of migrating granulocytes by 4 days after injection.

Within 3 hours of injecting indium-111 labelled granulocytes, the patient stands in front of an uncollimated gamma camera at a distance of 3–4 m and counts are recorded for 2 minutes. The counts are compared with a standard, containing a known amount of indium-111, counted from the same distance. This is repeated between 4 and 6 days later using the same standard. An uncollimated gamma camera is highly sensitive and, provided the patient is at a distance of at least 3 m, is almost insensitive to the vertical distribution of radioactivity within the body. Since the indium-111 may redistribute in the antero–posterior dimension between 3 hr and 4–6 days, the patient should be counted anteriorly and posteriorly and the geometric mean calculated. Provided no activity is lost from the body by 3 hr, the counts (relative to the standard) recorded at 4–6 days, expressed as a fraction of the counts recorded at 3 hours, gives the fraction of labelled granulocytes that have migrated and been excreted. Normal subjects lose about 1% of the indium-111 per day (through urine, saliva and faeces) (Saverymuttu *et al.* 1983) so the normal whole body retention (WBR) by this technique is 95% (with a lower 95% confidence limit of 90%). Counting the indium-111 in a four-day faecal collection is the 'gold-standard' method for quantifying the migration of indium-111 labelled granulocytes in IBD (Saverymuttu *et al.* 1983). All expectorated sputum would have to be added to the faeces for quantification of migration in bronchiectasis. WBR, as described above, is almost as accurate as supervised faecal collection, requires no patient compliance and has a useful role in clinical research, particularly for the evaluation of new drug therapies. The general technique of whole body counting with the un-collimated gamma camera has several other applications, including the quantification of bile salt loss (Section 9.5.2), serum amyloid P component (SAP) turnover in amyloidosis (Section 10.5), and gastro-intestinal protein loss in protein-losing enteropathy (Section 9.5.1).

10.4 Blood volume

The measurements of red cell volume (RCV) and plasma volume (PV) are both based on the dilution principle. For the adequate measurement of blood volume, it is usually necessary to measure both volumes separately and sum them for total blood volume.

10.4.1 Red cell volume

Several radionuclides are available to label red cells for the measurement of red cell volume (RCV), including technetium-99m, indium-111 and chromium-51. Chromium-51 and indium-111 have half-lives unnecessarily long for this application, unless mean red cell life-span is also measured, but their red cell binding is stable whereas technetium-99m shows some elution. Blood samples are taken at 10 and 20 minutes and, by extrapolating back to zero time, give the initial concentration of radioactivity C. RCV can then be calculated as follows:

$$\text{RCV} = \frac{\text{injected activity}}{C}. \qquad (10.41)$$

In a patient without unduly prolonged mixing times, the values based on the 10 and 20 minute samples should be identical, unless significant elution of label from the cells has occurred (as might be the case with technetium-99m). Patients with cardiac failure or particularly with splenomegaly have delayed mixing times and a sample at 30 or 60 minutes is required. The late sample should give a higher value of RCV than the earlier one. The most important clinical reason for measuring RCV is the investigation of polycythaemia and the exclusion of pseudo-anaemia, in which plasma volume is expanded but the RCV is normal.

10.4.2 Plasma volume

Plasma volume (PV) is measured, by tracer dilution, in much the same way as RCV, except that a labelled protein is given. This is usually iodine-125 labelled albumin, although indium-111-labelled transferrin and iodine-125 labelled immunoglobulin can also been used. There is an extravascular pool of albumin, so the albumin space is larger than PV (see Chapter 6). Samples are taken at 10, 20 and 30 minutes after injection and a disappearance curve is established. By assuming this to be monoexponential and extrapolating it to zero time, a correction can be made for the extravascular pool. Iodine-125 immunoglobulin gives a value for PV 0.95 that of iodine-125 albumin. The main indication for measuring PV is as an adjunct to the measurement of RCV for the separation of true polycythaemia from pseudopolycythaemia. The latter is associated with a normal RCV and a reduced PV.

10.5 Turnover of serum amyloid P component

Serum amyloid P component (SAP) is a normal circulating acute phase protein of molecular weight greater than 300 kDa, which, in the normal subject, has an intravascular half-life of several days. It has been shown to bind to all known forms of amyloidosis, deposits of which can therefore be imaged with iodine–123 labelled SAP. The existence of amyloid deposits binding SAP reduces the circulating half-life in proportion to the amyloid burden, down to values as low as a few minutes in extensive hepatosplenic amyloidosis. Measurement of the half-life in blood therefore provides a quantitative estimate of the extent of amyloidosis.

The whole body retention of iodine-131-labelled SAP provides another means of quantifying amyloidosis. In normal subjects, iodinated SAP is metabolised with release and excretion of the radioiodine. In amyloidosis, on the other hand, the whole body retention is prolonged as a result of stable binding to amyloid fibrils, and can be measured by whole body counting, using either a conventional whole body counter or an uncollimated gamma camera (Hawkins *et al.* 1990).

References

Allsop P, Peters AM, Arnot RN, Stuttle AWJ, Deenmama-mode M, Gwilliam ME, Myers MJ and Hall GM. Intrasplenic blood cell kinetics in man before and after brief maximal exercise. *Clinical Science* 1992, **83**: 47–54.

Athens JW, Mauer AM, Ashenbrucker H, Cartwright GE and Wintrobe MM. Leukokinetic studies III. The distribution of granulocytes in the blood of normal subjects. *Journal of Clinical Investigation* 1961, **40**, 159–64.

Carpani de Kaski M, Peters AM, Knight D, Stuttle AWJ, Lavender JP and Hodgson HJ. In-111 whole body retention: a new method for quantification of disease activity in inflammatory bowel disease. *Journal of Nuclear Medicine* 1992, **33**: 756–62.

Currie DC, Saverymuttu SH, Peters AM, Needham SG, George P, Dhillon DP, Lavender JP and Cole PJ. Indium-111 labelled granulocyte accumulation in respiratory tract of patients with bronchiectasis. *Lancet* 1987, **1**: 1335–9.

Dancey JT, Deubelbeiss KA, Harker LA and Finch CA. Neutrophil kinetics in man. *Journal of Clinical Investigation* 1976, **58**: 705–15.

Dornhorst AC. The interpretation of red cell survival curves. *Blood* 1961, **6**: 1284–92.

Dresch C, Najean Y and Bauchet J. Kinetic studies of ^{51}Cr and DF^{32}P labelled granulocytes. *British Journal of Haematology* 1975, **29**: 67–80.

Hawkins PN, Wootton R and Pepys MB. Metabolic studies of radioiodinated serum amyiod P component in normal subjects and patients with systemic amyloidosis. *Journal of Clinical Investigation* 1990, **86**: 1862–9.

Klausner MA, Hirsch LJ, Leblond PF, *et al.* (1975) Contrasting splenic mechanisms in the blood clearance of red blood cells and colloidal particles. *Blood*, **46**: 965–76.

Miles KA, Hayball M and Dixon AK. Colour perfusion imaging: a new application of computed tomography. *Lancet* 1991, **337**: 643–5.

Mills JN. The lifespan of the erythrocyte. *Journal of Physiology.* 1946, **105**: 16P–17P.

Murphy EA and Francis ME. The estimation of blood platelet survival 11. The multiple hit model. *Thrombotic. Diathesis. Haemorrhogica.* 1971, **25**: 53–80.

Peters AM, Klonizakis I, Lavender JP and Lewis SM. Use of indium-111 labelled platelets to measure spleen function. *British Journal of Haematology* 1980, **46**: 587–93.

Peters AM, Ryan PFJ, Klonizakis I, Elkon KB, Lewis SM, Hughes GRV and Lavender JP. Kinetics of heat damaged autologous red blood cells. Mechanisms of clearance from blood. *Scandinavian Journal of Haematology* 1982, **28**: 5–14.

Peters AM, Walport MJ, Bell RN and Lavender JP. Methods of measuring splenic blood flow and platelet transit time with In-111 labelled platelets. *Journal of Nuclear Medicine* 1984a, **25**: 86–90.

Peters AM, Walport MJ, Elkon KB, Reavy HJ, Ferjencik PP, Lavender JP and Hughes GRV. The comparative blood clearance kinetics of modified radiolabelled erythrocytes. *Clinical Science* 1984b, **66**: 55–62.

Peters AM, Saverymuttu SH, Wonke B, Lewis SM and Lavender JP. The interpretation of platelet kinetic studies for the identification of sites of abnormal platelet destruction. *British Journal of Haematology* 1984c, **57**: 637–49.

Peters AM, Saverymuttu SH, Keshavarzian A, Bell RN and Lavender JP. Splenic pooling of granulocytes. *Clinical Science* 1985, **68**: 283–9.

Peters AM, Gunasekera RD, Henderson BL, Brown J, Lavender JP, de Souza M, Ash JM and Gilday DL. Non-invasive measurement of blood flow and extraction fraction. *Nuclear Medicine Communications* 1987, **8**: 823–37.

Peters AM, Allsop P, Stuttle AWJ, Arnot RN, Gwilliam M and Hall GM. Granulocyte margination in the human lung and its response to strenuous exercise. *Clinical Science* 1992, **82**: 237–44.

Saverymuttu SH, Peters AM, Hodgson HJ, Chadwick VS and Lavender JP. Quantitative fecal In-111 leukocyte excretion in the assessment of disease activity in Crohn's disease. *Gastroenterology* 1983, **85**: 1333–9.

Saverymuttu SH, Peters AM, Keshavarzian A, Reavy HJ and Lavender JP. The kinetics of 111-indium distribution following injection of 111-indium labelled autologous granulocytes in man. *British Journal of Haematology* 1985, **61**: 675–85.

Slater DN, Trowbridge EA and Martin JF. The megakaryocyte in thrombocytopenia: a microscopic study which supports the theory that platelets are produced in the pulmonary circulation. *Thrombosis Research* 1983, **31**: 163–76.

Ussov Yu, Aktolun C, Myers MJ, Jamar F and Peters AM. Granulocyte margination in bone marrow. Comparison with margination in the spleen and liver. *Scandinavian Journal of Clinical Laboratory Investigation* 1995, **55**: 87–96.

Walport MJ, Peters AM, Elkon KB, Pusey CD, Lavender JP and Hughes GRV. The splenic extraction ratio of antibody coated erythrocytes and its response to plasma exchange and pulse methylprednisolone. *Clinical and Experimental Immunology* 1985, **65**, **465–73.**

Williams R, Condon RE, Williams HS, and Kreel L. Splenic blood flow in cirrhosis and portal hypertension. *Clinical Science* 1968, **34**: 441–52.

11 The genitourinary system

Introduction

The functional unit of the kidney is the nephron of which there are two types: cortical and juxtamedullary. Cortical nephrons are relatively short, with loops of Henle that extend into the medulla only as far as the outer medulla. Juxtamedullary nephrons, which comprise about 15% of the total nephron population, have long loops of Henle extending into the medulla almost as far as the papilla. The nephron starts at the glomerulus and finishes at the distal collecting tubule. Blood is carried into the glomerulus by the afferent arteriole and away from it by the efferent arteriole. Between the afferent and efferent arterioles is the glomerular papillary network, which is situated within Bowman's capsule, and through which filtration occurs to form the glomerular filtrate. The efferent arteriole then supplies blood to a second capillary network. In the cortical nephrons these capillary loops are numerous and form the peritubular capillary network. In juxtamedullary nephrons they penetrate to the inner medulla where they make hairpin bends before returning to the inner cortex; they are known as the vasa recta and are intimately concerned with the urinary concentrating mechanism. It is important to appreciate the structural and functional differences between cortical and juxtamedullary nephrons.

11.1 Renal haemodynamics

11.1.1 Renal blood flow

Each kidney receives 10–12% of the cardiac output, or 500–600 ml per min. Although a glomerulus is supplied by a single afferent arteriole and drained by a single efferent arteriole, the efferent arteriole subsequently breaks up into peritubular capillaries or vasa recta that supply neighbouring nephrons as well as the nephron from which they originate. About 85% of nephrons are of the cortical type.

Corresponding to this about 85% of renal blood flow supplies the cortex and about 10% the medulla.

Since the vasa recta are distributed throughout a relatively larger tissue volume than the peritubular capillaries, medullary blood flow is less than that of the cortex when expressed as a perfusion (i.e. flow per unit tissue volume). A lower perfusion in the medulla is of great importance for maintenance of the osmotic gradient that exists from outer to inner medulla.

The proportion of total renal blood flow respectively supplying cortex and medulla, or more precisely supplying cortical and juxtamedullary nephrons, varies under a number of physiological conditions, such as sodium intake and systemic blood pressure. The term redistribution of blood flow between cortex and medulla is somewhat misleading since the resistance of each of these two parallel circuits can be varied independently of each other. Thus flow to one does not occur at the expense of flow to the other; in contrast flow to either zone may change to a greater or lesser extent than flow to the other.

Blood flow to the kidneys displays the phenomenon of auto-regulation; thus renal blood flow (RBF) is held fairly constant over a wide range of perfusing pressures, about 80–180 mm Hg. For flow to remain constant, vascular resistance must vary in proportion to perfusion pressure. Several mechanisms explain the phenomenon. Since auto-regulation remains intact in the transplanted kidney, these mechanisms must be intrinsic to the kidney and, conversely, be virtually independent of neural regulation. One is the myogenic mechanism in which an increase in distension pressure in the arteriole directly results in smooth muscle contraction and a subsequent increase in resistance. Another, based on tubulo–glomerular feedback, is more subtle and described below in relation to the effects of renovascular disease on renal function.

Measurement of renal blood flow may be useful in several clinical circumstances, including renovascular disease, renal transplant rejection and nephrotoxicity from several chemotherapeutic agents such as cyclosporin. Essentially all of the techniques described in Chapter 3 are applicable to the kidney, the most important being plasma clearance of reno-specific agents like hippurate, fractionation of cardiac output and clearance from renal uptake measurement.

11.1.1.1 Hippuran clearance

RBF, or more specifically renal plasma flow (RPF), has historically been most frequently measured from plasma hippurate clearance, either radioiodinated ortho-iodohippurate (OIH) or para-amino hippurate (PAH). Two important assumptions are made: firstly, that there is no extra-renal hippuran uptake and, secondly, that the renal hippuran extraction efficiency approaches 100%. Because, in individual circumstances, extraction fraction is not as high as this, and because 3–5% of total RPF serves the connective tissue elements of the kidney, mainly the capsule, RPF measured in this way is usually described as effective renal plasma flow (ERPF). ERPF is therefore synonymous with hippuran clearance.

Following intravenous injection of a known quantity of the tracer, blood samples are taken from the arm opposite to that injected, initially at intervals of 5 minutes and then at intervals increasing to about 20 minutes up to a total of about 90 minutes. The radioactivity in each sample is counted in a well counter and corrected for physical decay with respect to injection time. After counting a standard (i.e. a sample with known radioactivity), a time–concentration curve can be constructed. A significant percentage of hippuran (variously estimated as 30–70%) is protein bound in plasma, so the effective volume of distribution is somewhere between plasma volume and extracellular fluid volume. Activity therefore simultaneously enters the kidney and extra-cellular fluid space, giving rise to a bi-exponential clearance curve, the first exponential of which is completed by about 30 minutes **(Fig. 11.1)**. Hippuran clearance, or ERPF, is then equal to injected activity divided by the area under the clearance curve; i.e.

$$\text{ERPF} = \frac{\text{injected activity}}{\text{area}}. \quad (11.1)$$

The area enclosed under a mono-exponential curve is the zero time intercept divided by the rate constant (Sections 1.2.4 and 2.2.1.2), so the area under a bi-

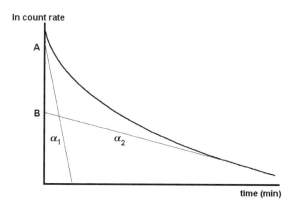

▮ **Fig. 11.1** Bi-exponential renal tracer (hippuran or DTPA) clearance from plasma. Plasma clearance is equal to injected activity divided by total area under the plasma curve. As the curve is bi-exponential, the total area is equal to the sum of the areas under the two exponentials. These areas are defined as intercept divided by rate constant so total area is $[A/\alpha_1 + B/\alpha_2]$. (N.B. A very early exponential is also present but its rate constant is so fast that it makes a negligible contribution to the total area under the curve).

exponential curve, like that representing hippuran clearance, is simply the sum of the ratios (intercept/rate constant) for each of the two exponentials. These two exponentials can be resolved by curve stripping or computer curve fitting. So

$$\text{ERPF} = \frac{\text{injected activity}}{A/\alpha_1 + B/\alpha_2} \quad (11.2)$$

where A and B are the zero time intercepts of the two exponentials and α_1 and α_2 are their corresponding rate constants.

The blood flow to each individual kidney can be measured from the rate of uptake (i.e. renal clearance) of OIH, preferably labelled with iodine-123, by gamma camera scintigraphy (Rutland 1979). The principles are the same as those for measuring individual kidney glomerular filtration rate (GFR) with technetium-99m DTPA (Section 11.1.2.3).

As mentioned above, ERPF can only be equal to true renal plasma flow if extraction fraction is unity. This requirement is almost satisfied by normal kidneys but unfortunately not in abnormal kidneys. In renal vascular disease, for example, hippuran extraction fraction has been shown to vary widely. It is also affected by certain drugs, for instance, angiotensin-converting enzyme inhibitors and cyclosporin.

Following its introduction as a technetium-99m labelled tubular agent, mercaptoacetyltriglycine (MAG_3) is being increasingly used to estimate ERPF. However, since its extraction fraction is no more than 50%, its plasma clearance is even further removed from RPF. A more recent technetium-99m labelled tubular agent is L,L-ethylenedicysteine (L,L-EC) which has a renal extraction efficiency intermediate between MAG_3 and hippuran — about 60%.

In order to simplify the measurement of ERPF for clinical use, several authors have described techniques, applicable to all three tubular agents, that give reasonably close estimates of RPF from a single blood sample taken at a specified time after injection. The concentration of tracer in the sample is expressed in relation to the injected activity, giving a value with units of volume. This imaginary volume is sometimes loosely called the distribution volume (at the sampling time). It has no relation to the anatomical distribution space, which for these tracers is the ECF space, or to the effective distribution volume, which, because of protein binding in plasma, is effectively less than the ECF volume. Regression equations relating the distribution volume at the sampling time (i.e. injected activity/ plasma concentration) and the 'true' ERPF, determined by multiple sampling, have been described for both hippuran and MAG_3. The timing of the single sample which gives the best estimate of ERPF is about 45 min for hippuran and 60 min for MAG_3 and L,L-EC, although the time is increased in the presence of reduced ERPF (Tauxe *et al.* 1982). It is important to appreciate that these approximations to ERPF are only intended for routine clinical use in patients with reasonable renal function and not for the more rigorous setting of clinical research (also see below for DTPA and GFR).

11.1.1.2 Xenon-133 washout

The technique of inert gas washout following intra-arterial injection has found widespread use in renal physiology and disease (Thorburn *et al.* 1963, Rosen *et al.* 1968, Blaufox *et al.* 1970). The washout curve is multi-exponential and up to four exponentials have been described. At least some of them represent perfusion in different vascular compartments within the kidney (**Fig. 11.2**). Perfusion in the outer cortex, for instance, is considerably greater than that of the

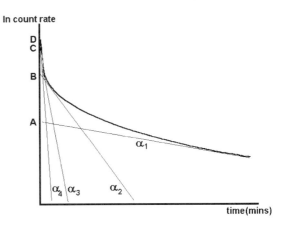

▮ **Fig. 11.2**   Xenon-133 washout from the kidney following renal arterial injection is multi-exponential, typically consisting of 4 exponentials. The fastest is renal cortical perfusion which is very high, approaching 400 ml/min/100 g.

medulla, although whether all exponentials correspond to particular 'compartments' is doubtful. Mean perfusion can be derived from the weighted harmonic mean of the exponentials, from initial height over area or, more simply, from the initial (or maximum) slope. Normal mean renal perfusion is quite torrential being in the region of 350 ml/min/ 100 ml. This corresponds to a half-time on the washout curve of only a few seconds, in contrast to resting muscle, for instance, which has a xenon-133 half time clearance of about 5 minutes. The general formula for calculating perfusion from xenon-133 washout curves, given in Section 3.1.1.1, is applicable to the kidney. The xenon-133 partition coefficient between blood and renal tissue is usually taken as 0.7.

11.1.1.3 Fractionation of cardiac output

The fraction of cardiac output (CO) supplying the kidney (*i.e. renal blood flow/cardiac output*) is, at least from a theoretical standpoint, most straightforwardly measured from the injection of radio-labelled microspheres directly into the left side of the heart. Assuming:

(1)   complete mixing of tracer in the cardiac chambers;

(2)   no elution of tracer from the microspheres;

(3)   no streamlining of tracer in the arterial tree;

(4) complete entrapment of microspheres in the renal vascular bed;

then the total quantity of activity entering (and being trapped) in the kidney, expressed as a fraction of the total injected activity, is equal to RBF/CO. So for an injected activity D

$$\frac{\text{RBF}}{\text{CO}} = \frac{\text{M}}{\text{D}} \qquad (11.3)$$

Now

$$M = \gamma R \qquad (11.4)$$

where M is the activity (MBq) delivered to the kidney, R is the count rate recorded from the kidney and γ a constant relating this count rate to MBq.

Several general methods are available for quantifying the total renal activity, in particular measuring γ, and these are covered in Section 5.4.3. The simplest is to measure the renal depth from a lateral image; cursors are placed on the digital image over the posterior abdominal wall (most readily identified by a radioactive pen marker) and the centre of the kidney. This then allows for correction of the attenuation of the photons emitted from within the kidney and detected on the posterior view. Another way to correct for attenuation is to calculate the geometric mean of counts from anterior and posterior projections (Section 5.4.3.2).

This technique for measuring RBF/CO was utilized by Crean *et al.* (1986) who obtained a value of 0.25 (both kidneys combined). It is however unsuitable for routine use. Furthermore it is not easy to measure the injected activity accurately because the radio-labelled microspheres readily adhere to the injection syringe and catheter, both of which have to be counted after injection in order to estimate the true activity injected.

The technique of cardiac output fractionation can be modified for non-invasive use (Peters *et al.* 1987) with almost any radio-pharmaceutical, as will now be described. If the time course of radio-labelled microsphere activity in arterial blood could be measured and then integrated it would have the same shape as the time activity curve recorded over the kidney, which essentially performs a 'biological', in contrast to mathematical, integration of the arterial time activity curve. Since the integrated arterial and kidney time–activity curves have the

same shape, the ratio of their maximum upslope gradients, g_a and g_k respectively, will be equal to the ratio of their plateau heights, A and R respectively (**Fig. 11.3**); i.e.

$$g_k/g_a = R/A$$

with units

$$\frac{\text{count/min/min}}{\text{counts/min}} = \frac{\text{counts/min}}{\text{counts}}$$

and

$$R = g_k/g_a \times A \qquad (11.5)$$

where A is equal to the total area under the non-integrated arterial curve and g_a is equal to its peak height. Here R is proportional to the total activity trapped in the kidney as in equation 11.3. For a recirculating tracer, given intravenously, the arterial curve will show a recirculation peak and the renal curve will fail to reach a plateau. However the arterial time activity curve will still reach its peak height before recirculation and so g_a can still be measured. Furthermore, the arterial curve can be corrected for recirculation (see cardiac output measurement, Section 7.2.1) and A obtained. Provided the renal upslope curve displays its maximum slope within the period of the minimum intravascular tracer transit time through the kidney, g_k can also be measured. Hence M can be calculated and inserted into equation 11.3. So

$$M = g_k/g_a \times A \times \gamma \qquad (11.6)$$
$$= \frac{\text{RBF}}{\text{CO}} \times D. \qquad (11.7)$$

It can be appreciated that, in essence, the arterial time activity curve is used to forward extrapolate the renal time activity curve to a plateau that it would have reached if the tracer, having entered the kidney, was completely trapped; i.e. had an infinite transit time, like a microsphere.

In practice, the arterial time activity curve can be recorded in several regions of interest: lung, left ventricle or upper abdominal aorta, and a family of extrapolated renal plateaux thereby derived (i.e. a family of values for R). Either the mean or median of these separate estimates of RBF can be taken. Alternatively, and more simply, RBF can be based on the lung curve alone. Although the lung curve would be expected to have a greater peak height to area ratio (reflecting less spreading of the bolus at

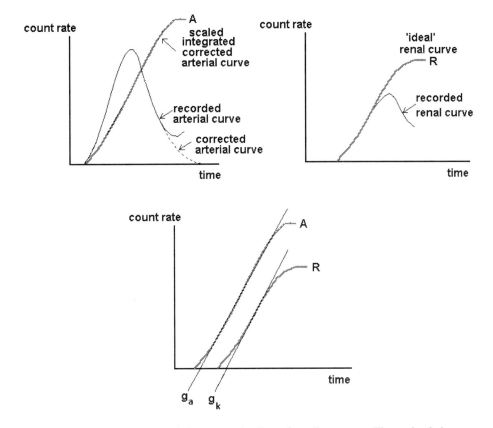

❙ **Fig. 11.3** Measurement of renal blood flow as a fraction of cardiac output. The recirculation-corrected curve generated from an arterial region of interest defines the width of the bolus and after integration can be scaled to have an upslope (g_a) parallel to the slope (g_k) of the recorded renal curve. The plateau (A) of the integrated arterial curve predicts the plateau that would have been reached by the renal curve (R) if the tracer had been completely retained by the kidney. Several arterial regions of interest can be used and should agree in their estimates of the plateau.

this point in the circulation), it is, to its advantage, much more clearly defined than the other arterial curves, and is easier to correct for recirculation. Its theoretical tendency to underestimate flow (because of the relatively high value of g_a) can be taken into account by multiplication by the empirically determined factor of 1.1.

If an intravascular tracer is used for measurement of RBF/CO by this approach, such as labelled protein or red cells, then by taking a blood sample at 5 minutes (as in the measurement of cardiac output), RBF can be derived in absolute units. Thus, rearranging equation 11.7,

$$\text{RBF/CO} = (g_k/g_a) \times (A/D) \times \gamma. \quad (11.8)$$

but

$$\text{CO} = \frac{D}{A \cdot \Gamma} \quad (11.9)$$

where Γ is a constant relating camera count rate to actual blood concentration in MBq/ml and which can be determined from the 5 min blood sample. So

$$\text{RBF} = \frac{g_k}{g_a} \times \frac{\gamma}{\Gamma}. \quad (11.10)$$

Note that injected activity is no longer needed, nor a correction for recirculation. Equation 11.10 indicates that absolute RBF is proportional to g_k/g_a. This provides a simple and convenient basis for quantifying changes in RBF in response to various interventions. If the arterial ROIs can be redrawn in the same position then the term γ/Γ cancels out when sequential studies are compared, so that

$$\frac{\text{RBF}_1}{\text{RBF}_2} = \frac{[g_k/g_a]_1}{[g_k/g_a]_2}. \quad (11.11)$$

11.1.1.4 Measurement of absolute renal blood flow by indicator dilution

This is included for the sake of illustration and completeness but is almost never employed in clinical practice. A venous time–concentration curve is constructed by renal venous sampling following injection of tracer into the renal artery: then

RBF = injected activity/area under curve. (11.12)

This is based on the indicator dilution principle and is analogous to the measurement of cardiac output, differing from it:

(a) in terms of the site of injection;
(b) the site of sampling.

11.1.1.5 Quantification of intra-renal blood flow distribution

There have been many attempts to quantify intrarenal distribution of blood flow using the inert gas washout technique and analysis of the exponentials thereby produced (see above). A non-invasive technique, based on iodine-123-hippuran and deconvolution analysis, has also been described (Gruenewald *et al.* 1981). Since the mean intrarenal transit time through cortical nephrons is faster than through juxtamedullary nephrons, there is a bimodal distribution of global renal transit times. By distinguishing and comparing transit time spectra for the two nephron populations, the fractionation of blood flow between them can be measured. ROIs are placed respectively over the outer cortex, containing cortical nephrons only, and the middle to outer cortex, containing both types of nephrons, and the subsequent renograms subjected to deconvolution analysis. By differentiating the retention function curves, outflow curves are generated for the two ROI (as explained in Section 2.1.1). After scaling the outflow curves so that their leading (i.e. left) edges are superimposed, they are subtracted from each other, thereby generating an outflow curve for juxtamedullary nephrons only. Provided the extraction fraction of the tracer is the same for the two types of nephron, the respective areas under the two outflow curves reflect relative blood flows to the two nephron populations. This gave a value of 83% of blood flow to cortical nephrons, corresponding well to the fraction of nephrons that are normally cortical, and lower values in hypertensives without necessarily a reduction in total renal blood flow.

11.1.2 Glomerular filtration

The barrier between the blood in the glomerular capillary and the tubular fluid in Bowman's capsule is composed of three elements; the capillary endothelium, the epithelium of Bowman's capsule (which is continuous with tubular epithelium) and a basement membrane between them. About 20% of the incoming water of the renal plasma flow is transferred across this barrier, and this is the glomerular filtrate. This water is accompanied by the same percentage of incoming solutes up to a molecular weight of about 5000 Da. With respect to such solutes therefore the composition of the filtrate and plasma is identical. For substances with molecular weights between 5000 and 70 000 Da however the concentration in the filtrate is less than that in plasma with filtrate plasma concentration ratios decreasing rapidly with increasing molecular size. Molecules above 70 000 Da are not normally filtered. Since substances with high molecular weight are not filtered, the filtrate is more correctly called an ultra-filtrate.

The volume of glomerular filtrate formed per unit of time, expressed as a fraction of renal plasma flow, is the filtration fraction (FF); i.e.

$$FF = GFR/RPF. \qquad (11.13)$$

There are several fundamental differences between glomerular capillaries and extra-renal capillaries with respect to water and solute transfer. Thus, in the glomerulus, bulk fluid transfer with the contained solutes takes place by filtration. In contrast, in extrarenal capillaries, water and solutes cross predominantly by diffusion, independently of each other. Only a small fraction of fluid transfer takes place by filtration. As a result of filtration in glomerular capillaries, only 20% of plasma water is transferred across the glomerular capillary and this is accompanied by 20% of small solutes. In contrast, in one pass through an extra-renal capillary, such as in muscle or skin, virtually 100% of the water enters the extra-vascular space by diffusion and almost all of it re-enters the plasma by the venous end of the capillary (see Chapter 6).

Glomerular filtration is held relatively constant in the face of changes in renal blood flow and extracellular fluid (ECF) volume, although it increases following volume expansion by saline infusion and decreases as part of the anti-natriuretic response to sodium deprivation. This results in a relative constancy in GFR when expressed in relation to ECF volume which can therefore be utilized as an alternative to body surface area for the normalisation of GFR (see below). Nevertheless the kidney is also able to maintain sodium excretion constant in spite of primary changes in GFR, as the kidney will continue to excrete sodium following saline infusion, even when GFR and RBF are reduced by means of an aortic clamp (and mineralocorticoid status held constant). This ability of the kidney to maintain sodium excretion, called *glomerular–tubular balance*, is probably controlled by intra-renal mediators. *Tubulo–glomerular feedback* is a separate intra-renal homeostatic mechanism whereby renal blood flow is influenced by sodium delivery to the macula densa. Its mediator is the renin-angiotensin system. Renin is contained in the secretory granules of the granular cells of the juxtaglomerular apparatus (JGA), a specialized structure found in the region where the tubule makes contact with the glomerulus from which it originated. The granular cells are part of the afferent arteriole while the specialized cells of the tubule in the JGA comprise a structure called the macula densa. The latter 'senses' the tubular sodium chloride content and by a poorly understood mechanism regulates the secretion of renin by the granular cells. Renin is a proteolytic enzyme which acts locally on angiotensinogen, a circulating protein synthesised in the liver, converting it to angiotensin 1 (A1). A1 is almost immediately converted to A2 by angiotensin converting enzyme (ACE). A2 is a powerful vaso-constrictor on both the afferent and efferent arterioles and is present in maximal concentration in the efferent arteriole. Since intra-renal A2 predominantly acts on the efferent arteriole while A2 of extra-renal origin predominantly acts on the afferent arteriole, the overall differential effect of A2 on the two arterioles regulates both renal blood flow and filtration fraction, especially in juxtamedullary nephrons. If sodium chloride delivery to the macula densa is decreased, renin output increases. Although renal blood flow is consequently reduced, GFR is defended by an increase in filtration fraction as a result of selective efferent arteriolar vaso-constriction. Systemic arterial pressure is also defended by the action of A2 on (1) peripheral arterioles and (2) on the adrenal cortex to increase aldosterone excretion, which in turn promotes tubular sodium reabsorbtion.

In renal vascular hypertension (RVH), renin output is inappropriately increased as a result of renal ischaemia. In functionally significant renal artery stenosis for example, glomerular filtration pressure is reduced, and the kidney 'thinks' that systemic hypotension is present, partly by virtue of the decreased delivery of sodium chloride to the macula densa. It was the classic experiments of Goldblatt which first clearly focused on the role of renal ischaemia in hypertension.

There are two variations to the Goldblatt model of reno–vascular hypertension; the two kidney one clip (KKC) model and the KC model. Unilateral nephrectomy is first performed to produce the KC model. The two clip two kidney (KKCC) model is essentially the same as the KC model in that no normal kidney is present to respond to alterations in fluid and sodium balance resulting from renal ischaemia. As pointed out above, the raised renin levels induce sodium retention via increased aldosterone production with a resulting expansion in plasma volume. This volume expansion and sodium retention depress renin levels by negative feedback but themselves sustain hypertension. The point at which renin returns to normal divides the hypertension into the initial renin-dependent and later renin-independent phases. It is only during the renin-dependent phase that the blood pressure will respond to ACE inhibition. Sodium restriction during the renin-independent phase will however restore the blood pressure responsiveness to ACE inhibition. This is because the peripheral renin level becomes elevated again as a result of sodium restriction and maintains the hypertension. In other words, during the renin-independent phase blood pressure is maintained at an elevated level either by high renin levels or by volume expansion. This applies to both KKC and KC models. The main difference between the two models is the duration of the renin-dependent phase which is much shorter in the KC model because of the absence of a normal kidney with which to deal with the sodium and fluid retention resulting from the elevated peripheral renin level.

The screening methods for renal vascular hypertension are based on the above physiology: for example high peripheral renin and high renal vein to inferior vena caval renin ratios are found in RVH. Furthermore the GFR, although supported by efferent arteriolar vaso-constriction, is reduced. It is not reduced as much as renal blood flow however so filtration fraction increases. As a result of an increase in oncotic pressure and a decrease in hydrostatic pressure in the peritubular capillaries, this leads to an exaggerated proximal reabsorbtion of tubular fluid and a consequent prolongation of the parenchymal transit time which is the basis of the delayed peak in the isotope renogram and the persistent nephrogram of the intravenous urogram. In addition, function on the stenotic side is usually less than on the normal side.

The individual kidney haemodynamic responses to inhibition of ACE are rather confusing both in the experimental situation and in human RVH. They depend on the phase of the hypertension, the functional state of the contralateral kidney and whether or not it is also stenosed, the volume status and sodium balance (and hence degree of activation of the renin angiotensin system), the differential effect of ACE inhibition on local and on peripheral A2 levels, the magnitude of the systemic hypotensive response and the severity of the renal artery stenosis. They are also affected by certain drugs, particularly for anti-hypertensive therapy. Systemic hypotension induced by ACE inhibition results in reduced renal perfusion pressure which, in the presence of severe renal artery stenosis, may place renal blood flow outside the autoregulatory range of the kidney. This results in renal shutdown and possible irreversible nephron loss and is more likely to occur in the presence of sodium depletion.

Although the A2 level falls after ACE inhibition, the peripheral renin level increases further as a result of the abolition of negative feedback. In the captopril test, developed to detect a renovascular cause of hypertension, a positive result is an increase in peripheral venous renin concentration in response to a single dose of a short-acting ACE inhibitor, such as captopril. The captopril renogram, an extension of the captopril test, is radionuclide imaging study which aims to determine the individual kidney haemodynamic responses to ACE inhibition and therefore to assess the functional impact of renal ischaemia and identify a kidney responsible for hypertension (**Fig. 11.4**). Clinically, it aims to predict the blood pressure response to renal revascularisation and to determine the impact on renal function of antihypertensive treatment with an ACE inhibitor which, in patients with bilateral renal artery stenosis or stenosis in a solitary kidney, may

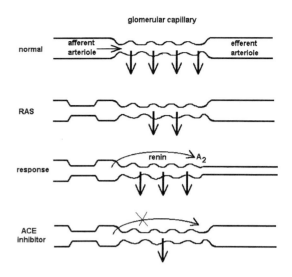

∎ **Fig. 11.4** Scheme explaining the effect of an ACE inhibitor on GFR of a single kidney with functionally significant renovascular disease. As a result of stenosis proximal to the glomerulus, filtration pressure decreases with a fall in GFR. The kidney defends GFR at the expense of a further reduction in RBF by producing renin which acts locally via the generation of angiotensin 2 to induce efferent (post-glomerular) arteriolar vasoconstriction. Because a greater proportion of the pressure gradient across the kidney is now dissipated through the post-glomerular resistance vessels, filtration pressure is elevated. Administration of a single dose of an ACE inhibitor, by blocking the defence mechanism, results in an increase in RBF and a fall or complete abolition of GFR in the kidney.

induce acute renal failure. Two renograms are performed on separate occasions, one of them one hour after a single oral dose of captopril. In haemodynamically significant renal artery stenosis, the homeostatic defence of GFR is abolished by ACE inhibition, resulting in a fall in GFR. This is manifest in a DTPA renogram as a decrease in function of the kidney, and in a MAG3 renogram as a progressively rising curve with no or delayed appearance of tracer in the collecting system (**Figs 11.5 and 11.6**). The inhibition of the intrarenal effects of A2 on the glomerular arterioles leads also to an increase in renal blood flow. A secondary effect of the reduced GFR is a further prolongation of the renal parenchymal transit time, which is manifested as a further delay in the peak of the renogram curve. A fall in individual kidney GFR (or

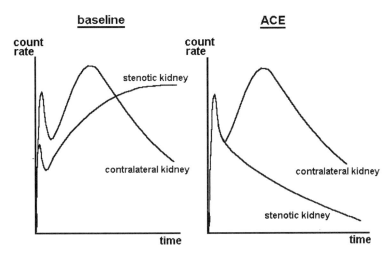

▌ **Fig. 11.5** Effect of ACE inhibition on DTPA renography in a patient with functionally significant unilateral renal artery stenosis. Functionally significant RAS gives (1) reduced RBF, (2) reduced GFR and (3) increased parenchymal transit time, thereby affecting all 3 phases of the renogram. ACE blockade results in (1) increased RBF, (2) reduced or absent GFR and (3) further prolongation of parenchymal transit time if any filtration is maintained. In the example shown here, GFR is abolished completely and the recorded renal curve would reflect the blood pool. The increase in RBF is non-specific, occurring also in the opposite kidney or in the complete absence of any renal disease.

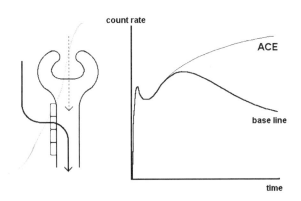

▌ **Fig. 11.6** Effect of ACE inhibition on MAG3 or hippuran renography in a patient with functionally significant renal artery stenosis. Because these agents are tubularly secreted, they are 'trapped' in the tubule in the absence of filtration. If some filtration continues, parenchymal transit time is prolonged as a result of decreased tubular fluid flow (which is accentuated by increased proximal tubular fluid absorption) and so a positive result is still seen as an abnormally rising curve since almost no MAG3 is filtered. Differential function does not change; the affected kidney may even improve slightly as a result of the non-specific increase in RBF.

increase in parenchymal transit time) following ACE inhibition is therefore interpreted as a positive captopril renogram, indicating the presence of functionally significant renal ischaemia. There is evidence to suggest that unless there is significantly reduced renal function, it is satisfactory to perform only the captopril study which, if normal, rules out functional renal ischaemia.

From the physiological considerations above, it can be appreciated that other responses (including an entirely negative response) may occur, giving rise to false negative results for RVH. The least desirable response from the point of view of the patient is renal shutdown. With this complication in mind, the patient should be well hydrated, sodium replete, off diuretics and maintained in the supine position with regular blood pressure measurements during the captopril arm of the study. The reliability with which captopril renography predicts the response to revascularization decreases with decreasing baseline renal function because the changes which constitute a positive captopril renogram primarily depend on a reduction in GFR by ACE inhibition.

In clinical practice, measurement of GFR has many uses, including the overall assessment of renal function, the diagnosis of renovascular hypertension and the impact of potentially nephrotoxic drugs on renal function. Measurement of GFR is essentially the same as measurement of the clearance of substances which are exclusively eliminated from the body by glomerular filtration — so called filtration markers — and can be based on any of the techniques described in Section 2.2.1.

11.1.2.1 Measurement of GFR from plasma clearance

Urinary inulin clearance is the gold standard for global GFR. Methods using radionuclides are generally based on the so-called single shot technique, in which the plasma clearance of a radio-pharmaceutical handled exclusively by glomerular filtration is measured from blood sampling. Filtration markers which give a reliable estimate of GFR by this approach include chromium-51 EDTA, technetium-99m DTPA and iodine-125 iothalamate, the latter better known as a radiological contrast agent. In principle, the single shot technique is identical to the measurement of ERPF. Thus the clearance of the agent is equated with GFR, analogous to equating hippuran clearance with RPF.

Samples are taken from the arm opposite the one injected. Filtration markers are confined to the extracellular space and do not enter red cells. The plasma disappearance curve is constructed after measuring radioactivity in the blood samples in a well counter. It is adequate to count 1 ml aliquots of whole blood and then apply a correction factor based on the sample haematocrit. As for hippuran clearance, a bi-exponential clearance curve is obtained. However, since filtration markers are not protein-bound in plasma, and because their extraction fraction by the kidney is only 20% (the filtration fraction) compared with about 80% for hippuran, it takes the body much longer to excrete them. The disappearance curve is therefore 'stretched out' over a longer period of time and it is necessary to take samples up to four hours. The curve is bi-exponential between 10 minutes and 4 hours.[†] The

first of the two exponentials is completed by 2 hours so the second can be seen from samples between 2 and 4 hours. Six samples, taken at 10, 20 and 30 minutes and 2, 3 and 4 hours are recommended. Then

$$\text{GFR} = \frac{\text{injected activity}}{\text{total area under plasma clearance curve}}$$

$$= \frac{\text{injected activity}}{A/\alpha_1 + B/\alpha_2} \tag{11.14}$$

where A and B are the zero time intercepts of the two exponentials and α_1 and α_2 their respective rate constants. The units are

$$\frac{\text{MBq}}{\text{MBq/ml} \times 1/\text{min}^{-1}} = \text{ml/min}.$$

A more convenient, but less accurate, method is to use only the second exponential for the calculation; i.e. the samples between 2 and 4 hours. This effectively assumes that the area under the first exponential, A/α_1, makes a negligible contribution to the total area under the disappearance curve. That is

$$\text{GFR} = \frac{\alpha_2 \times \text{injected activity}}{B}. \tag{11.15}$$

The denominator in equation 11.14 is therefore underestimated and GFR correspondingly overestimated. Since with poor renal function α_2 is small, and B/α_2 therefore large, the error produced from ignoring the first exponential is less in the presence of poor renal function (**Fig. 11.7**). Alternatively, it can be assumed that although ignoring A/α_1 will produce an error, it is nonetheless relatively constant, for which there is some support (Brochner–Mortensen 1972), and a correction factor applied to take it into account. What is often not recognized however, but obvious from an understanding of these kinetics and particularly of equation 11.14, is that the magnitude of the correction factor is inversely proportional to the level of filtration function (**Fig. 11.8**).

[†]The extracellular fluid space consists essentially of three compartments in series, two of which make up the extravascular extracellular space (see Sections 6.2.2.4.4 and 3.1.1.2). Equilibration between plasma and the fluid phase of the interstitial space is completed by about 20 min and gives an exponential which is so fast that it is visible only on arterial sampling; it is not seen on venous sampling because of tracer exchange in the extracellular space of the forearm from which venous blood is sampled. Exchange of tracer between the spaces of the interstitial fluid is slower and gives rise to a second slower clearance curve exponential, which on venous sampling is conventionally regarded as the first exponential. The terminal exponential, which represents turnover by glomerular filtration of the well-mixed ECF space, is seen from about two hours. Although having a substantial amplitude, the first exponential, invisible on venous sampling, has a fast rate constant and therefore makes only a very small contribution to the total area under the plasma clearance curve.

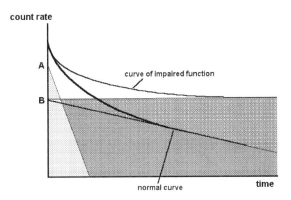

▌ Fig. 11.7 Effect of GFR on error generated in GFR by ignoring the first exponential in equation 11.14. When α_2 approaches zero, the area under the second exponential becomes very large. Consequently the area under the first exponential becomes negligible. A/α_1 is relatively independent of renal function and so a correction factor can be applied to the simplified term, (injected activity $\times \alpha_2$)/B, for measurement of GFR. The simplified term overestimates true GFR (as defined in equation 11.14) by about 15% at normal GFR, requiring a correction factor of 0.85 (and indicating that α_1 contributes 15% to the total area under the clearance curve). This overestimate disappears when GFR decreases to less than about 40 ml/min/1.73 m^2 corresponding to an α_2 value of about 0.003 min^{-1}.

The constants A and B are effectively converted to variables with units of concentration (MBq/ml) by counting a standard along with the blood samples, as for ERPF measurement. Appropriate corrections for physical decay of the isotope are applied which depend on the time interval between calibration of the dose and counting the samples.

Technetium-99m DTPA, although generally thought to be less accurate than chromium-51 EDTA or iodine-125 iothalamate, nevertheless gives total GFR with good precision and accuracy. A potential source of error is protein binding which has been shown to vary between commercial sources of technetium-99m DTPA. Plasma protein binding leads to an underestimation of GFR because the extraction fraction falls below filtration fraction. The presence of technetium-99m which is not bound to DTPA also results in a small error.

In order to account for variations in body size (especially to compare children with adults), GFR is conventionally expressed in relation to body surface area and normalized to 1.73 m^2 (i.e. GFR/1.73 m^2). The rationale for this is that basal metabolic rate and kidney weight are both proportional to body surface area. However some authorities have questioned the validity of this and suggested other variables against which to normalize or 'factor' GFR, such as total body water, extracellular fluid volume (ECF) or

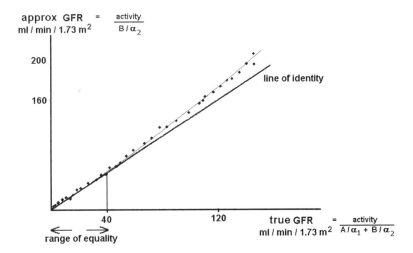

▌ Fig. 11.8 The relationship between GFR based on equation 11.15, which ignores the first exponential, and 'true' GFR based on equation 11.14, which includes the first exponential. The relationship is well fitted by a second order polynomial, values for which have been reported in the literature by several groups and can be used to convert a value obtained by the simplified method to the 'true' value.

plasma volume. It is easy to appreciate the difficulties imposed by such alternative variables, because they would require separate measurement if GFR was measured by the classical technique of urinary inulin clearance. In contrast, when measuring GFR from single shot plasma clearance, ECF volume is effectively measured at the same time and can be used as an alternative to surface area.

It is especially appealing to normalize GFR against ECF volume (ECV) because firstly, the filtration function of the kidney is to filter and regulate the composition of the ECF and secondly, the rate constant of the second exponential is a close approximation to the fraction of ECF filtered in unit time (in ml/min per litre of ECF). The ratio ECV/ GFR is equal to the mean 'waiting' time (i.e. residence, transit time) of a filtration marker (whose distribution volume is ECV) before filtration. This is an appropriate measure of filtration function just as one would be more likely to judge the efficiency of a customs hall from one's own waiting time rather than the rate of passenger clearance. Thus

$$T = \text{ECV}/\text{GFR}$$
$$= \frac{A/\alpha_1^2 + B/\alpha_2^2}{A/\alpha_1 + B/\alpha_2} \qquad (11.16)$$

(see Section 2.1.1).

As already mentioned, α_2 closely approximates $1/T$ although, as with GFR itself based on samples between only 2 and 4 hr, becomes further removed from it with increasing filtration function. Inspection of equation 11.16 shows that when A and α_1 are ignored, the right-hand side reduces to α_2, which becomes equal to $1/T$ when α_2 becomes low. Whereas GFR based on 2–4 hr progressively overestimates true GFR as filtration function increases, α_2 progressively *underestimates* true GFR/ ECV as filtration increases, although the error is always less than that of GFR based on 2–4 hr, as can be shown as follows.

For clarity, let A/α_1 be x, B/α_2 be y, and α_2/α_1 be z. Then, from equations 11.14 and 11.15,

$$\text{GFR}_{2-4\,\text{hr}}/\text{GFR}_{\text{true}} = 1 + (x/y) \qquad (11.17)$$

i.e. $\text{GFR}_{2-4\text{hr}}$ is always greater than GFR_{true} **(Fig. 11.8)**.

From equation 11.16, and denoting $1/\alpha_2$ as $T_{2-4\text{hr}}$ (in effect, an approximate estimate of T_{true}),

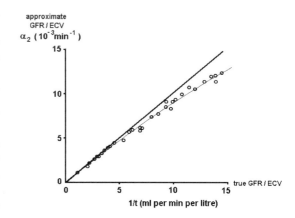

∎ **Fig. 11.9** The relationship between α_2 and 'true' GFR/ ECV (which is the reciprocal of the mean residence time of DTPA in the ECF space before filtration). In contrast to the relationship between true GFR and GFR based only on the second exponential, the approximate method α_2 for GFR/ ECV underestimates true GFR/ECV. Again α_2 can be converted to a true value of GFR/ECV using a second order polynomial based on a population of patients.

$$\frac{T_{2-4\,\text{hr}}}{T_{\text{true}}} = 1 + \frac{1-z}{z+(y/x)}, \qquad (11.18)$$

i.e. $T_{2-4\text{hr}}$ is always greater than T_{true} (because z, by definition, is less than 1) and therefore α_2 always less than $1/T_{\text{true}}$ **(Fig. 11.9)**. The ratio $\text{GFR}_{2-4\text{hr}}/\text{GFR}_{\text{true}}$ must always be greater than $T_{\text{true}}/T_{2-4\text{hr}}$ because, by combining equations 11.17 and 11.18, we find that

$$\frac{\text{GFR}_{2-4\,\text{hr}}}{\text{GFR}_{\text{true}}} \times \frac{T_{\text{true}}}{T_{2-4\,\text{hr}}} = 1 + \frac{zx}{y}. \qquad (11.19)$$

There are several conditions which illustrate the validity of normalizing GFR to ECF volume, rather than say to body surface area (BSA). For example, GFR/BSA is increased in acromegaly, suggesting significant hyperfiltration, while it is reduced in hypopituitarism, suggesting underfiltration. The ratio GFR/ECV however is normal in both conditions, indicating that the ECF volumes are abnormal and that the kidney responds appropriately. Furthermore, whilst normal adult males have a slightly but significantly higher GFR/BSA than normal adult females, their respective values of GFR/ECV are identical. Reassuringly, the α_2 for inulin is very similar to that for Tc-99m DTPA (Gunasekera *et al.* 1996) or slightly less (Rehling *et al.* 1984), indicating that GFR/ECV based on α_2 is not dependent on the filtration marker used to measure it.

A scaling factor based on α_2 can be applied to α_2 to obtain true GFR/ECV. Such a factor has been determined for adults (Peters 1992) and infants (Peters *et al.* 1994a) and for dogs and horses (Gleadhill *et al.* 1995). In the case of human infants, it is noteworthy that whilst GFR/BSA is subnormal up to about 12 years of age compared with adults, GFR/ECV reaches adult levels by age 2 yr. This is a reflection of the relatively high body surface area of small children. In this population, GFR factored for total body water (McCance and Widdowson 1952), lean body mass (Kurtin 1989) or body weight (Friis-Hansen 1961) are all more in line with GFR/ECV than GFR/BSA. Measurement of GFR/ECV (as α_2) offers the opportunity to measure GFR in 'real time' by external probe monitoring (Rossing *et al.* 1978, Rabito *et al.* 1993).

As in the measurement of ERPF, several formulae have been described for the measurement of global GFR from a single blood sample taken about 2 hr after injection of DTPA (Waller *et al.* 1987, Bubeck 1993). In one such method the patient's ECF is assumed from height and weight and used along with injected activity to derive the zero-time plasma concentration. Combined with the measured late concentration, this gives a two-point clearance curve from which GFR can be calculated from equation 11.15. The assumed ECF volume should however be modified to account for the error produced when it is measured by extrapolation of the second exponential to zero time (see Section 13.1). This error is fractionally identical to the error produced in GFR by ignoring the first exponential. Bubeck (1993) has pointed out that the apparent volume of distribution of tracer at a specified time bears a non-linear relationship to the true clearance of the tracer. However, by normalizing the apparent volume of distribution to a body surface area of 1.73 m^2, a linear relationship is generated with the clearance similarly normalized. This makes such algorithms equally applicable to children.

It is instructive to compare the GFR calculated from two points on the second exponential (sometimes called the *C*-slope method — Chantler and Barratt 1972) with the one sample method. Since α_2 and B are respectively the numerator and denominator for calculation of GFR in equation 11.15, and

because a change in α_2 results in a directionally similar change in B, any error in α_2 is counterbalanced by an opposing error in B. The effect of this is that for any value of C_1 (the concentration in the first of the *two* samples taken at time *t*), there is a maximum value of GFR from a two-sample GFR measurement, as will now be shown.

For a plasma clearance of technetium-99m DTPA with terminal rate constant α_2 the concentration in the first blood sample C_1 taken at time *t* is given by

$$C_1 = Be^{-\alpha_2 t} \qquad (11.20)$$

where B is the zero time intercept. Restating equation 11.15,

$$\text{GFR} = \frac{\alpha_2 \times M_0}{B}.$$

Substituting for B gives

$$\text{GFR} = \frac{M_0 \alpha_2 e^{-\alpha_2 t}}{C_1}. \qquad (11.21)$$

The apparent volume of distribution of DTPA V_1 at the time of the first sample is given by

$$V_1 = \frac{M_0}{C_1}$$

so

$$\text{GFR} = V_1 \alpha_2 e^{-\alpha_2 t}. \qquad (11.22)$$

A maximum value of GFR is found by differentiating equation 11.22 with respect to α_2 and setting the result to zero. That is

$$\frac{d(\text{GFR})}{d\alpha_2} = V_1\, e^{-\alpha_2 t} - V_1 \alpha_2 t e^{-\alpha_2 t}.$$

When $\dfrac{d(\text{GFR})}{d\alpha_2} = 0$,

$$V_1 e^{-\alpha_2 t} = V_1 \alpha_2 t e^{-\alpha_2 t}.$$

and

$$\alpha_2 t = 1.$$

This yields a maximum value of $\alpha_2 e^{-\alpha_2 t}$ for a given volume of distribution V_1 when $\alpha_2 = 1/t$. When $\alpha_2 e^{-\alpha_2 t}$ is plotted against α_2, a family of curves is produced of the form illustrated in Fig. 11.10, in which it can be seen that the maximum value of $\alpha_2 e^{-\alpha_2 t}$ occurs at a time the reciprocal of which is equal to α_2 (Waller *et al.* 1987).

From Fig. 11.10 it can be seen that as C_1 is based on later values of *t*, the value of α_2 at which GFR is

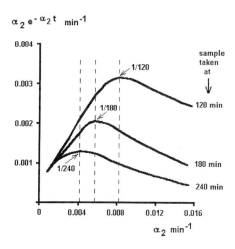

▮ **Fig. 11.10** The relationship between one-sample and two-sample GFR. The one-sample GFR compares the injected activity with the concentration in a sample obtained at a particular time after injection (usually between 2 and 4 hr) and expresses the result as a 'volume of distribution' (V_1), high values reflecting low GFR. GFR measured from two samples using equation 11.22, where the first sample is used to determine V_1, is given by $V_1 \cdot \alpha_2 \cdot e^{-\alpha_2 t}$. A plot of $\alpha_2 e^{-\alpha_2 t}$ against α_2 shows a maximum value at a value of α_2 equal to the reciprocal of the time of the first sample. This mathematical outcome has implications for the accuracy of one-sample GFR measurement and the relationship between one-sample and two-sample GFR values simultaneously measured in a given population of patients.

maximal from a two-sample GFR decreases. Several authors have validated one-sample GFR against two-sample GFR, and used the relationship between them to derive formulae which give GFR from one sample. Often the sample for the one-sample method has been the same as the first sample in the two-sample method. The resulting relationship between the distribution volume V_1 (x-axis) based on the single sample (i.e. dose/C_1) and GFR from two samples (y-axis) predictably shows the following features (Fawdry and Gruenwald 1987) (Fig. 11.11). Firstly, for any value of C_1 and therefore for any distribution volume, there is a maximal two-sample GFR value, giving rise to a boundary to the left of the scatter plot. Secondly, this maximal value, i.e. the boundary, shows a linear correlation with

volume of distribution; thus, if say t is 120 min for all points, maximal α_2 is 0.008 min^{-1}, so GFR is equal to 0.008/C_1, which correlated with injected activity/C_1 (i.e. volume of distribution) obviously gives a straight line passing through the origin. Thirdly, low volumes of distribution tend to be associated with low values of α_2 and high volumes with high α_2 values. So at either side of a mid-range of α_2 values, it can be seen from Figs. 11.10 and 11.11 that there is greater variation in GFR for unit change in α_2. The effect of this is to give more scatter at the extremes of the relationship between volume of distribution and two-sample GFR than in the middle, where the correlation is spuriously tight. Thus at values of α_2 approaching the reciprocal of the time of the first sample, the variation in α_2 is more constrained. The single sample GFR will give its greatest accuracy (least variation) when the reciprocal of the rate constant is equal to the time of sampling.

The implication of these kinetics is that, for greatest accuracy, patient populations with higher than normal rate constants would require a sampling time that is shorter than the standard nominal sampling time, while patient populations with smaller than normal rate constants would require a longer sampling time. Since the sampling time has to be fixed to some reasonable value (say between 2 and 4 hours) then, faced with a patient with an unknown GFR, there is no guarantee that the measurement will have the highest accuracy, and a method of GFR assessment based on that patient alone, such as the two-sample method, may be preferred. Furthermore, a single-sample GFR based on the best fit of a regression of distribution volumes on two sample GFR will only apply to the population on which that regression was based and may not be suitable for a prospective measurement of GFR in an individual patient.

11.1.2.2 Differential renal function

Differential renal function is defined as the function in each kidney expressed as a percentage of the total function of the two kidneys. The meaning of differential function depends on the particular renal agent used to measure it and the renal functions that contribute to its uptake. DTPA is a filtration marker, so differential function with this agent is specifically differential GFR. Uptake of DMSA depends on renal blood flow, GFR, tubular extraction efficiency (both for tracer directly removed from peritubular capillary blood and for filtered tracer) and the avidity with which cortical proteins bind and retain DMSA. So, in acute outflow obstruction, differential function based on DTPA may be different to that based on DMSA.

Differential function is most easily measured by expressing the counts (whatever agent is used) accumulated in one kidney as a percentage of the counts accumulated by both kidneys. 'Background' counts contribute to the counts recorded over the kidney and should be first subtracted. Background correction is discussed in more detail below. Images are acquired up to a time at which it can be reliably assumed that no activity that has entered either kidney has yet left it. For excreted agents like DTPA, MAG$_3$ and hippuran, this assumption holds good only up to the minimum intra-tubular transit time, which is the shortest time the agent can traverse the tubule between its point of entry and the collecting system. More precisely, it is the minimum transit time of the agent through the region of interest drawn around the kidney, and is longer for a whole kidney region of interest than for one which includes only the parenchyma.

It is usually assumed that this time restriction does not apply to differential function based on DMSA since it remains fixed in the kidney, thereby allowing differential function to be based upon images taken at almost any time. However an appreciable percentage (10–20%) of DMSA is excreted in the urine, compared with 50% retained in the kidneys. This urinary DMSA nevertheless represents 'renal handling'.

11.1.2.3 Differential GFR and single kidney GFR

These are best considered together as the techniques for measuring them are closely related. Probably the most accurate way of measuring single kidney GFR is to measure total GFR and divide it between two kidneys using the differential function obtained from technetium-99m DTPA renography (based on the same administered injected activity of DTPA). The other method for measuring single kidney GFR uses

the first few minutes of the renogram itself and requires only one blood sample (see below).

The simplest way to measure differential GFR is to compare the uptakes of technetium-99m DTPA in regions of interest drawn around the two kidneys in images acquired over 2–3 minutes following injection and to apply some form of background correction. A more elaborate approach is based on the following differential equation (Piepsz *et al.* 1977) which states that the rate of accumulation of activity in the kidney at any time is proportional to the simultaneous plasma activity:

$$dR/dt = \alpha \cdot P(t)$$

which rearranged is

$$\alpha = dR/dt \times 1/P(t). \qquad (11.23)$$

Here R is the background-corrected renal count rate, $P(t)$ is the count rate from a cardiac region of interest at time t less than the minimum renal tubular transit time and α is a constant of proportionality with units of min^{-1} which represents the GFR of the kidney (**Fig. 11.11**). Since $P(t)$ is the same for each kidney, relative function of the two kidneys is the same as the relative values for dR/dt. In other words, differential function is given by the relative gradients of the respective second phases of the background-corrected renograms. Since α is constant, dR/dt divided by $P(t)$ must be constant and is said to be the uptake function of the kidney. Differential function therefore is equal to the relative values of α for each side. Since the kidneys may be at different depths, and therefore subject to unequal photon attenuation, depth correction improves accuracy. This requires lateral views to establish the depth of each kidney. However, unless one or both kidneys are ectopic or markedly hydronephrotic, or the patient has kyphoscoliosis, ignoring depth correction results in little error.

Integration of equation 11.23 (**Fig. 11.11**) gives[†]

$$R(t) = \alpha \int P(t) \, dt. \qquad (11.24)$$

Since $\int P(t)$ is the same for both kidneys,

$$\frac{R(t)_{\text{left}}}{R(t)_{\text{right}}} = \frac{\alpha_{\text{left}}}{\alpha_{\text{right}}}. \qquad (11.25)$$

[†]If an image is continuously acquired over say two minutes for measurement of differential renal function, then the image represents a double integral of the plasma activity. Thus the number of counts accumulated in the image is proportional to the sum of all the $R(t)$ values between 0 and 2 min, i.e. $\int R(t)dt = \alpha \int [\int P(t)dt]dt$ (see Section 12.1.6.1 and Fig. 12.4).

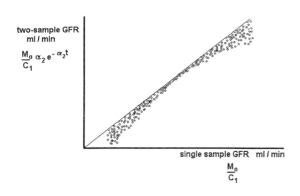

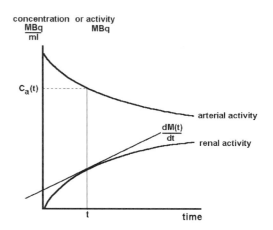

∎ **Fig 11.11** Relationship between one-sample GFR (ie M_0/C_1 and 2-sample GFR (ie $[M_0/C_1] \cdot \alpha_2 e^{-\alpha_2 t}$ [see equation 11.21]). For any value of C_1 (based on time t), 2-sample GFR has a maximal value when $\alpha_2 e^{-\alpha_2 t}$ is maximal, as illustrated in Fig. 11.10, thereby producing a boundary to the right of which all points must lie. The regression of maximal 2-sample GFR on one-sample GFR (ie the boundary) must be a straight line, passing through the origin, with slope t (since the term $\alpha_2 e^{-\alpha_2 t}$ reduces to e^{-1}/t when $1/\alpha_2 = t$). A third feature of the relationship is a spuriously close correlation in the mid-range of GFR where α_2 is close to $1/t$.

∎ **Fig. 11.12** The rate of increase $dM(t)/dt$ of renal activity at time t following injection of technetium-99m DTPA is proportional to the arterial activity $C_a(t)$ at time t, with a constant of proportionality equal to the GFR of the kidney. The relationship breaks down when t exceeds the minimum intrarenal transit time of the tracer (about 2.5 minutes). If the tracer was MAG3 or hippuran then $dM(t)/dt$ would be proportional to individual kidney tracer clearance.

Probably the best method to estimate differential function is based on a graphical technique of analysis which although more widely known as the Patlak plot was first applied to isotope renography by Rutland (1979). The technique calculates the uptake function α and simultaneously corrects for background activity — at least the intravascular component of background (see also Section 6.2.2.4.2). Ignoring the extravascular component for the time being, the 'raw' renal curves (i.e. those recorded in the renal region of interest without any background subtraction) represents the sum of 'filtered' counts (from equation 11.24) and background counts; i.e.

$$R(t) + I(t) = \alpha \int P(t) \cdot dt + I(t) \qquad (11.26)$$

where $I(t)$ is the intravascular background signal. Note that for the derivation of equation 11.26, $I(t)$ has been added to both sides of equation 11.24. As $I(t)$ is proportional to $P(t)$,

$$R(t) + I(t) = \alpha \int P(t) \cdot dt + k \cdot P(t) \qquad (11.27)$$

where k is a constant of proportionality. Dividing throughout by $P(t)$

$$\frac{R(t) + I(t)}{P(t)} = \alpha \frac{\int P(t) dt}{P(t)} + k. \qquad (11.28)$$

Equation 11.28 is a simple linear regression equation in which $[R(t) + I(t)]/P(t)$ is the y-axis co-ordinate and $\int P(t) \cdot dt/P(t)$ is the x-axis co-ordinate. The plot of $[R(t)+I(t)]/P(t)$ against $\int P(t) \cdot dt/P(t)$ has slope α and intercept k (**Fig. 11.14c**). Based on regions of interest over kidney and blood pool, the units of equation 11.28 are camera counts. They cancel out on the left side of equation 11.28. On the right, $\int P(t) \cdot dt/P(t)$ has units of time and so α must have units of the reciprocal of time. Inspection of the units in equations 11.23 and 11.24 also shows that α has units of min.$^{-1}$

The attraction of equation 11.28 compared with equations 11.23 and 11.24 is that it eliminates intravascular background, as α and k are derived separately. Here k represents intravascular background since it describes that fraction of the cardiac blood pool signal that is seen within the renal region of interest and is unitless. Equation 11.28 does not however remove the extravascular component of background which predominates in the skin and muscle of 'background tissue'. Movement of tracer

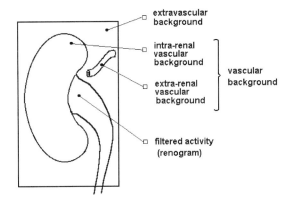

extravascular
background

intra-renal
vascular
background

extra-renal
vascular
background

} vascular
background

filtered activity
(renogram)

▌ **Fig. 11.13** Sources of signals originating from an ROI over the kidney during the first 3 minutes of a DTPA renogram. The signals arising from the kidney itself are from (1) intra-renal blood and (2) filtered activity. The signals arising from the extra-renal tissue are from (1) blood vessels and (2) interstitial tissue. The 'background' signal in a renogram therefore arises from intra- and extra-renal blood and extra-renal interstitial tissue. The interstitial signal in the kidney is negligible. Over the first 2–3 minutes, the intravascular background signal falls (i.e. it has a negative 'GFR equivalent' tending to decrease the recorded GFR) while the extravascular background signal rises (i.e. has a positive 'GFR equivalent').

from intravascular to extravascular spaces can be visualized as clearance of technetium-99m DTPA across the microvasculature of background tissue. It is therefore virtually impossible to separate the simultaneous clearances of technetium-99m DTPA from the intravascular space into the proximal tubule on the one hand and into the extravascular space of background tissues on the other **(Fig. 11.13)**. The Rutland approach therefore, whilst not requiring background subtraction with respect to intravascular background, requires subtraction for correction of extravascular background. Background is handled differently by the other two analytical approaches to single kidney GFR **(Fig. 11.14)**.

Single kidney GFR is proportional to α, which can be transformed to single kidney GFR (with units of ml/min) as follows. Whether using equations 11.23, 11.24 or 11.28, $P(t)$ has to be converted from its camera units of counts/min to units of radionuclide concentration (MBq/ml), and $R/(t)$ from units of counts/minute to units of quantity, MBq. The parameter α then has units of ml/min and k (equation 11.28) units of ml.

The value of R is calibrated from camera sensitivity (in counts/MBq/min) and then corrected for kidney depth, and P is calibrated from a single timed blood sample taken at a time, about 15–20 minutes, when the blood level of technetium-99m DTPA is relatively stable. This is then counted in a well counter alongside a standard in order to derive the technetium-99m DTPA concentration (MBq/ml). The gamma camera count rate recorded from the cardiac blood pool region of interest at the time at which the blood sample is taken corresponds with this calculated technetium-99m DTPA blood concentration and so the entire gamma camera blood pool curve can be calibrated in units of MBq/ml.

Although the calibration of R is relatively straightforward, that of P faces a fundamental difficulty related to the assumption that the signal detected in the cardiac blood pool region of interest exclusively represents a blood pool signal and that the amount of DTPA in the extravascular space of the chest wall in the cardiac region of interest is negligible. Although probably negligible up to 3 minutes after injection (when it is about 10% of the total signal) it is about 35% of the total signal at 15 minutes, and cannot therefore be ignored. It can be accounted for by placing a region of interest over the chest on the opposite side and subtracting the resulting time–activity curve from the cardiac curve. Unfortunately this results in a corrected curve with low counts and which is therefore noisy. Omitting the correction results in a systematic overestimation of single kidney GFR of about 15%.

As with global GFR, single kidney GFR is usually scaled for body size by normalization against body surface area. However an alternative whole body variable which is especially applicable to single kidney (SK) GFR determined from renography is another fluid volume — plasma volume (PV). Like GFR/ECV, measurement of GFR in relation to PV does not require separate measurement of either GFR or the fluid volume. If it is assumed that no DTPA leaves the plasma space within 3 min of injection, then the slope of the renogram, up to 3 minutes after injection, divided by the injected activity is directly proportional to SKGFR/PV:

$$\frac{\text{slope}}{\text{injected activity}} = \frac{\text{SKGFR}}{\text{PV}}$$

with units

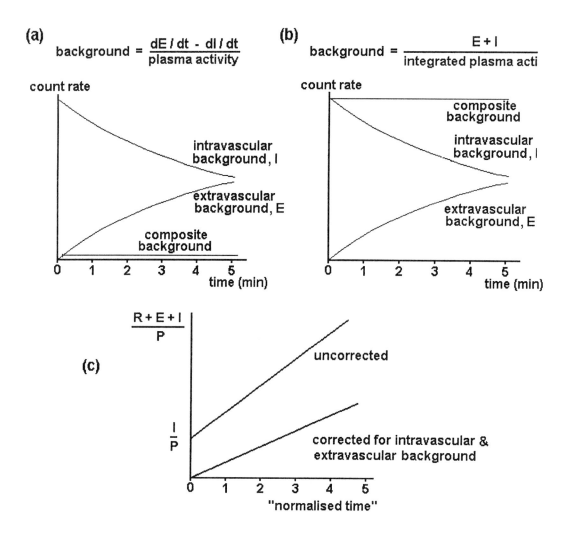

∎ **Fig. 11.14** Different ways in which gamma camera techniques for measuring GFR (represented by α, equation 11.23) treat background (BG), expressed as a "GFR equivalent". If R = renal activity, I = intravascular background, E = extravascular background, P = plasma activity:

(a) $\alpha = \dfrac{dR(t)/dt}{P(t)}$ BG (GFR equivalent) $= \dfrac{dE/dt - dI/dt}{P(t)}$

The intravascular and extravascular background signals are changing in opposite directions so the effect of background is minimized.

(b) $\alpha = \dfrac{R(t)}{\int P(t)dt}$ BG (GFR equivalent) $= \dfrac{E(t) + I(t)}{\int P(t)dt}$.

The intravascular and extravascular background signals summate and the effect of background is maximized. Rearranging equation (b), adding E and I to both sides and dividing throughout by P we obtain:

(c) Patlak–Rutland plot

$$\frac{R + E + I}{P} = \frac{\alpha \int Pdt + E}{P} + \frac{I}{P}$$

where I and P are both blood pool signals, so I/P is a constant and is identifiable separately from GFR as the intercept of the plot. The GFR equivalent of extravascular background E/P is added to the slope of the plot.

$$\frac{\text{MBq/min}}{\text{MBq}} = \frac{\text{ml/min}}{\text{ml}}.$$

This is how Zubal and Caride (1992) have measured GFR from DTPA renography. They work out plasma volume from tables of height and weight in order to obtain absolute SKGFR. This is rather circular however since in order to scale the GFR for body size, the same height and weight would be applied. The assumption of no losses of DTPA from the plasma volume over the first 3 min is also questionable since as a result of substantial early diffusion into the interstitial space of the whole body, the plasma concentration of DTPA at 3 min is only about 50% of the zero time concentration. (Since the slope of the renogram from 0–3 min is used in the calculation, the error is not in fact as large as 50%, since at times earlier than 3 min, the plasma concentration will be somewhere between 50 and 100% of the starting concentration.) The assumption and resulting error can be dealt with by measuring the gradient of the renogram at zero time. It is however difficult to do this directly (i.e. from the renogram) but an alternative approach is as follows (Peters *et al.* 1994b).

Thus

$$dM(t)dt = SKGFR \cdot C_a(t) \quad (11.29)$$

where M is amount of activity in the kidney and C_a is arterial DTPA concentration. At $t = 0$, when all tracer is confined to the plasma volume PV,

$$dM(0)/dt = SKGFR \cdot C_a(0). \quad (11.30)$$

Assuming rapid intravascular mixing,

$$C_a(0) = \frac{\text{injected activity}}{\text{PV}}. \quad (11.31)$$

Substituting for $C_a(0)$ in equation 11.30

$$\frac{dM(0)/dt}{\text{injected activity}} = \frac{SKGFR}{PV}. \quad (11.32)$$

As already stated, it is difficult to directly measure $dM(0)/dt$, but it can be obtained as follows:

$$\Gamma \cdot P(t) = C_a(t), \quad (11.33)$$

and

$$\gamma \cdot R = M \quad (11.34)$$

where P is the count rate over a cardiac region, Γ is the proportionality constant relating $C_a(t)$ to $P(t)$, R

is count rate over the kidney and γ is the proportionality constant relating camera count rate to MBq. The constant Γ has units of MBq/ml/counts/min and γ units of MBq/counts/min. Then, from equations 11.31, 11.32 and 11.33,

$$dR(0)/dt = \frac{\Gamma}{\gamma} \cdot SKGFR \cdot P(0) \quad (11.35)$$

Taking $[\Gamma/\gamma \cdot SKGFR]$ as a 'lumped' constant α which is identical to α in equations 11.23, 11.24 and 11.28,

$$dR(0)/dt = \alpha \cdot P(0)$$

and $\quad dM(0)/dt = \alpha \cdot \gamma \cdot P(0). \quad (11.36)$

where $P(0)$ can be measured by extrapolation of the cardiac curve; α can be calculated from a Patlak–Rutland plot applied to the renal and cardiac ROI (equation 11.28); and γ from renal depth measurement. SKGFR/PV is then obtained from equation 11.32.

11.1.3 Filtration fraction

Filtration fraction is the ratio of glomerular filtration rate (GFR) to renal plasma flow (RPF) and can be measured from simultaneous measurements of GFR and ERPF as the ratio of the clearances of inulin (or chromium-51 EDTA) and PAH (or radio-iodinated hippuran). Single kidney filtration fraction can be obtained by scintigraphic detection of the respective renal uptake rates of technetium-99m DTPA and radio-iodinated OIH; i.e.

$$\text{filtration fraction} = \frac{\alpha_{DTPA}}{\alpha_{hippuran}} \quad (11.37)$$

where α is the same as in equation 11.28.

This approach however, like the measurement of ERPF with hippuran, suffers from the questionable assumption of a renal hippuran extraction efficiency of 100%. Measurement of renal blood flow by fractionation of cardiac output, as described above, avoids this assumption but then, in order to obtain filtration fraction, requires conversion to an absolute value; i.e. cardiac output, needs to be known. Alternatively, the rate constant of plasma DTPA clearance (after equilibration; i.e. α_2 of equation 11.15) and RBF as a fraction of cardiac output may both be normalised to standard values for extracellular fluid volume and cardiac output, respectively. Thus, as described above, the rate constant of plasma DTPA clearance from the time of completion of equilibration between intravascular and extravascular spaces is nearly equal to the rate at which the extracellular fluid volume is turned over by GFR. Normally, ECF volume is 12–13 litres, so a value of 0.01 min^{-1} for GFR/ECV, obtainable from α_2, corresponds to a GFR of 120–130 ml/minute. Cardiac output is normally 5 litres/minute at rest which corresponds to a cardiac plasma output of about 3 litres/minute. If RBF/CO was, say, 0.1, then RPF normalized for a cardiac output of 5 litres/minute would be 300 ml/minute. The attraction of this dual normalization approach is that changes in fluid balance and variations in body dimensions (including those with age) would result in broadly parallel changes in ECF volume and cardiac output.

Regional filtration fraction may be portrayed as an image by taking the ratio of the images summed over the filtration phase of the technetium-99m DTPA renogram (representing GFR) and the image summed over the initial frames of the flow phase. By analogy with the quantitative argument in Section 8.2.3 *concerning lung blood volume, the flow phase* image must be terminated at the time of minimum intravascular transit time through the kidney, otherwise the image would become weighted by kidney blood volume.

This approach can be used to quantify filtration fraction within a single kidney or region within the kidney (Peters *et al.* 1989). Thus from Section 11.1.1.3,

$$RPF = \frac{g_k}{g_a} \times \frac{\gamma}{\Gamma}. \qquad (11.38)$$

where Γ is now the constant relating counts to MBq per ml of *plasma* instead of blood.

Consider α from Section 11.1.2.3, which represents single kidney (or regional GFR):

$$\alpha = \frac{R(t)}{\int P(t) \cdot dt}$$

so

$$GFR = \frac{R(t)}{\int P(t) dt} \times \frac{\gamma}{\Gamma}. \qquad (11.39)$$

In other words, α is converted to GFR by applying the same depth and camera sensitivity corrections (collectively represented by γ/Γ) as for RBF measurement.

Now

$$\text{filtration fraction} = \frac{GFR}{RPF}$$

$$= \alpha \times \frac{\gamma}{\Gamma} \bigg/ \frac{g_k}{g_a} \times \frac{\gamma}{\Gamma} \qquad (11.40)$$

$$= \frac{g_a}{g_k} \times \alpha \qquad (11.41)$$

Note that equation 11.41 needs no correction for recirculation: g_a and α have to be based on the same region of interest over blood pool and this is a major drawback. This region of interest cannot be placed over the left ventricle since, on the posterior view, some lung is placed between the left ventricle and the camera. The temporal displacement of activity in left ventricle and lung on first pass but not during the filtration phase therefore invalidates the use of the left ventricle.

An alternative region of interest is the right lung, but this faces the problem of extravascular chest wall activity present during the filtration phase but not during the flow phase. The effect of this is to reduce the value for filtration fraction but at least the error is systematic, and normal filtration fraction by this approach is about 10%. Although imperfect at this stage of technical development, the technique could be more accurate if dynamic SPECT was used, with the facility for three-dimensional imaging of filtration fraction. Furthermore, 11.41 is a general equation for extraction fraction, and for tracers such as DMSA, the error is minimized by protein binding in plasma. Thus the renal extraction fraction of DMSA is about 6% by this approach, similar to values based on renal vein catheterization.

Regional three-dimensional filtration fraction can also be imaged with PET, performed sequentially during flow and filtration phases. Renal perfusion can be imaged with rubidium-82, a potassium analogue with a half-life of 75 seconds, using either the principle of fractionation of cardiac output or continuous infusion, as described for the myocardium in Section 7.1.1.3. Filtration can be imaged with gallium-68 EDTA.

Another three-dimensional approach to measurement of both single kidney GFR and filtration fraction is dynamic computed tomography (CT) (Dawson and Peters 1993). This is analogous to PET because, in CT, X-ray attenuation is a linear function of tissue iodine concentration (one Hounsfield Unit being equivalent to an iodine concentration of 25 mg/ml). Similarly to radionuclide concentration in PET, CT expresses the iodine concentration per ml of 'whole tissue' even though contrast remains in the extracellular space, so that single kidney GFR comes out in units of ml/min/100 ml of renal tissue within the tomographic slice. The same is true for single kidney GFR measured by dynamic PET using gallium-68 EDTA.

11.2 Tubular function

In addition to important synthetic functions, such as erythropoetin production, tubular function involves a highly complex exchange of materials in both directions between tubular cell and tubular lumen, and the generation of osmotic gradients in the control of water concentration and excretion. Tubular reabsorbtion is the process whereby a substance is actively taken up by the tubular cell from the lumen. Some substances undergo tubular secretion; i.e. are actively taken up from peritubular blood by the tubular cell and transported by a carrier-mediated process into the tubular lumen. They include para-amino-hippurate (PAH) and penicillin. Some substances undergo bi-directional transport between peri-tubular blood and tubular lumen, for example potassium, uric acid and possibly DMSA. In either direction, a transport maximum (Tm) exists. At high plasma glucose levels, for example, filtered glucose exceeds Tm and produces glycosuria. At increasing plasma levels of PAH, the secreted load eventually becomes constant at the Tm, although the total excretion continues to increase as a result of increasing glomerular filtration of non-protein-bound PAH.

In the proximal tubule, there are two separate non-selective carrier systems for the respective secretion of weak organic acids (organic anions, $HB \rightleftharpoons H^+ + B^-$) and weak organic bases (organic cations, $HB^+ \rightleftharpoons H^+ + B$). PAH, OIH, penicillin and probenecid are organic anions which share the same carrier system. It is possible therefore for administered drugs to competitively inhibit PAH and OIH secretion in the same way that probenecid inhibits penicillin secretion. Routine agents like OIH, PAH and MAG-3 are organic anions, but there are no established cations for renal imaging. It may however be worthwhile to develop one since several

nephrotoxic drugs, such as cyclosporin, injure the kidney by selectively damaging the cationic transport system. A cationic renal agent that has been explored is DACH. Its clearance is about 160 ml/min, higher than GFR but not as high as MAG-3 clearance. It is competitively but weakly inhibited by thiamine, a cation which shares the same transport pathway, in a manner analogous to the inhibition of PAH secretion by probenecid.

Whereas renal blood flow and GFR can be measured with some precision, there are no established physiological techniques to measure the functional status of the tubule. Many insults to the kidney are selective for the tubule, such as ischaemia (especially in the transplant) and cyclosporin nephrotoxicity. In acute tubular necrosis (ATN), for example, renal blood flow may be relatively normal in spite of an essentially zero GFR. This is the result of passive diffusion of solutes and water through the damaged tubule, which is normally completely impermeable to substances such as inulin and DTPA. So although a filtrate continues to be produced, it returns to blood before reaching the collecting ducts. This has divergent effects on the renal handling of DTPA and MAG3 in ATN. In the case of DTPA, the second phase of the renogram is absent because the solute diffuses back into blood, whereas in the case of MAG3, the second phase is prolonged because although MAG3 continues to accumulate in the tubular cell, there is no tubular fluid for distal luminal transport and the tracer is effectively trapped. (The same divergence is seen in a positive captopril renogram although here filtration itself is abolished.) Cyclosporin, in addition to effects on renal blood flow, is capable of producing an ATN-like picture. It may also cause more subtle tubular damage which, whilst insufficient to completely abolish tubular solute impermeability, nevertheless reduces it so that GFR is apparently reduced out of proportion to renal blood flow, i.e. produces an apparent reduction in filtration fraction. Indeed, it is worth remembering that measurement of GFR with inulin or DTPA assumes no loss of this absolute tubular solute impermeability.

Clearly a means of identifying tubular damage short of ATN would be potentially useful. One approach is to measure the extraction fraction of a radiopharmaceutical which is tubular-specific, using the technique described in Section 11.1.3, and renal clearance in order to derive *PS* product. High plasma protein binding would be an advantage by reducing accumulation in the interstitial space and thereby improving the cardiac blood pool signal for the measurement of extraction fraction. A low extraction fraction would also be an advantage so that the renal uptake was relatively blood flow independent and renal clearance close to *PS* product. It is noteworthy that with respect to renal agents, there has been little attention paid to steady-state *PS* product in comparison say to myocardial perfusion agents. There may be several reasons for this:

(i) according to the intact nephron hypothesis, individual nephron blood flow should be maintained in disease;

(ii) Whereas the principal aim of perfusion imaging in the myocardium is to detect regional abnormalities, this has not hitherto been a prime aim in renal imaging;

(iii) instead, renal agents have been used more for the measurement of global function (including the individual kidney).

MAG3 and hippuran have extraction fractions that render their renal uptake critically blood flow dependent. Thus assuming a renal cortical plasma flow of 200 ml/min/100 ml, the steady-state *PS* product for hippuran is about 350 ml/min/100 ml, and for MAG3 about 150 ml/min/100 ml. For DMSA, on the other hand, it is about 15 ml/min/ 100 ml. At a perfusion of 100 ml/min/100 ml, extraction of DMSA would be about 25% and of MAG3, about 80% if there were no changes in *PS* product. So for DMSA, clearance would remain close to *PS* product over perfusion ranging from 100–200 ml/min/100 ml, whilst for MAG3, clearance would fall well short of *PS* product. It would therefore be more rational to use DMSA as a marker of tubular integrity than MAG3. Although using a different carrier, one which is targeted by cyclosporin, DACH is less attractive because it is weakly protein bound in plasma and a large component of its renal excretion is therefore via glomerular filtration.

Another potential approach to assessing tubular integrity is to compare the simultaneous plasma and urinary concentration ratios of two filtration markers of dissimilar molecular size. If the tubular epithelium is submaximally damaged, it may display widely disparate permeabilities to the two solutes on the basis of molecular size. If the respective filtration

rates remain similar then the urinary concentration ratio will be out of proportion to the plasma ratio. The success of this idea is likely to depend on critical molecular sizing — chromium-51 EDTA (360 Da) is an obvious candidate for the small molecule; the larger is more difficult but should perhaps exceed 6000 Da (the size of inulin).

Two thirds of the tubular fluid is re-absorbed in the proximal tubule. Because of high permeability to water, the osmolality of the proximal tubular fluid remains essentially identical to that of plasma. The tubular concentration of solutes such as inulin and DTPA, to which the tubular epithelium is impermeable, therefore increases threefold after passing through the proximal tubule; i.e. the tubular fluid to plasma inulin concentration ratio (TF_{in}/P_{in}), is 3 at the beginning of the loop of Henle. The TF_{in}/P_{in} ratio in the tubule gives an indication of the amount of water that has been reabsorbed from the tubule. The mechanism of urine concentration and dilution which takes place in the remainder of the nephron is one of the most interesting examples of the way structure and function complement each other and now will be briefly reviewed. It is of relevance to nuclear medicine because of the use of frusemide in renography. The crucial energy-expending process which leads to the development of both a concentration gradient within the medulla (for urinary concentration) and a dilute (hypotonic) urine, is the active re-absorption of sodium and chloride from the thick ascending limb of the loop of Henle. It is this process that is blocked by frusemide, which is an example of a loop diuretic. The loop of Henle is the structure responsible for counter current multiplication and the vasa recta for counter current exchange. The medullary concentration gradient developed by counter current multiplication could not be maintained without countercurrent exchange. In both instances, the phrase 'countercurrent' refers to the opposing directions of flow in descending versus ascending portions of the loop of Henle and vasa recta respectively, and not to opposing directions of flow between tubule and vasa.

Multiplication is primarily achieved by active re-absorption of sodium and chloride against a concentration gradient by the thick ascending limb of the loop of Henle. Since the descending limb is highly permeable to water but impermeable to solute, and since in the ascending limb these permeabilities are reversed, the combination of active sodium and chloride reabsorbtion and counter current direction of flow in the loop results in progressively increasing osmolality in tubular and peritubular fluid towards the papilla. Juxta-medullary nephrons, which are responsible for the generation of a concentrated urine, have ascending limbs which are thick only in their upper third, at the level of the outer zone of the medulla, yet the gradient extends to the inner medulla. The thin ascending limb does not have an active uptake mechanism, so how is the gradient multiplied at this level? The answer is urea. The collecting tubule is permeable to water but impermeable to urea in both the cortex and medulla, whereas it is highly permeable to urea in the papilla. This is why the distal convoluted tubule, with its ability to generate a hypotonic tubular fluid by active reabsorbtion of sodium and chloride, is important. It delivers a hypotonic urine to the collecting tubule and in the presence of anti-diuretic hormone there is passive water reabsorbtion from the collecting tubule as it descends. Urea is therefore delivered to the papillary collecting tubule in a very high concentration from where it diffuses passively into the innermost medulla and provides the osmotic drive for passive water reabsorbtion from the lower end of the thin descending loop of Henle. Frusemide abolishes the concentration gradient within minutes as a result of inhibiting the active reabsorbtion of sodium chloride, and thereby, somewhat paradoxically, interfering with the development of a hypotonic distal tubular fluid.

Ultimately the water reabsorbed under the influence of anti-diuretic hormone from the collecting tubule has to be removed without being allowed to dilute the gradient. This is the function of countercurrent exchange, an entirely passive process provided by the vasa recta. The system works because blood flow in the vasa recta is fast enough that equilibration of water and solutes between plasma and peritubular fluid is never quite achieved as the plasma flows down the descending limb of the vasa recta. This means that as plasma descends into the medulla it has an osmolality always slightly less than the peritubular fluid at the same horizontal level and, as it ascends back towards the cortex, it has a slightly higher osmolality than surrounding peritubular fluid. In order to carry away the water removed from the collecting tubule under the influence of the osmotic gradient, flow in the ascending vasa recta

must slightly exceed flow in the descending vasa recta. This is achieved by the oncotic pressure of plasma protein, which opposes water loss from the descending vasa recta but supports water gain in the ascending portion. Because of the removal of the filtrate from the plasma at the glomerulus, the concentration of plasma proteins is higher in peritubular capillaries and vasa recta than in extra-renal capillaries. This means that the oncotic pressure driving these fluid movements is correspondingly greater. As already mentioned, about two thirds of the water in the glomerular filtrate is re-absorbed by the proximal tubule. At the tip of the loop of Henle in cortical nephrons the TF_{in}/P_{in} ratio reaches 6 and in the tip of the loop of Henle in juxtamedullary nephrons reaches a ratio of about 12. This means that by the time the tip is reached about 92% of the water has been re-absorbed. The TF_{in}/P_{in} ratio remains unchanged throughout the distal tubule and starts to rise again as the collecting tubule descends through the medulla. In the production of a maximally concentrated urine, the final urine flow rate is about 1 ml/min. This means that the maximal variation in water reabsorbtion as a result of the concentration gradient is between 93 and 99% of the water initially delivered to the nephron.

11.2.1 Parenchymal and whole kidney transit time

Renal transit times (parenchymal and whole kidney) can be measured routinely during renography by deconvolution analysis. As described in Section 1.5., deconvolution analysis in principle predicts the renogram that would be obtained if the agent was injected as an infinitely narrow bolus into the renal artery and there was no recirculation of unextracted agent. The shape of the retention (impulse response) curve so predicted reflects the three phases of the renogram — blood flow, uptake and excretion. If background is not subtracted from the renogram curve before deconvolution analysis, then a very early spike is seen, representing the inflowing bolus of tracer followed by a plateau, which represents the minimum transit time of tracer through the region of interest. The final falling phase is a manifestation of variable nephron transit times and transit through the collecting system **(Fig. 11.15)**. Transit times can be measured from the kidney retention function curve

impulse retention function

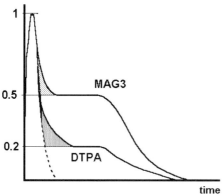

∎ **Fig. 11.15** Impulse retention function curves produced by deconvolution analysis applied to background-uncorrected MAG3 and DTPA renograms. Each curve shows 3 phases: (i) an early spike corresponding to arterial inflow; (ii) a plateau with a duration corresponding to minimum intra-renal transit time and (iii) a falling phase corresponding to tracer leaving the kidney. The height of the plateau is proportional to the renal extraction fraction of the tracer, higher for MAG3 than DTPA, and compared between the two kidneys can be used to express differential function. The shaded areas represent the effect of bi-directional diffusion of tracer between plasma and interstitial fluid, larger for DTPA because, unlike MAG3, it is not protein bound.

intravascular transit time of a few seconds would then be included.

Deconvolution analysis applied to background unsubtracted renograms provides a retention function curve that not only includes an initial spike of intravascular activity but also a component that represents clearance of tracer from intravascular to extravascular spaces (i.e. the extravascular component of background). This is added to the plateau representing tracer which is filtered or extracted into the tubules, and will be greater for agents, like DTPA, that are not protein bound in plasma. In theory, this component should not be flat like that due to filtration/extraction (**Fig. 11.16**), since tracer immediately returns to the intravascular space in proportion to the extravascular concentration and should produce a retention function curve of its own which decreases mono-exponentially to its baseline (the plateau). With sufficiently accurate deconvolution techniques and good quality data, it should be possible to identify the extravascular component of background and subtract it without the need for a separate background region of interest.

(after subtraction of the initial spike) by dividing the area under the curve by the plateau height, a ratio which must have the same units as the *x*-axis; i.e. time. If the region of interest is confined to the renal parenchyma, then the transit times are those through the parenchyma, whereas if it includes the pelvis they are those of the whole kidney. After subtraction of the initial spike, the height of the plateau is proportional to single kidney GFR; the ratio of heights of the two plateaux therefore gives differential function. With technetium-99m DTPA, the initial height, representing flow, is about 5 times the height of the plateau which reflects the 20% of the DTPA that is extracted (filtration fraction). The plateau is a higher fraction of the height of the initial spike for tracers like MAG-3 and hippuran which have higher extraction fractions (50 and 80% respectively). If the area is divided by the spike height, then mean transit time would be much shorter since tracer (80% in the case of DTPA) which never reaches the tubules and has an

impulse retention function

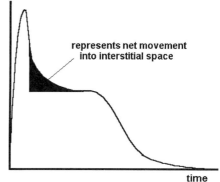

∎ **Fig. 11.16** Retentive function curve to show the effect of extra-renal extravascular background. DTPA diffuses in both directions across the endothelium of background tissues. Initially there is net movement into the interstitial space but this, which can be regarded as DTPA clearance into the interstitial space, decreases with equilibration by about 10–15 minutes after injection. The process manifests as a shoulder on the retention function between the blood flow spike and the plateau. It tends to disappear after accurate background subtraction and the plateau becomes more obvious.

The mean transit time of tracer entering the tubules that is actually measured by this technique is that of the tracer through the region of interest. Thus if the region of interest includes the pelvis, the mean transit time through the region of interest will include the time taken for the tracer to move through the pelvis. If, on the other hand, the region of interest is limited to parenchyma, then the mean transit time through the region of interest approximates to mean parenchymal transit time. The difference between whole kidney transit time and parenchymal transit time approximates the transit time of tracer through the pelvis (including whatever part of the proximal ureter is included within the region of interest). If urine flow rate was known, then pelvic volume could be calculated from pelvic transit time using the transit time equation, $T = V/Q$ (equation 5.3). The parenchymal transit time of tracers like MAG-3 or hippuran, which are secreted into the tubules, should be somewhat less than that of DTPA since they gain access to the tubule 'downstream' from the glomerulus. There is little difference however since the speed of transit in the proximal tubule is fast relative to sampling time (i.e. frame rate — 10 seconds for example).

Transit time measurement from deconvolution analysis is routinely performed in renal nuclear medicine, although in the experience of some, is generally of rather limited clinical value because of the statistical quality of the generated curves. Its main use is in the distinction between urinary tract obstruction and dilatation without obstruction (see below) for which there is some evidence that it is better than diuretic renography. Its other main use is in the assessment of functionally significant renal artery stenosis, which results in increased tubular fluid reabsorbtion and therefore decreased tubular flow. Since it is inversely related to flow, mean transit time increases under these circumstances and can be measured by deconvolution analysis. Parenchymal transit time measurements are technically easier in the absence of a dilated pelvis which otherwise tends to overlap the parenchymal region of interest. Mean parenchymal transit time as an index of renal vascular hypertension has the potential advantage over captopril renography of requiring only one study. After ACE inhibition in patients with reno–vascular hypertension, parenchymal transit time increases further.

11.2.2 Quantifying pelvic drainage

Defining outflow tract obstruction is difficult. There are several possible definitions, each peculiar to the discipline interested in it. Thus there is a clinical definition — loin pain, especially in relation to a diuresis, with or without urinary infection; a physiological definition — the intrapelvic pressure required to achieve a given flow rate; a pathological definition — loss of renal function; and a renographic definition — a failure to drain adequately after a diuretic stimulus or a prolonged parenchymal transit time. Although the pathological definition is the only indisputable one, it is retrospective. The physiological and renographic definitions are difficult to interpret in the face of variations in urine production and flow rates. Thus urine flow in a well-functioning kidney may be obstructed at a level which might not result in obstruction in a poorly functioning kidney. If the flow rate producing a critical pelvic pressure in a given kidney could be determined at antegrade pyelography (the Whitaker test), it may be possible to identify or exclude obstruction in that kidney on contemporaneous renography if single kidney urine flow rate could be renographically measured. Unfortunately however the renographic definition of obstruction is perhaps the loosest of all since, unlike the physiological definition, it is difficult to measure urine flow rates and impossible to measure pressures. The renographic criteria are, in other words, based essentially on transit times.

There are three approaches to quantifying drainage from renography, all aimed at the exclusion of outflow tract obstruction. The first is deconvolution analysis, based on regions of interest placed respectively over the parenchyma and the whole kidney, including the pelvis. In a dilated non-obstructed system, parenchymal transit time is normal while whole kidney transit time is increased. The difference between parenchymal transit time and whole kidney transit time is pelvic transit time. The latter however is rather irrelevant in the clinical setting of obstruction/dilatation since the exclusion or otherwise of obstruction is based on the parenchymal transit time.

The second approach is the diuretic renogram. The response to a diuretic, usually Frusemide, has been quantified in several ways, all based on indices like the T75 or T50 (the times to a 75% or 50%

reduction in kidney counts) or maximum downslope gradient on the renal time activity curve. They will not be further discussed here except to emphasise that the response to a diuretic may be incomplete if the bladder is full. If the index does not exclude obstruction, then micturation is mandatory and a further index applied to the kidneys' response to micturation. One such post-micturation index is the percentage decrease in renal counts in the immediate post micturation view compared with the count rate at 20 minutes after injection of the tracer. A cut-off point that has been suggested is 50%.

The third approach is to plot a curve representing cumulative pelvic outflow starting from the time of injection of the radiopharmaceutical. This technique is reminiscent of the measurement of renal blood flow described in Section 11.1.1.3. Thus, the curve recorded from a region of interest over the left ventricle, integrated up to a time t represents the total amount of activity made available to the kidney for filtration up to the time t (**Fig. 11.17**). For the first 2–3 minutes after injection, the kidney also 'integrates' the activity since none leaves the kidney up to this time. So the renal time activity curve and integrated ventricular time activity curve can be scaled and superimposed on each other over the duration of the minimum intra-renal transit time. After the completion of this time, the two curves diverge and the difference between them represents the cumulative outflow curve. An attraction of this technique is that it takes into account the prevailing level of renal function, except that reduced glomerular filtration is not necessarily associated with reduced urine flow rate.

11.3 Ureteric function

11.3.1 Ureteric motility

The dynamics of urine movement in the ureter can be assessed using a so-called space–time matrix or compressed image (Muller-Schauenburg *et al.* 1987). Several regions of interest are placed one above the other over the length of the ureter, and a time activity curve, in frame mode, constructed for each. The y-axis of the space time matrix is the region of interest number with the region nearest the pelvis at the top. The x-axis is time. The matrix can

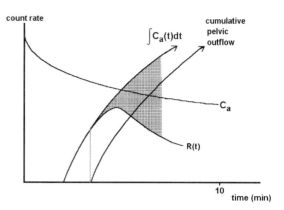

∎ **Fig. 11.17** Quantification of pelvic drainage. The plasma curve (recorded for an ROI over the cardiac blood pool) is integrated, scaled and moved so that it is superimposed on the upslope of the background-corrected renogram curve. The rising integrated curve then defines the relative amount of radioactivity that would accumulate in the kidney in the absence of any drainage. The difference between this and the recorded renal curve represents activity that has drained from the kidney. Compare this figure with Fig. 3.12, 7.2, 8.8 and 11.3.

be imagined to be divided into grids or pixels. Each matrix is gray scale or colour coded for the counts recorded in the corresponding region of interest during a particular time frame. The results are expressed in the form illustrated schematically in **Fig. 11.18**, from which the 'waves' or radioactive urine passing down the ureter, i.e., ureteric peristalsis, can be identified. Flow in the reverse direction (i.e., reflux) can also be appreciated.

11.3.2 Vesico–ureteric reflux

Although, as the name implies, the refluxed urine in vesico-ureteric reflux (VUR) originates from the bladder, it is important to realise that 'yoyo' reflux may occur in the ureter. Thus urine pooling at the distal end of the ureter may flow back up towards the pelvis. It is difficult to quantify this as such because the refluxing urine, originating from the ureter behind the bladder, looks as though it has come from the bladder, and this is also reflected in the time activity curve placed over the bladder. 'Yoyo' reflux is recognized to occur in duplex systems which fuse into a single ureter before entry into the bladder. The movement of fluid down one limb and up the other can readily be identified during contrast micturating

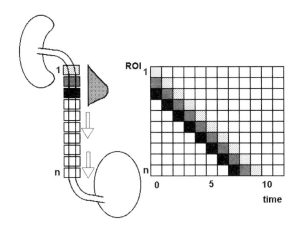

∎ **Fig. 11.18** Space–time matrix technique applied to the ureter. Each ROI corresponds to a horizontal row of squares in the matrix. The vertical columns correspond to time. The grey scale within a square in the matrix is proportional to the activity in the corresponding ROI at the time defined by the column. Peristaltic velocity and rate can be visualized, and retrograde peristalsis shows 'hot squares' moving from left to right and *upwards* instead of downwards.

cystourethrography (MCU), in contrast to the 'yoyo' reflux in the single ureter, which because of the unphysiological nature of the examination, cannot be recognized on MCU.

The volume V of urine refluxing into the kidney as a result of VUR can be quantified by calibrating the time–activity curve recorded over the kidney into volume units (Godley *et al.* 1990). This requires quantification of the activity M_k reaching the kidney (in MBq) and dividing it by the concentration of radioactivity C_u measured in a urine sample obtained at the same time; i.e.

$$V = \frac{M_k}{C_u}. \qquad (11.42)$$

After conversion of the kidney time–activity curve resulting from reflux into a volume curve, it is then possible to measure the maximum volume of reflux (the peak of the curve), the maximum rate of reflux (the gradient of the upslope of the curve) and the rate of subsequent pelvic drainage. Measurement of VUR can be combined with bladder urodynamics by catheterization of the bladder and insertion of a pressure gauge in the rectum for respective measurement of intravesical and intra-abdominal pressures and

their difference, which is the transvesical pressure.

Another approach to VUR is the measurement of the rate of reflux–episodes by plotting a space–time matrix (**Fig. 11.18**). This is identical in principle to the application of a space–time matrix to the ureter for quantification of ureteric peristalsis except, of course, in the case of VUR the fluid movement is in the opposite direction. The matrix can be miniaturised with respect to the time axis to produce a so-called compressed image.

11.4 Genital system

11.4.1 Penile blood flow

The penis is unusual in that, when active, its blood flow is reduced compared with the inactive state. Erection is initiated by the parasympathetic nervous supply, which initially causes an increase in arterial inflow to the corpora. There is relaxation of the smooth muscle of the corporeal lacunae, which become engorged with blood. Venous outflow is impeded by an intra-corporeal valve mechanism and, as a result of the increasing intracorporal pressure, also by compression of subtunical veins against the inflexible tunica albuginea. With maximal arterial dilatation, systemic arterial pressure is then transmitted to the corpora.

Measurement of penile blood flow is aimed at investigating impotence, of which there are three fundamental causes:

(1) neurological or psychogenic;
(2) arterial disease;
(3) venous leak.

The latter two are together known as vasculogenic impotence. The papaverine test distinguishes psychogenic from vasculogenic impotence. Intracorporeal papaverine or prostaglandin E produces smooth muscle relaxation and arterial dilatation and, if erection ensues, then impotence cannot be vasculogenic. If papaverine fails to induce erection, or the erection cannot be sustained, then investigation of penile haemodynamics after intra-corporeal papaverine may distinguish arteriopathic impotence from a venous leak. The presence of a venous leak can be most dramatically demonstrated by contrast cavernosography in which intracorporeal contrast shows tortuous dilated veins. The technique however is difficult, uncomfortable and not without risk.

11.4.1.1 Penile plethysmography

Penile haemodynamics may be assessed by scintigraphic penile plethysmography using an intravascular agent such as technetium-99m labelled red cells. The count rate in a region of interest around the normal penis increases during the induction of erection, reaching a plateau which reflects penile blood volume at the completion of erection (Siraj *et al.* 1986). The rate of increase of penile volume at any time from flaccid through to erect states is equal to the difference between arterial inflow and venous outflow. Using technetium-99m labelled red cells, brief episodes of arterial inflow can be observed in the flaccid penis of normal subjects but not those with vasculogenic impotence, producing spikes on the continuously recorded time–activity curve. A development of blood pool phallography is the sequential direct injection of technetium-99m labelled red cells into the corpora, first when the penis is flaccid and then after papverine-induced erection. The washout rate during erection in normal subjects is consistently reduced compared with that in the flaccid state, whereas in patients with a venous leak, the washout rate is increased compared with flaccid (Grosher *et al.* 1992).

11.4.1.2 Penile xenon-133 washout

Following papaverine stimulation, penile blood flow (PBF) can be measured from tracer washout in the flaccid, through tumescent, to erect state. The clearance half-times of intracorporeal xenon-133 is a measure of venous outflow from the penis (Miraldi *et al.* 1992). Assuming a partition co-efficient of unity for xenon-133, then $PBF/V = \ln 2/t_{1/2}$, where V is the volume of distribution. In the absence of a venous leak, pharmacological induction of erection decreases the $t_{1/2}$, indicating, a reduction in venous outflow during erection. In the presence of a venous leak, papaverine fails to reduce venous outflow, which may substantially increase. In arteriopathic impotence, an increase in venous outflow is not seen.

The gradient on the downslope of the xenon-133 washout curve at any time between flaccid and erect states is equal to the ratio of venous outflow to penile volume *at that time*. So by simultaneously measuring venous outflow from the xenon-133 washout curve and the time course of penile volume (from technetium-99m red cells), the arterial inflow can be measured. Maximal arterial inflow (and maximal venous outflow) are both abnormally low in arteriopathic impotence. There is no difference between arteriopaths and normals with respect to venous outflow, whereas patients with a venous leak have an increased peak venous flow.

The theory underlying this technique can be summarised as follows.

$$V(t) = \frac{\gamma}{C_{Tc}} N_{Tc}(t) \qquad (11.43)$$

where V is penile blood volume, N_{Tc} is the technetium-99m count rate, C_{Tc} is the technetium-99m concentration in blood and γ is a constant relating count rate to radioactivity. The parameter t, in brackets, is to remind the reader that V, usually a constant, is a function of time here. Now

$$dV/dt = Q_a(t) - Q_v(t) \qquad (11.44)$$

where Q_a and Q_v are arterial inflow and venous outflow, respectively.

Assuming the additional extravascular volume within which xenon-133 is distributed is negligible,

$$Q_v(t) = \alpha(t) \cdot V(t) \qquad (11.45)$$

where $\alpha(t)$ is the instantaneous gradient of the semi-logarithmic plot of xenon-133 time–activity curve at time t. This is an interesting and complex situation in which the rate of xenon-133 washout is being progressively retarded by its expanding volume of distribution.

11.4.2 Fallopian tube transit time

A novel technique recently described for the investigation of female infertility is the measurement of the transit time of a radiotracer from upper vagina to the fallopian fimbriae. The tracer is technetium-99m radiolabelled albumin microspheres (Itturalde and Venter 1991). In order to facilitate the passage of spermatozoa, the fallopian tubes are ciliated. It has been shown that cigarette smoking may delay the transit of microspheres. Cigarette smoking also impairs the action of cilia in the bronchial tree, but what is interesting about the fallopian cilia is that the effect of smoking seems to be systemic rather than local.

References

Blaufox MD, Fromowitz A, Gruskin A, Meng C-H and Elkin M. Validation of use of xenon-133 to measure intrarenal distribution of blood flow. *American Journal of Physiology* 1970, **219**: 440–4.

Brochner-Mortensen J. A simple method for the determination of glomerular filtration rate. *Scandinavian Journal of Clinical and Laboratory Investigation*, 1972, **30**: 271–4.

Bubeck B. Renal clearance determination with one blood sample: improved accuracy and universal applicability by a new calculation principle. *Seminars in Nuclear Medicine* 1993, **23**: 73–86.

Chantler C and Barratt TM. Estimation of glomerular filtration rate from plasma clearance of 51-Cr-EDTA. *Archives of Diseases of Children* 1972, **47**: 613–7.

Crean PA, Pratt T, Davies GJ, Myers MJ, Lavender JP and Maseri A. The fractional distribution of the cardiac output in man using microspheres labelled with technetium-99m. *British Journal of Radiology* 1986, **59**: 209–15.

Dawson P and Peters AM. Dynamic contrast bolus computed tomography for the assessment of renal function. *Investigative Radiology* 1993, **11**: 1039–42.

Fawdry RM and Gruenewald SM. Three-hour volume of distribution method: an accurate simplified glomerular filtration rate measurement. *Journal of Nuclear Medicine* 1987, **28**: 510–3.

Friis-Hansen B. Body water compartments in children: changes during growth and related changes in body composition. *Pediatrics* 1961, **28**: 69–75.

Gleadhill A, Peters AM and Michell AR. A simple, minimally invasive and clinically acceptable method of measuring glomerular filtration rate in dogs. *Research in Veterinary Science* 1995, **59**: 118–23.

Godley M, Ransley PG, Parkhouse HF, Gordon 1, Evans K and Peters AM. Quantitation of vesico–ureteric reflux by radionuclide cystography and urodynamics. *Paediatric Nephrology* 1990, **4**: 485–90.

Groshar D, Lidgi S, Frenkel A and Vardi Y. Radionuclide assessment of penile corporal venous leak using technetium-99m-labeled red blood cells. *Journal of Nuclear Medicine* 1992, **33**: 49–51.

Gruenewald SM, Nimmon CC, Nawaz MK and Britton KE. A non-invasive gamma camera technique for the assessment of intrarenal flow distribution in man. *Clinical Science* 1981, **61**: 385–9.

Gunasekera RD, Allison DJ and Peters AM. Glomerular filtration rate in relation to extracellular fluid volume: similarity between Tc-99m-DTPA and inulin. *European Journal of Nuclear Medicine* 1996, **23**: 49–54.

Iturralde MP and Venter PF. Radionuclide studies of ciliary function in infertile smoking females. *European Journal of Nuclear Medicine* 1991, **18**: 623.

Kurtin PS. Standardization of renal function measurements in children: kidney size versus metabolic rate. *Clinical Nephrology and Urology* 1989, **9**: 337–9.

McCance RA and Widdowson EM. The correct physiological basis on which to compare infant and adult renal function. *Lancet* 1952, **1**: 860–2.

Miraldi F, Nelson AD, Jones WT, Thompson S and Kursh ED. A dual-radioisotope technique for the evaluation of penile blood flow during tumescence. *Journal of Nuclear Medicine* 1992, **33**: 41–6.

Muller-Schauenburg W, Hofmann U, Feine U, Flach A and Erdmann W. Criteria for ureteral obstruction by functional imaging of the upper urinary tract. *Contributions to Nephrology*; Radionuclides in Nephrology eds Bischof Delaloye, Blaufox MD. Karger, Basel 1987, **56**: 225–31.

Peters AM. Expressing glomerular filtration rate in terms of extracellular fluid volume. *Nephrology Dialysis and Transplantation* 1992, **7**: 205–10.

Peters AM, Gunasekera RD, Henderson BL, Brown J, Lavender JP, de Souza M, Ash JM and Gilday DL. Non-invasive measurement of blood flow and extraction fraction. *Nuclear Medicine Communications* 1987, **8**: 823–37.

Peters AM, George P, Brown J and Lavender JP. Filtration fraction: Non-invasive measurement with Tc-99m DTPA and changes induced by angiotensin — converting enzyme inhibition in hypertension. *Nephron* 1989, **51**: 470–3.

Peters AM, Heckmatt JZ, Hasson N, Henderson BL, El-Meleigy D, Rose ML and Dubovitz V. Renal haemodynamics of cyclosporin nephrotoxicity in children with juvenile dermatomyositis. *Clinical Science* 1991, **8**: 153–9.

Peters AM, Allison H and Ussov WY. Measurement of the ratio of glomerular filtration rate to plasma volume from the Tc-99m DTPA renogram. *European Journal of Nuclear Medicine* 1994, **21**: 322–7.

Peters AM, Gordon I and Sixt R. Normalization of glomerular filtration rate in children: body surface area, body weight or extracellular fluid volume? *Journal of Nuclear Medicine* 1994, **35**: 438–44.

Piepsz A, Dobbeleir A and Erbsmann F. Measurement of separate kidney clearance by means of Tc-99m DTPA complex and a scintillation camera. *European Journal of Nuclear Medicine* 1977, **2**: 173–7.

Rabito C, Moore RH, Bougas C and Dragotakes C. Non-invasive, real-time monitoring of renal function: the ambulatory renal monitor. *Journal of Nuclear Medicine* 1993, **34**: 199–207.

Rehling M, Moller ML, Thamdrup B, Lund O and Trap-Jensen J. Simultaneous measurement of renal clearance and plasma clearance of Tc-99m labelled DTPA, Cr-51 labelled EDTA and inulin in man. *Clinical Science* 1984, **66**: 61 3–9.

Rossing N, Bojsen J and Frederiksen PL. The glomerular filtration rate determined with Tc-99m DTPA and a portable cadmium telluride detector. *Scandinavian Journal of Clinical and Laboratory Investigation* 1978, **38**: 23–8.

Rehling M, Moller ML, Lund JO, Jensen KD, Thamdrup B and Trap-Jensen J. Tc99m DTPA gamma camera renography: normal values and rapid determination of single kidney glomerular filtration rate. *European Journal of Nuclear Medicine* 1985, **II**: 1–6.

Rosen SM, Hollenberg NK, Dealy JB and Merrill JP. Measurement of the distribution of blood flow in the human kidney using the intra-arterial injection of xenon-133. *Clinical Science* 1968, **34**: 287–302.

Russell CD, Taylor A and Eshima D. Estimation of technetium-99m-MAG3 plasma clearance in adults from one or two blood samples. *Journal of Nuclear Medicine* 1989, **30**: 1955–9.

Rutland MD. A comprehensive analysis of DTPA renal studies. *Nuclear Medicine Communications* 1985, **6**: 11–30.

Rutland MD. A single injection technique for subtraction of blood background in [131]1-hippuran renograms. *British Journal of Radiology* 1979, **52**: 134–7.

Siraj QH, Hilson AJW, Townell NH, Morgan RJ and Cottral MF. The role of the radioisotope phallogram in the investigation of vasculogenic impotence. *Nuclear Medicine Communications* 1986, **7**: 173–82.

Stoffel M, Jamar F, Van Nerom CG, Verbruggen A, Besse T, Squifflet J-P and Beckers C. Estimation of Tc- 99m-L,L-ethylene dicysteine clearance by simplified methods and correlation with iodine-125- orthoiodohippurate for the determination of effective renal plasma flow. *European Journal of Nuclear Medicine* 1996, **23**: 365–70.

Tauxe WN, Dubovsky EV, Kidd T, Diaz F and Smith LR. New formulas for the calculation of effective renal plasma flow. *European Journal of Nuclear Medicine* 1982, **7**: 51–4.

Thorburn GD, Kopald HH, Herd A, Hollenburg M, O'Morchoe CC and Barger AC. Intra-renal distribution of nutrient blood flow detected with krypton-85 in the anaesthetised dog. *Circulation Research* 1963, **13**: 290–307.

Waller DG, Keast CM, Fleming JS and Ackery DM. Measurement of glomerular filtration rate with technetium-99m-DTPA: comparison of plasma clearance techniques. *Journal of Nuclear Medicine* 1987, **28**: 372–7.

Zubal IG and Caride VJ. The technetium-99m-DTPA renal uptake-plasma volume product: a quantitative estimation of glomerular filtration rate. *Journal of Nuclear Medicine* 1992, **33**: 1712–6.

12 The brain

12.1 Cerebral blood flow

Like renal blood flow, cerebral blood flow is autoregulated. Thus changes in arterial perfusion pressure are met by corresponding changes in cerebrovascular resistance. Normal mean cerebral blood flow is about 55 ml/100 g/min and falls during hypotension only when arterial pressure falls below 60 mm Hg. Between about 25 and 55 ml/100 g/min, perfusion is said to be in the *oligaemic* zone but no functional disturbances ensue because the brain is able to maintain its oxygen requirements by increasing oxygen extraction efficiency. The *ischaemic* zone extends over a perfusion range of about 10 to 25 ml/100 g/min within which there are functional neuronal disturbances but they are reversible if oxygen delivery is restored. Cerebral blood flow shows a prominent response to tissue carbon dioxide levels, increasing by up to 50% in the presence of hypercapnia and showing a corresponding decrease in response to hypocapnia. Tissue acidosis can be induced by acetazolamide which blocks carbonic anhydrase. This is a convenient way to reproducibly increase cerebral blood flow.

There are several approaches to the measurement of cerebral blood flow, both global, expressed as ml/min, and regional, expressed as ml/100 g/min or ml/100 ml/min. The areas of clinical interest with respect to cerebral blood flow include cerebrovascular disease and stroke, dementias, especially Alzheimer's disease, temporal lobe epilepsy, migraine and, more recently, myalgic encephalomyelitis. Although the development of technetium-99m HMPAO for imaging the distribution of cerebral blood flow has given impetus to clinical interest in cerebral blood flow measurement, technetium-99m HMPAO SPECT is only semi-quantitative giving a 'map' of regional cerebral blood flow distribution. The classical inert gas technique therefore remains important insofar as its theoretical basis forms a platform for the understanding of contemporary techniques for quantitative imaging of cerebral blood flow based on SPECT and PET.

12.1.1 Measurement of cerebral perfusion using inert gases

12.1.1.1 Measurement by desaturation

There is an extensive literature going back several decades on the use of inert gases, especially xenon-133 and krypton-85, for the measurement of cerebral blood flow by the inert gas washout technique (reviewed by Lassen *et al.* 1983). Because of its discrete confines, the brain lends itself well to this and related techniques.

The kinetic theory is similar to that described earlier for other organs. The inert gas washout curve is essentially biexponential following bolus injection into the carotid artery; the first and second exponentials are thought to represent washout from grey and white matter, respectively. The cerebral concentration–time curve can therefore be described by the following equation:

$$C_\tau = Ae^{-\alpha_1 t} + Be^{-\alpha_2 t} \qquad (12.1)$$

where $\alpha_1 = (Q/\lambda V)_{grey}$ and $\alpha_2 = (Q/\lambda V)_{white}$.

Since the white matter is rich in lipid, and λ_{white} therefore high (usually taken as 1.5), the rate constant of the second exponential is low in relation to white matter perfusion. In other words, the effective distribution volume is high. The value of λ_{grey} is usually taken as 0.8. Since white matter density is significantly less than unity, perfusion is higher when expressed in terms of tissue mass rather than tissue volume. As in most other tissues, further exponentials, which may have anatomical counterparts, may be identified by extending the recording time. A third exponential in a cerebral washout curve may, for example, correspond to clearance from extracerebral (mainly scalp) tissue.

The partition of total cerebral inflow between grey and white matter can be derived from the ratio of the zero time intercepts of the corresponding exponentials before there has been any washout. If A is the zero time intercept of the fast exponential, representing grey matter perfusion, and B is the zero time intercept of the slow exponential, representing grey matter perfusion,

$$\frac{\text{total grey matter flow}}{\text{total white matter flow}} = \frac{A}{B}$$

with units

$$\frac{\text{ml/min}}{\text{ml/min}}. \qquad (12.2)$$

This calculation assumes that the detecting geometry is the same for both tissues or, in other words, that the two tissues are effectively grossly anatomically inseparable.

Mean cerebral perfusion; i.e. total flow: total mass (or volume) can be derived from the weighted harmonic mean of grey and white matter perfusions. Since this technique essentially measures total height divided by total area, contributed by each exponential, mean values for λ and ρ (tissue density) have to be applied. An alternative approach is to derive separate perfusion values for grey and white matter using their appropriate λ and ρ values and the absolute blood flow ratio (i.e. $A/[A+B]$ or $B/[A+B]$), as follows.

Of 50 ml/min supplying cerebral tissue, a fraction $[A/A + B] \cdot 50$ ml/min supplies grey matter. Therefore if grey matter perfusion is $(Q/V)_{\text{grey}}$ ml/100 g/min, then this blood flow serves $[A/(A+B)] \cdot 50$ divided by $(Q/V)_{\text{grey}}$ grams of grey matter. Similarly, $[B/(A+B)] \cdot 50$ divided by $(Q/V)_{\text{white}}$ grams of white matter are supplied by $[B/(A+B)] \cdot 50$ ml/min. The sum of these two masses of cerebral tissue are served by 50 ml/min from which mean perfusion can be calculated (see worked example, Section 14.5).

As an alternative to intra-arterial injection, xenon-133 can be given intravenously for measurement of cerebral perfusion (Veal and Mallet 1965). The signal from the brain is then based on the 5% that escapes extraction in the lung. A problem with this approach is that there is a continuous but declining input of xenon-133 into the brain resulting from the presence of xenon-133 in the alveolar spaces, which is in equilibrium with xenon-133 in pulmonary venous (and therefore systemic arterial) blood. The mathematical form of this input is also influenced by xenon-133 returning to the lung from all the tissues of the body. There is therefore a complex model consisting of three compartments: the lung, the brain

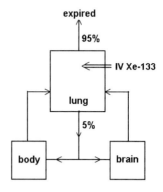

∎ **Fig. 12.1** Model representing kinetics of an intravenous bolus of xenon-133 in saline. 95% of the activity enters the alveolar gas in the lungs while 5% enters the systemic circulation. The alveolar xenon-133 equilibrates with pulmonary capillary blood with a partition coefficient hugely in favour of alveolar gas. The lungs retain a large reservoir of xenon, some of which is recirculated to the systemic circulation.

(treating it for the time being as one compartment) and the rest of the body from which xenon-133 is returning to the lung **(Fig. 12.1)**. The time course of activity in the brain compartment is given by the resultant of the exponentials representing cerebral washout, ventilatory turnover and washout from the rest of the body (see Section 1.3.3). The washout curve over the brain would only approach an exponential reflecting cerebral washout if the other two exponentials were substantially faster, which is unlikely to be the case. This therefore dictates continuous monitoring of the lung activity with a second detector. Since alveolar xenon-133 is in equilibrium with pulmonary venous blood, this gives a continuous record of the time course of arterial xenon concentration; i.e. the input function. The cerebral tissue time–activity curves C_{τ} are, for both grey and white matter, the convolution of the arterial concentration C_{a} on the corresponding cerebral washout rates; i.e.

$$C_{\tau}(t) = \frac{Q}{V}\int C_{\text{a}}(t)^{*}e^{-(Q/\lambda V)t} \cdot \mathrm{d}t \qquad (12.3)$$

(see equation 3.35) and the cerebral washout curve can be obtained by deconvolution analysis. If the patient rebreaths xenon-133 from a closed circuit, then a continuous arterial infusion will effectively be established. The curve recorded over the brain will then become a saturation curve of the type described below for continuous nitrous oxide arterial infusion. The mathematics are essentially the same as for an intravenous injection. This approach has been used by Lassen (1985) for tomographic imaging of regional cerebral perfusion with xenon-133 and dynamic SPECT as described below. Although cerebral perfusion is seldom measured clinically using intra-arterial techniques, there is a substantial literature on the intravenous and inhalation techniques.

12.1.1.2 Measurement by saturation

The forerunner of xenon-133 washout for measurement of cerebral perfusion is a technique based on stable nitrous oxide which, in principle, is very similar, but requires cerebral venous outflow sampling as well as continuous arterial infusion of nitrous oxide. Like xenon, krypton and water, nitrous oxide is highly diffusible through cells, and equilibrates rapidly crosses the blood brain barrier. Following commencement of infusion therefore the concentration within the brain increases. Because of rapid equilibration between cerebral tissue and cerebral venous blood, the jugular venous nitrous oxide concentration follows the same time course as the cerebral tissue concentration, which increases and eventually becomes equal to the arterial concentration. This approach represents measurement of perfusion from tracer *saturation*, in contrast to measurement by desaturation. For a homogeneously perfused zone of tissue, the cerebral venous nitrous oxide level increases exponentially with a rate constant α which can be shown to be proportional to the perfusion, Q/V of the zone, analogously to a desaturation rate constant, which is also proportional to perfusion (**Fig. 12.2**).

Thus, starting from the Fick principle,

$$\frac{dC_\tau}{dt} = \frac{Q \cdot C_a}{V} - \frac{Q \cdot C_v}{V}$$

$$= \frac{Q}{V} \cdot C_a - \frac{Q}{\lambda V} \cdot C_\tau. \quad (12.4)$$

Let $\qquad dC_\tau/dt = x$

where x is an arbitrary variable used to simplify the equation, so

$$x = \frac{Q}{V} \cdot C_a - \frac{Q}{\lambda V} \cdot C_\tau. \quad (12.5)$$

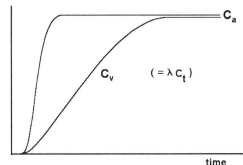

concentration

∎ **Fig. 12.2** Saturation curve of inert gas in an organ during continuous intra-arterial infusion (with a constant arterial concentration C_a). The curve is the inverse of a desaturation curve and can be treated as such (see Figs 12.3 and 6.11).

Now $Q \cdot C_a/V$ is constant so

$$\frac{dx}{dt} = \frac{-Q}{\lambda V} \cdot \frac{dC_\tau}{dt} \quad (12.6)$$

$$= \frac{-Q}{\lambda V} \cdot x. \quad (12.7)$$

The standard solution to equation 12.7 (see Section 1.4) is

$$x = x(0) \cdot e^{-(Q/\lambda V)t} \quad (12.8)$$

where $x(0)$ is the value of x at $t = 0$. From equation 12.5,

$$\frac{Q}{V} \cdot C_a - \frac{Q \cdot C_\tau}{\lambda V} = x(0) \cdot e^{-(Q/\lambda V)t} \quad (12.9)$$

At $t = 0$, $C_\tau = 0$, so

$$x(0) = \frac{Q}{V} \cdot C_a. \quad (12.10)$$

Substituting for $x(0)$ in equation 12.9, followed by re-arrangement

$$C_\tau = \lambda C_a(1 - e^{-[Q/\lambda V]t}). \quad (12.11)$$

In other words, C_τ rises exponentially to a plateau of λC_a with rate constant $Q/\lambda V$.

As nitrous oxide is not radioactive, venous concentrations are measured in contrast to tissue concentrations (or in other words, transit time measurement is based on outflow detection in contrast to residue detection — see Section 5.4). Also since like xenon and krypton, nitrous oxide is a gas and therefore does not recirculate, the arterial level remains constant during a constant infusion.

The xenon-133 technique for measuring cerebral perfusion circumvented the need for cerebral venous sampling by enabling the time course of cerebral tissue gas concentration to be measured by external probe (residue) detection.

As discussed in Section 3.1.1.1, mean perfusion can be obtained from the xenon washout curve by dividing the initial height of the washout curve by the area under it (height over area method), using a mean partition coefficient value. From inspection of Fig. 12.2, which shows an inert gas uptake (i.e. saturation) curve, it can be seen that the difference in height of the uptake curve and the height of the constant arterial input concentration divided by the area between the arterial and cerebral venous concentration–time curves is also equal to perfusion. (Turn the figure upside down and this saturation curve becomes a desaturation curve (**Fig. 12.3**)).

It should also be noted that it is not necessary to continue the infusion until venous and tissue levels become equal to the arterial concentration, as shown in Fig. 12.3

Depending on the time interval chosen, Q/V will be weighted in a non-homogeneously perfused tissue like the brain to a higher or lower perfusion value and so this approach gives a value which is not mean perfusion. It is nevertheless reminiscent of the use of the initial slope of a washout curve which although used as an approximation to mean perfusion is more closely related to the compartment with the highest perfusion (see Section 3.1.1.1).

12.1.2 Measurement of cerebral blood flow at steady state

Cerebral perfusion can be measured at steady state during the continuous infusion of short-lived lipophilic tracers (Section 3.1.1.2). The principle underlying the use of these tracers is essentially to 'titrate' the half-time of physical decay against the half-times of washout from cerebral tissue. Ideally, the half-life of the radionuclides should be much shorter than the half-time of washout, as shown in Fig. 3.6. The relationship between arterial and tissue concentrations of tracer is given in the following equation:

$$\frac{C_\tau}{C_a} = \frac{Q/V}{\dfrac{Q}{\lambda V} + \delta} \qquad (12.12)$$

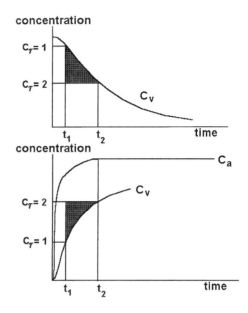

∎ Fig. 12.3 Similarity between a desaturation curve (obtained following bolus intra-arterial injection of inert gas) and a saturation curve (obtained during continuous intra-arterial infusion of an inert gas). They can be analysed in an analogous way; for example, applying the height over area approach, perfusion can be calculated from the desaturation curve by initial height over area, using the whole area (for mean perfusion) or a segment, or from the saturation curve by height of equilibrium (C_a) over area between tissue curve and arterial concentration curve, or a segment.

which can be rearranged for Q/V:

$$\frac{Q}{V} = \frac{\delta \cdot C_\tau}{C_a - C_\tau/\lambda}. \qquad (12.13)$$

Thus mean values should be used for λ and, if perfusion is expressed in relation to tissue mass, for tissue density ρ. Krypton-81m is highly diffusible (but insoluble in water, thereby disqualifying intravenous or inhalation routes of administration) and meets the requirement of instantaneous equilibration with cerebral tissue in one capillary pass. The diffusibility of water however is somewhat slower and equilibrium is not quite achieved, especially at high levels of cerebral perfusion. Furthermore the relatively long half-life of oxygen-15 renders labelled water insensitive to increased levels of perfusion and so the tracer is better adapted to the detection of abnormally low values of cerebral perfusion. Alternatively, the single bolus technique can be used, relying on different principles, as in the measurement of myocardial tissue perfusion (Section 7.1.1.4).

Cerebral blood flow measurement with labelled water is frequently combined with the quantification of cerebral oxygen-15 extraction, oxygen utilization and cerebral blood volume (based on oxygen-15 labelled carbon monoxide) in the same slice. It is then possible to produce tomographic images of oxygen utilization rate and extraction fraction, and of intravascular transit time (Frackowiak *et al.* 1980). Cerebral blood flow can also be combined with glucose utilization rate (based on fluorine-18 deoxy-glucose) to determine glucose extraction fraction (Alavi *et al.* 1986).

12.1.3 Cerebral blood volume

Regional cerebral blood volume measurement is useful in several circumstances:

(1) to correct for the component of tissue volume that is occupied by blood in the measurement of cerebral perfusion using lipophilic tracers and water;

(2) to correct for unextracted oxygen-15-labelled oxygen in the cerebral blood pool during PET measurement of the cerebral utilization rate of oxygen;

(3) as part of the measurement of mean cerebral intravascular transit time, which, through the transit time equation (see below), is related to cerebral blood flow.

Cerebral blood volume (CBV) can be measured with autologous erythrocytes labelled with technetium-99m or, for PET, with carbon-11 or oxygen-15-labelled carboxy-haemoglobin. The detected signal can be related to volume by measuring the absolute tracer concentration C_v in a venous blood sample taken after complete mixing of the labelled red cells throughout the vascular space. Cerebral haematocrit is less than peripheral haematocrit, for which a correction has to made. Therefore

$$\text{CBV} = \frac{N \cdot \gamma}{C_v} \times \frac{1}{R} \qquad (12.14)$$

where R is the ratio of cerebral to peripheral haematocrit, N is recorded count rate and γ is a constant converting N to tracer content (MBq). Here

R has a value of about 0.7. For PET, the corresponding equation is

$$\text{CBV} = \frac{C_{\text{brain}}}{C_v} \times \frac{1}{R} \qquad (12.15)$$

with units of ml/100 ml.

12.1.4 Cerebral intravascular transit time

Mean cerebral intravascular transit time is an important haemodynamic variable in its own right since under conditions of ischaemia, when blood flow decreases, cerebral vasodilatation amplifies the corresponding increase in transit time by increasing blood volume.

Regional cerebral transit time can be measured from separate derivations of regional blood flow and blood volume by PET. In single photon scintigraphy it is usually measured directly and used with measurement of cerebral blood volume to derive an estimate of cerebral blood flow using the transit time equation. Since it is an important variable in its own right it is useful to derive regional estimates of transit time. Although this can be readily performed using PET, regional transit time 'maps' can also be derived using simple photon techniques. Two approaches have been described: first to obtain a residue curve function based on an intravascular tracer and deconvolution analysis and second to obtain regional time–activity curves fitted to a gamma variate from which mean transit time can be 'directly' calculated.

12.1.5 Cerebral blood flow from the transit time equation

Since $Q = V/T$, blood flow can be derived if volume and tracer transit time through that volume are known. This is essentially how blood flow is measured with lipophilic inert gases, the residence time of which is recorded externally while the volume of distribution is the entire tissue volume of the brain. The latter need not be measured if flow is expressed in relation to tissue volume, as in perfusion. If the transit time of an intravascular tracer, such as labelled red blood cells, is measured, the blood flow can be expressed in terms of cerebral blood volume. If cerebral blood volume is also measured, and this is relatively easy following injection of labelled red cells, then absolute cerebral blood flow, in ml/min, can be obtained. The brain lends itself well to this approach (Granowska *et al.* 1980).

Applying deconvolution analysis to the aortic and cerebral curves, the residue curve over the brain is obtained from which T is calculated as height over area. Following mixing of the red cells throughout the circulation and stabilization of the count rate over the brain, cerebral blood volume V is measured from the count rate recorded over the brain and the simultaneous activity in a blood sample. Thus

$$V = \frac{\text{brain count rate}}{\text{blood sample count rate}} \times \frac{\gamma}{\Gamma} \quad (12.16)$$

where γ and Γ are constants, relating to the gamma camera and well-counter sensitivities, respectively, for converting brain counts to MBq and sample counts to MBq/ml. Assumptions have to be made about the shape of the brain in comparison with a phantom, filled with radioactivity and designed to be the same shape as the brain, and corrections made for non-cerebral counts recorded from the scalp.

12.1.6 Quantification of the regional distribution of cerebral blood flow

Radiolabelled lipophilic agents are highly extracted by the brain and can therefore be used to generate tomographic images depicting the regional distribution of cerebral blood flow. These agents include technetium-99m labelled hexamethylpropylene-amine oxime (HMPAO), iodine-123 labelled amines, xenon-133, krypton-81m and positron-labelled water. As for other tissues, the myocardium for example, a fundamental assumption for any such perfusion image is that the regional extraction fraction of the tracer is constant. Partly because of this limitation, SPECT images based on HMPAO and iodinated amines, although giving images of the distribution of perfusion, are not truly quantitative insofar as regional count rates are directly proportional to regional perfusion. Nevertheless the generation of images with regional count rates that are more directly and linearly proportional to regional cerebral blood flow can be achieved with oxygen-15-labelled water and xenon-133 SPECT.

12.1.6.1 Xenon-133 SPECT

This technique was developed by Lassen and his group (Lassen 1985) and is based on the recirculation of inhaled xenon-133. The patient continuously inhales the gas from a suitable circuit while tomographic images are acquired. The arterial xenon-133 concentration (C_a) is determined by the alveolar xenon-133 concentration (C_{alv}) such that

$$C_a = n \cdot C_{alv} \quad (12.17)$$

The parameter n is a simple proportionality constant which depends on attenuation and counting geometry, and, as will be clear from below, does not need to be known. The time course of C_{alv} is continuously monitored with a scintillation probe over the lung. Various tomographic detector systems have been developed for the purpose of imaging the xenon-133 concentration in the brain, including multiple rotating or fixed scintillation probes, but their details will not be further discussed.

The tracer kinetics underlying the technique are in general similar to those of other lipophilic tracers displaying single pass extraction fractions in the brain approaching unity. The equation describing the amount of tracer in a region of cerebral tissue at any time t after the start of inhalation is similar to equation 12.3 and to the equation describing labelled water concentration after intravenous bolus injection:

$$M_\tau = Q \int C_a(t)^* e^{-(Q/\lambda V)t} \cdot dt. \quad (12.18)$$

It states that the amount of xenon-133 in a region is determined by the regional arterial blood flow and would be directly proportional to the area under the arterial tracer concentration time curve recorded up to t if tracer was not, at the same time, being continuously washed out of the brain at rate determined by $Q/\lambda V$. In other words the amount of tracer in the brain is determined by the convolution (denoted by*) of tracer washout on the arterial input function. Combining equations 12.17 and 12.18,

$$M_\tau = Q n \int C_{alv}(t)^* e^{-(Q/\lambda V)t} \cdot dt. \quad (12.19)$$

Dividing both sides by V gives

$$C_\tau = \frac{Q}{V} n \int C_{alv}(t)^* e^{-(Q/\lambda V)t} \cdot dt. \quad (12.20)$$
$$= N\gamma$$

thereby obtaining an expression relating count rate N to cerebral perfusion Q/V.

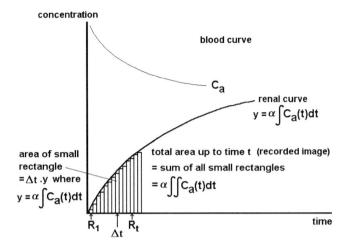

▌ **Fig. 12.4** An example of double integration routinely used in nuclear medicine. Differential renal function is often calculated from dynamic renography by a comparison of images continuously acquired over a period of about 2 minutes following injection of tracer. The image represents the integral of counts acquired in each frame (typically over 10 seconds) of which there may be 15 or so, each one of which is itself the integral of the arterial activity up to the corresponding time, i.e. $\int C_a(t)\, dt$. (See exercise 19b.)

In practice, the period of inhalation, a total of 4.5 min, is divided into four phases, the first of 1.5 min and then three of 1 min, and separate tomographic images acquired during each phase. Since the images acquired during each phase represent an integration of the counts recorded in the phase, the equation describing the image is the integral of equation 12.20; i.e. a double integral:

$$\gamma \int N = \frac{Q}{V}\gamma \int [\int C_{\mathrm{alv}}(t)^* e^{-(Q/\lambda V)t} \cdot dt] dt \qquad (12.21)$$

Then $\int N$, the total counts acquired in the region during a phase, is computed for each phase and represents the acquired image[†]. It should be noted that γ varies from one region of brain to another, as does the corresponding proportionality constant in a technetium-99m HMPAO brain SPECT scan.

Each phase of acquisition is relatively short and the assumption is made that t in equation 12.21 is negligible and so the term $e^{-(Q/\lambda V)t}$ is effectively equal to unity (i.e. no washout); therefore

$$\gamma \int N = \frac{Q}{V} n \int [\int C_{\mathrm{alv}}(t) \cdot dt] dt \qquad (12.22)$$

Since C_{alv} is constant for all regions of the brain,

$$\gamma \int N = \frac{Q}{V} n C_{\mathrm{alv}} \cdot \frac{t^2}{2}. \qquad (12.23)$$

The tomographic image depicts regional cerebral perfusion. Note that the image does not depict regional washout of xenon-133. Indeed, a claimed advantage of the technique is that the effects of uncertainties in λ are minimized. The assumption that $e^{-(Q/\lambda V)t}$ is equal to unity may seem ambitious given that normal mean cerebral blood flow is about 55 ml/100 ml/min. With a mean λ value of 1.2, $Q/\lambda V$ will be about 0.45 min^{-1}, indicating that of a discrete bolus of xenon-133 arriving in a region of brain, about 36% (i.e. $e^{-0.45} = 0.64$) will have washed out in one minute. However the effect of the double integration, firstly as performed by the brain and secondly by the detector, is to minimize this apparent error (see Question 19 Chapter 14).

[†]Double integration, complicated as it sounds, is in fact a mathematical operation carried out in routine nuclear medicine perhaps more frequently than realized. It is, for instance, frequently applied in the measurement of differential renal function from dynamic renography when an image is generated from the first 3 minutes of data. The first integration is performed by the kidney itself as it accumulates tracer; the second is performed by the gamma camera as it sums the counts recorded up to 3 minutes (**Fig. 12.4**). The dependence of the image on t^2 rather than t may appear surprising, but as the image is acquired it is not simply a situation in which a count rate is multiplied by time, since as the image builds up so too does the count rate, itself a function of time.

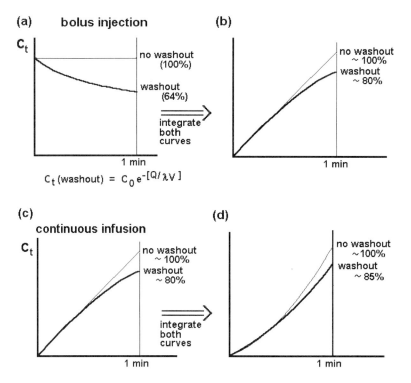

$$C_t \text{(washout)} = C_0 e^{-[Q/\lambda V]}$$

❙ **Fig. 12.5** Minimization by integration of the error generated in the parametric imaging of regional cerebral perfusion by assuming no xenon-133 washout during an acquisition interval of one minute. If the xenon was given by intra-arterial bolus injection the washout curve would fall to 64% of the initial value by one minute for a normal CBF (a). The area under the washout curve would however be 82% of the area under the curve had there been no washout (b). The xenon is effectively given by continuous arterial infusion which can be imagined to represent a series of bolus injections (c) which over a period of image acquisition the brain itself would 'integrate' in the same way as the kidney does in Fig. 12.4 (d). (See exercise 19a.)

Thus, although the count rate from a discrete bolus would fall to 64% the initial value after one minute, the area under the washout curve (i.e. the first integration) would be about 80% of the area under the hypothetical rectangle corresponding to no washout. A second integration reduces the difference further to less than 20% **(Fig. 12.5)**. The tomographic image of the brain essentially depicts the regional distribution of tracer to the brain and is analogous to the SPECT image produced by technetium-99m HMPAO. The regional determination of the factors relating to counting geometry and attenuation, γ (equation 12.20), need to be considered. The slice thickness in xenon-133 SPECT is greater than in PET and so the resolution is inferior, but the technique has nevertheless been useful for experimental studies in man on the effects of several physiological interventions on the distribution of regional cerebral blood flow.

12.1.6.2 Regional intravascular transit time

A technique for quantifying regional intravascular transit time, based on the gamma function equation, has been developed by Merrick and his group (Merrick *et al.* 1991). An image of the brain which depicts regional intravascular transit time can be generated by recording a first-pass time–activity curve in each image pixel following bolus intravenous injection of a tracer which does not penetrate the blood brain barrier. The importance of transit time as a variable in its own right was emphasized above. In principle, the curve in each pixel can be subjected to any one of several different analytical approaches including the generation of an impulse retention function by deconvolution analysis. An alternative approach, (Merrick *et al.* 1991) is to correct all individual pixel curves for tracer recirculation by fitting them to a gamma function. The equation which defines a gamma function,

$$N(t) = \kappa \cdot t^\alpha \cdot e^{-\beta t} \qquad (12.24)$$

or more precisely in the current situation,

$$N(t) = \kappa \cdot (t - AT)^\alpha \cdot e^{-\beta(t-AT)} \qquad (12.25)$$

(where AT is the minimum transit time from the injection site to the brain [arrival time]) is then used to calculate mean cerebral transit time T for each pixel from

$$T + AT = \frac{1}{\beta}(\alpha + 1). \qquad (12.26)$$

(Note that, since a gamma function is based on the concept of multiple 'mixing chambers', the number of which is $\alpha + 1$, the curve becomes monoexponential when $\alpha = 0$, since equation 12.24 reduces to $N(t) = \kappa \cdot e^{-\beta t}$.) The time of arrival ($AT$) from the intravenous injection site to the brain is significant compared with cerebral intravascular transit time and is measured with a scintillation probe over the arch of the aorta; the arrival time between arch and brain is assumed to be negligible. Since the variation in individual tracer molecule arrival times is what actually influences the shape of the recorded time–activity curve, the assumption that is effectively required is that there is no further 'spreading' of the bolus between aortic arch and cerebral artery.

By fitting a gamma function to the curve recorded over the aortic arch and all the individual pixel curves recorded over the brain, then for each pixel

$$T_{IV-arch} = (1/\beta_a) \cdot (\alpha_a + 1) - AT \qquad (12.27)$$

and

$$T_{IV-brain} = (1/\beta_b) \cdot (\alpha_b + 1) - AT \qquad (12.28)$$

where subscripts a and be refer respectively to aortic arch and brain. Therefore

$$T_{brain} = T_{IV-brain} - T_{IV-arch}$$

$$= [(1/\beta_a) \cdot (\alpha_a + 1) - AT] - [(1/\beta_b) \cdot (\alpha_b + 1) - AT]$$

$$= [(1/\beta_a) \cdot (\alpha_a + 1)] - [(1/\beta_b) \cdot (\alpha_b + 1)]. \qquad (12.29)$$

By performing this calculation for every pixel, an image of regional intravascular transit times is generated. An attraction of the technique is that the fitting of a gamma function minimizes noise in the resulting curve in contrast, say, to deconvolution analysis which generates retention functions with substantial noise. The gamma function technique is therefore well-suited to pixel-by-pixel analysis and the generation of a parametric image. When cerebral transit time is significantly increased as a result of disease, or when a narrow bolus is difficult to achieve, for example in cardiopulmonary disease, none of these techniques work well. Furthermore, although, in general, pertechnetate is an adequate tracer, regional cerebral disease may result in a breakdown of the blood brain barrier, necessitating the use of a large molecule, for example albumin, with a higher certainty of remaining intravascular during the first pass.

12.2 Cerebral oxygen consumption

Energy metabolism in the brain is exclusively aerobic and glucose is the only energy substrate. The oxygen consumption of oxidative metabolism is sufficiently rapid compared with the half-life of oxygen-15 to make this a useful tracer of oxygen metabolism. Normally, the fraction of incoming oxygen extracted by the brain is relatively low, thereby providing a large functional reserve such that under conditions of reduced cerebral blood flow the brain can maintain a normal oxygen utilization rate by increasing oxygen extraction fraction.

Following uptake from cerebral capillary blood oxygen-15 labelled oxygen is rapidly utilized for metabolism, with the production of oxygen-15 labelled water, which is then washed out of the brain according to the well-described rules of tissue clearance of lipophilic tracers such as inert gases. Because inhaled or injected labelled oxygen does not therefore progressively accumulate in the brain (in contrast to fluoro-deoxyglucose, see below), the rate of oxygen utilization by the brain ($CMRO_2$) is more easily measured or imaged by first determining oxygen extraction fraction (E) and combining it with cerebral blood flow (CBF); i.e.

$$CMRO_2 = E \times CBF. \qquad (12.30)$$

This approach holds because the brain does not store oxygen; i.e. all the oxygen required is immediately used following uptake. The kinetics involved in the measurement of cerebral oxygen extraction fraction are rather complicated and revolve around the separation of oxygen-15 signals arising from native oxygen and from the metabolite, oxygen-15 labelled water. The contribution of unextracted labelled oxygen in the cerebral blood volume is a further confounding factor.

Oxygen extraction fraction is most simply measured, from a theoretical standpoint, by recording a time–activity curve over the brain following the intra-carotid injection of labelled oxygen bound as oxyhaemoglobin (Ter-Pogossian and Herscovitch 1985). The resulting time–activity curve, which can be recorded by highly collimated scintillation probes placed over the vertex, rises to an immediate peak and then falls within seconds to a slowly declining plateau (**Fig. 12.6**). The height of the plateau, extrapolated to the time of the peak and expressed as a fraction of the peak, is a measure of the oxygen extraction fraction. A contemporaneous injection of oxygen-15 labelled water can be used to measure CBF, from which $CMRO_2$ can be obtained. PET techniques for measuring $CMRO_2$ are based on inhalation of labelled oxygen but require more complex kinetic analysis. As in the measurement of cerebral perfusion with oxygen-15 labelled water, two approaches are possible; firstly, the steady-state method based on continuous inhalation which exploits the short half-life of the isotope and, secondly, a method based on a discrete period of inhalation in which the counts recorded from the brain are corrected for isotope physical decay.

When a subject inhales oxygen-15 labelled oxygen, the signal from the brain arises initially from unextracted and extracted labelled oxygen but is soon supplemented by oxygen-15 in the water of metabolism which is formed almost immediately following tissue extraction and subsequent oxidative metabolism of labelled oxygen. With either approach, a relatively simple model can be formulated in which there are simultaneous cerebral inputs of oxygen-15 labelled oxygen and oxygen-15-labelled water. The unextracted labelled oxygen and the labelled water recirculate, the latter after washout from the tissue at a rate governed by tissue perfusion.

12.2.1 Steady-state method

Consider first only radioactivity in the extravascular tissue of the brain. The derivation of the steady-state equation defining this activity is identical to those defining labelled water in the brain for the measure-

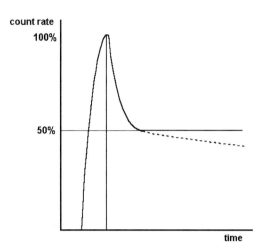

∎ **Fig. 12.6** Cerebral oxygen extraction fraction determined from the time activity curve recorded over the brain following bolus intravenous injection of oxygen-15 labelled oxyhaemoglobin. In this case, the extraction fraction is 50%. The curve falls more slowly after the initial 'spike' as a result of conversion to oxygen-15 labelled water which is immediately also washed out of the brain.

ment of cerebral perfusion and krypton-81m in tissue or pulmonary alveoli for measurement of perfusion or regional pulmonary ventilation. Thus the amount of activity M_t changes as a result of the difference between the rate of tracer delivery on the one hand and the sum of tracer washout and tracer physical decay on the other. Therefore in a region of brain we can say

$$\frac{dM_\tau}{dt} = Q \cdot E \cdot C_a^o(t) + QC_a^w(t) - \frac{M_\tau Q}{\lambda V} - M_\tau \cdot \delta$$

$$(12.31)$$

where C_a^o and C_a^w are the arterial oxygen-15 labelled oxygen and water concentrations respectively, Q and V are tissue blood flow and volume respectively, and λ is the partition coefficient of water between blood and brain (Jones *et al.* 1976, Frackowiak *et al.* 1980).

At steady state

$$\frac{dM_\tau}{dt} = 0 \qquad (12.32)$$

so, after re-arrangement of equation 12.31,

$$M_\tau = \frac{Q \cdot E \cdot C_a^o + QC_a^w}{Q/\lambda V + \delta} \qquad (12.33)$$

and

$$E = \frac{[M_\tau(Q/\lambda V + \delta)] - Q \cdot C_a^w}{Q \cdot C_a^o}. \qquad (12.34)$$

In equation 12.34, a feature of practical importance which is not encountered in the measurement of perfusion with labelled water is the presence of two arterial oxygen-15 concentrations. These can be resolved in an arterial blood sample because virtually all the labelled oxygen is bound to red cells as oxyhaemoglobin. The labelled water however is distributed between red cells and plasma water. Nevertheless, at the time of contemporaneous measurement of cerebral perfusion, which is required for the measurement of oxygen utilization, the distribution of labelled water between arterial blood and plasma can be determined. Arterial plasma oxygen-15 concentration, recorded at the time of measurement of CMRO$_2$, indicates labelled water concentration. The concentration of labelled water in red cells can then be calculated from the preceding measurement of the distribution of labelled water between plasma and red cells, made at the time of cerebral blood flow measurement.

Since an appreciable fraction of incoming oxygen-15 labelled oxygen is not extracted there is an additional signal from oxygen-15 in the cerebral blood volume. There are grounds for ignoring this because the blood volume of the brain is only about 4% of total tissue volume. Nevertheless this signal can be taken into account by using a similar approach to that which addresses the amount of tracer in the tissue compartment M_τ. Thus the rate of change of blood oxygen-15 is the difference between the input rate and the sum of washout and decay rates. The input rate is the product of blood flow and unextracted arterial oxygen-15 concentration (i.e. 1-E). The rate of washout is governed by the reciprocal of the transit time in the vascular compartment; i.e. Q/V_b (where V_b is the vascular volume). If V_b is 4% of total tissue volume, then mean transit time through the vascular compartment will be 25 times faster than mean transit time of labelled water through the total tissue volume.

Thus,

$$\frac{dM_b}{dt} = Q \cdot (1 - E) \cdot C_a^o - M_b \cdot \frac{Q}{V_b} - M_b \cdot \delta \qquad (12.35)$$

and

$$M_b = \frac{Q \cdot (1 - E) \cdot C_a^o}{Q/V_b + \delta}. \qquad (12.36)$$

The total oxygen-15 (oxygen itself and water) content of the brain, which is actually measured by PET, will therefore be the sum of equations 12.33 and 12.36:

$$M_\tau + M_b = \frac{Q \cdot E \cdot C_a^o + Q \cdot C_a^w}{Q/\lambda V + \delta} + \frac{Q \cdot (1 - E) \cdot C_a^o}{Q/V_b + \delta}$$

or in terms of tissue concentration

$$C_\tau + C_b = \frac{Q/V \cdot E \cdot C_a^o + Q \cdot C_a^w}{Q/\lambda V + \delta} + \frac{Q/V \cdot (1 - E) \cdot C_a^o}{Q/V_b + \delta} \qquad (12.37)$$

from which E can be solved. Cerebral blood volume can be separately measured using oxygen-15 labelled carbon monoxide.

The effects of ignoring the cerebral vascular unextracted oxygen-15 on measurement of oxygen extraction fraction can be explored by inserting ranges of values for the variables in equation 12.37. The error is obviously greater for low values of E, since $1 - E$ will be higher and the cerebral vascular oxygen concentration higher. Under normal circumstances the arterial oxygen-15 is two-thirds oxygen (in red cells) and one-third water (distributed between plasma and red cells). The extent to which a steady-state PET image is linearly proportional to regional oxygen utilization depends on the prevailing levels of the variables in equation 12.37.

12.2.2 Non-steady-state method

In the non-steady-state method, the patient inhales gaseous oxygen-15 and PET images are acquired over the brain for a period of about one minute (Mintun *et al.* 1984, Herscovitch *et al.* 1985). The signal component due to labelled water at time t after the start of inhalation is given by

$$C_\tau^w = \frac{Q}{V} \int C_a^w(t)^* e^{-kt} \cdot dt \qquad (12.38)$$

where $k = Q/\lambda V$. This equation is identical to equation 3.35 and is an example of the mass over area equation for clearance or flow, except in this case the area of the arterial curve is modified by continuing washout of tracer from the tissue; i.e. the tissue signal is proportional to the arterial curve convolved (denoted by*) on the washout (or retention function) curve.

The signal component due to oxygen itself is proportional to the regional oxygen clearance, $E \cdot Q/V$, and the area under the arterial oxygen-15 labelled oxygen curve. The latter is also modified by tracer washout but, because of rapid conversion of extracted oxygen-15 to labelled water, it is also convolved on the brain water retention curve, with a rate constant of clearance of $Q/\lambda V$. So

$$C_\tau^o = E \cdot \frac{Q}{V} \int C_a^o(t)^* e^{-kt} \cdot \mathrm{d}t. \qquad (12.39)$$

Note $E.Q$ rather than Q in equation 12.41; this is because, unlike water, oxygen is only partly extracted in one pass through the brain while water is assumed to be completely extracted so $E = 1$.

Therefore the total extravascular tissue oxygen-15 concentration is the sum of equations 12.38 and 12.39

$$C_\tau = \frac{Q}{V} \int C_a^w(t)^* e^{-kt} \cdot \mathrm{d}t. + E \cdot \frac{Q}{V} \int C_a^o(t)^* e^{-kt} \cdot \mathrm{d}t. \qquad (12.40)$$

Re-arranging

$$E = \frac{C_\tau - Q/V \int C_a^w(t)^* e^{-kt} \mathrm{d}t}{Q/V \int C_a^o(t)^* e^{-kt} \mathrm{d}t}. \qquad (12.41)$$

As in the steady-state method, CBF has to be measured in order to solve for E.

No account has been taken in equation 12.41 of unextracted labelled oxygen in cerebral blood. This can be taken into account by assuming that the blood pool signal arises from unextracted oxygen, giving rise to an average tissue blood concentration of C_b, which can be expressed thus

$$C_b = \frac{C_a^o V_b}{V} - \frac{E \cdot C_a^o \cdot V_b}{V}. \qquad (12.42)$$

Adding equation 12.42 to the right hand side of equation 12.39 followed by re-arrangement gives

$$E = \frac{C_\tau - [Q/V \int C_a^w(t)^* e^{-kt} \mathrm{d}t] - [C_a^o V_b]}{[Q/V \int C_a^o(t)^* e^{-kt} \mathrm{d}t] - [C_a^o V_b]}. \qquad (12.43)$$

It can be seen therefore that in addition to CBF it is also necessary to measure regional cerebral blood volume and this is usually achieved by PET following the administration of carbon monoxide labelled with carbon-11 or oxygen-15.

CMRO$_2$ is a valuable measurement in patients with cerebral ischaemia, particularly as the maintenance of CMRO$_2$ in the face of falling CBF is required for normal neuronal function. It is therefore almost always performed in association with measurement of CBF and, by necessity, oxygen extraction fraction.

12.3 Cerebral glucose utilization

The brain uses glucose exclusively for its energy requirements. Under anaerobic conditions, lactate production ensues and this is toxic to brain cells. Regional glucose utilization can be quantified by PET using fluorine-18 labelled deoxyglucose (FDG) (Lucignani *et al.* 1993). The brain takes up this glucose analogue using the same facilitated transport mechanism as for glucose (see Section 7.4.2). It cannot however be further incorporated into the glycolytic pathway and, as the brain lacks glucose-6-phos-phatase, remains metabolically trapped within the cell.

The cerebral tissue FDG concentration C_τ can be recorded by PET following intravenous injection. By taking arterial blood samples to obtain an arterial concentration (C_a)–time curve, the cerebral clearance of FDG, Z_{FDG}, can be measured. Since FDG is trapped, without backflow into blood, a Patlak plot is a convenient analytical approach. Thus

$$\frac{C_\tau(t)}{C_a(t)} = \frac{Z_{FDG}}{V} \frac{\int C_a(t) \cdot \mathrm{d}t}{C_a(t)} + \frac{V_i}{V}, \qquad (12.44)$$

with units that all cancel

$$\frac{\mathrm{MBq/ml}}{\mathrm{MBq/ml}} = \frac{\mathrm{ml/min}}{\mathrm{ml}} \times \frac{\mathrm{MBq/ml}}{\mathrm{MBq/ml}} \times \mathrm{min} + \frac{\mathrm{ml}}{\mathrm{ml}},$$

where V_i is the blood volume seen within the slice and the other symbols are the same as for cerebral blood flow measurement.

When $C_\tau(t)/C_a(t)$ is plotted against $\int C_a(t) \, \mathrm{d}t C_a(t)$, a straight line is obtained with slope Z_{FDG}/V and intercept V_i/V.

The term Z_{FDG}/V is the cerebral clearance of FDG/unit volume of brain tissue which explains why, like perfusion, it has units of the reciprocal of time. By measuring the arterial native glucose concentration, Glu$_a$, the rate of cerebral glucose utilization per unit volume of brain, CMR_{glu} can be calculated from Z_{FDG}; i.e.

$$CMR_{glu} = \frac{Z_{FDG}}{V} \cdot Glu_a \qquad (12.45)$$

with units

$$\frac{g}{min \cdot ml} = \frac{ml}{min \cdot ml} \cdot \frac{g}{ml}$$

Equation 12.45 assumes equal cerebral clearance rates for FDG and native glucose; i.e. assumes a 'lumped' constant of unity (see Section 7.4.2.) Extraction fraction is equal to the ratio, clearance/flow, so the regional cerebral glucose extraction fraction can also be obtained from Z_{FDG} and cerebral perfusion (using labelled water). A functional image generated by performing a mathematical operation on two separate images is called a parametric image[†] (Section 5.5.1). So dividing an image of regional glucose clearance by an image of regional cerebral blood flow gives an image of regional glucose extraction fraction. Similarly oxygen extraction fraction can be portrayed on a three dimensional image by dividing a blood flow image with an oxygen image. An image of intravascular cerebral transit time can be portrayed by dividing a flow image with a cerebral blood volume image obtained with oxygen-15 labelled carbon monoxide labelled red cells.

12.4 Radio-ligand uptake by cerebral receptors

Several saturable neuronal receptors for neurotransmitters and their antagonists have been imaged with specific radiolabeled ligands, by both SPECT and PET (Martin *et al.* 1989). By providing tissue tracer concentrations, PET permits the application of Scatchard analysis to tomographic images for the calculation of ligand- receptor binding affinity (or dissociation constant K_d) and of tissue receptor density. The basis of the Scatchard plot was developed in Section 5.6:

$$[L - R] = [R]_{max} - \frac{K_d[L - R]}{[L]} \qquad (12.46)$$

where L is free ligand, R is receptor, $L - R$ receptor-bound ligand and the square brackets indicate concentration. Since the ligand is radioactive, $[L - R]$ is measured from PET in the cerebral region of interest (i.e. bearing the relevant receptors), while $[L]$, the concentration of unbound ligand, can be measured from an irrelevant region of the brain where the specific receptors are known to be absent, often the cerebellum. Plotting $[L - R]$ on the y-axis against $[L - R]/[L]$ on the x-axis generates a negative regression line with a slope equal to K_d and a y-axis intercept (at $x = 0$) equal to $[R_{max}]$, the total number of receptors present (**Fig. 5.20**).

Measurement of the rate of fluorine-18 labelled DOPA uptake in the basal ganglia in the assessment of patients with movement disorders such as Parkinson's disease is a variant of this approach (Brooks *et al.* 1990). Following dynamic acquisition, time–activity curves are constructed from regions of interest over the caudate nuclei and over a reference tissue (i.e. one not actively accumulating the tracer, for example occipital cortex). Since DOPA is irreversibly accumulated in the caudate nuclei, Patlak, rather than Scatchard analysis, can be used to generate values for regional tracer clearance, using the signal from the reference tissue to provide the input function. Such an input function is no less appropriate for a Patlak plot than one based on arterial tracer concentration. For example, it incorporates the component in the output curve which is the result of vascular dispersion, insofar as dispersions in the two regions are comparable. Thus recalling the Patlak equation and using more conventional notation,

$$C_\tau(t) = Z \int C_a(t) \cdot dt \qquad (12.47)$$

and adding 'capillary blood background', $C_p(t)$, to both sides

$$C_\tau(t) + C_p(t) = Z \int C_a(t) \cdot dt + C_p(t) \qquad (12.48)$$

followed by division of both sides by $C_a(t)$,

$$\frac{C_\tau(t) + C_p(t)}{C_a(t)} = Z \frac{\int C_a(t) \cdot dt}{C_a(t)} + \frac{C_p(t)}{C_a(t)} \qquad (12.49)$$

$$= Z \frac{\int C_a(t) \cdot dt}{C_a(t)} + k. \qquad (12.50)$$

[†] Such parametric images can also be obtained by manipulating sets of single photon images; for example, parametric images of renal transit time or images of extraction fraction (produced by dividing a clearance image such as a renal parenchymal DTPA image by a flow image).

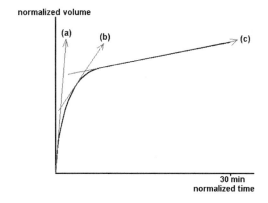

█ **Fig. 12.7** A Patlak-Rutland plot based on an arterial time-activity curve as the input potentially contains 3 components: (a) an initial phase which represents vascular dispersion (ie replacement of non-radioactive plasma with radioactive plasma); (b) a second phase which represents tracer clearance from plasma to interstitial fluid; and (c) a third phase which represents unidirectional active tracer uptake. By taking an irrelevant tissue region instead of arterial blood for the input, the first 2 phases tend to disappear.

Until there is complete mixing of tracer between arterial and capillary blood, k is not equal to $C_p(t)/C_a(t)$, and the early gradient of the Patlak slope based on arterial blood therefore includes a positive component which represents replacement of non-radioactive blood in the capillaries of the tissue with radioactive blood (**Fig. 12.7**). The input (from the reference region of interest) and output (from the cerebral region of interest) functions are both expressed per pixel, so the gradient of the regression has units of min^{-1} and is called the input constant. The input function soon includes not only intravascular activity but also DOPA in the interstitial space of the brain. Again, however, since it is the intracellular uptake of DOPA that is of primary interest, it is appropriate to include extracellular activity in the input function and, as a consequence, eliminate the early gradient in the Patlak–Rutland regression slope due to exchange between intravascular and interstitial tracer.

References

Alavi A, Dann R, Chawluk J, Alavi J, Kushner M and Reivich M. Positron emission tomography imaging of regional cerebral glucose metabolism. *Seminars in Nuclear Medicine* 1986, **16**: 2–34.

Brooks DJ, Salmon EP, Mathias CJ, Quinn N, Leenders KL, Bannister R, Marsden CD and Frackowiak RSJ. The relationship between locomotor disability, autonomic dysfunction, and integrity of the striatal dopaminergic system in patients with multiple system atrophy, pure autonomic failure, and Parkinson's disease, studied with PET. *Brain* 1990, **113**: 1539–52.

Frackowiak RSJ, Lenzi G-L, Jones T and Heather JD. Quantitative measurement of regional cerebral blood flow and oxidative metabolism in man using ^{15}O and positron emission tomography: theory, procedure, and normal values. *Journal of Computer Assisted Tomography* 1980, **4**: 727–36.

Granowska M, Britton KE, Afshar F, Wright CW, Smyth RRJ, Lee TY and Nimmon CC. Global and regional cerebral blood flow, non-invasive quantitation in patients with sub-arachnoid haemorrhage. *Journal of Neurosurgery* 1980, **53**: 153–9.

Herscovitch P, Mintun MA and Raichle ME. Brain oxygen utilization measured with oxygen-15 radiotracers and positron emission tomography: generation of metabolic images. *Journal of Nuclear Medicine* 1985, **26**: 41 6–7.

Jones T, Chesler DA and Ter-Pogossian MM. The continuous inhalation of oxygen-15 for assessing regional oxygen extraction in the brain of man. *British Journal of Radiology* 1976, **49**: 339–43.

Lassen NA, Henriksen O and Sejrsen P. Indicator methods for measurement of organ and tissue blood flow. In: Shepherd JT, Abboud FM, (eds) *Handbook of physiology*, section 2: The cardiovascular system 111. American Physiological Society, Bethesda, Maryland: 1983, 21–63.

Lassen NA. Cerebral blood flow tomography with xenon-133. *Seminars in Nuclear Medicine* 1985, **15**: 347–56.

Lucignani G, Schmidt KC, Moresco RM, Striano G, Colombo F, Sokoloff L and Fazio F. Measurement of regional cerebral glucose utilization with fluorine-18-FDG and PET in heterogeneous tissues: theoretical considerations and practical procedure. *Journal of Nuclear Medicine* 1993, **34**: 360–9.

Martin WRW, Palmer MR, Peppard RF and Calne DB. Quantitation of presynaptic dopaminergic function with positron emission tomography. *Neurology* 1989, **39**: (suppl 1), 1–63.

Merrick MV, Ferrington CM and Cowen SJ. Parametric imaging of cerebral vascular reserves. 1. Theory, validation and normal values. *European Journal of Nuclear Medicine* 1991, **18**: 171–7.

Mintun MA, Raichle ME, Martin WRW and Herscovitch P. Brain oxygen utilization measured with oxygen-15 radiotracers and positron emission tomography. *Journal of Nuclear Medicine* 1984, **25**: 177–87.

Ter-Pogossian M and Herscovitch P. Radioactive oxygen-15 in the study of cerebral blood flow, blood volume and oxygen metabolism. *Seminars in Nuclear Medicine* 1985, **15**: 377–94.

Veal N and Mallett BL. Regional cerebral blood flow determination by 133-xenon inhalation and external recording: the effect of arterial recirculation. *Clinical Science* 1965, **30**: 353–69.

13 Body fluids, electrolytes and bone

13.1 Fluid distribution

Body water is either intracellular or extracellular. The extracellular fluid (ECF) is divided between plasma and interstitial fluid. In terms of electrolyte composition, the ECF differs from the intracellular fluid mainly with respect to potassium, sodium and chloride. The solutes of the ECF exchange relatively rapidly between plasma and interstitial fluid, although with some fluids, the turnover is slow. These include ocular fluid, cerebrospinal fluid, and serosal fluids such as in the pleura and peritoneum. Exchange is slow because these fluids are separated from plasma by an epithelial layer. They make up a minor sub-compartment of the ECF called the transcellular fluid.

The volume and composition of the body fluids is under the control of several sensor and effector mechanisms. Important sensors are osmo-receptors, baro-receptors and chemo-receptors. The osmo-receptors are responsive to osmolality, the chemo-receptors to pH and the baro-receptors, indirectly, to volume. The effector mechanisms include the thirst centre, which regulates water intake, and several hormones, including a) anti-diuretic hormone, the control of which primarily responds to osmo-receptors, b) atrial naturietic peptide (ANP), which responds to atrial baro-receptors, and c) the renin-angiotensin axis, the activation of which responds indirectly to baro-receptors in the carotid and pulmonary arteries and directly to mechanisms intrinsic to the renal vasculature. A detailed description of the interplay of these afferent and efferent factors is outside the aims of this text. Nevertheless, certain aspects of the control of body fluid volumes are important insofar as they relate to the relevance of expressing glomerular filtration rate in terms of body fluid volumes in comparison with indices of body size, such as surface area and weight.

13.1.1 Extracellular fluid volumes

13.1.1.1 Measurement of extracellular fluid volume

Measurement of extracellular fluid (ECF) volume is based on the dilution of tracers which are not protein bound in plasma and which diffuse freely between plasma and the ECF but do not penetrate the intracellular space. Such tracers inevitably undergo glomerular filtration. The principle of plasma volume measurement by dilution of tracer that remains within the plasma compartment is described in Section 10.4.2. Measurement of ECF volume is more complex because of:

(a) the delay in the mixing of the appropriate tracers;
(b) their simultaneous clearance through filtration at the glomerulus.

This means that one cannot inject the tracer and simply wait for it to mix throughout the ECF since losses via urine will occur in the meantime. No problem would arise if mixing of the tracer was instantaneous throughout the ECF or there were no urinary losses but, as described in the measurement of GFR, it takes about two hours for these tracers to mix or equilibrate throughout the ECF. Despite this, a commonly used technique for the measurement of ECF volume is to take two or three plasma samples after mixing has been completed and extrapolate the decreasing plasma concentration–time curve back to zero time (**Fig. 13.1**). Measurement of dilution is then based on the extrapolated zero time plasma concentration $C(0)$ in relation to the injected activity $M(0)$; i.e.

$$V_{\text{ECF}} = \frac{M(0)}{C(0)} \tag{13.1}$$

Equation 13.1 overestimates ECF volume since $C(0)$ is less than it would be if the tracer fell instanta-

In plasma concentration

$$V_{ECF} = \frac{M(0)}{C(0)} = \frac{MBq}{MBq\,/\,ml} = ml$$

▌ **Fig. 13.1** Measurement of the extracellular fluid volume using a filtration marker. Once the tracer has equilibrated throughout its distribution volume (close to ECF volume), it disappears from plasma as a single exponential. The zero-time intercept of this exponential is an approximation to the concentration of the tracer in the ECF that would have been reached in the absence of any excretion and therefore gives the volume of the ECF when divided *into* the injected activity. This approach effectively assumes no losses from the ECF compartment during the period of complete mixing throughout the ECF, an assumption which is valid only in the presence of poor or no renal function, and which otherwise leads to an over-estimation of the volume. As in the measurement of GFR using only the second exponential, the over-estimation is positively related to renal function in a non-linear manner that can be well fitted by a second-order polynomial.

neously to its monoexponential rate of loss.[†] The overestimation is exactly the same as the over-estimation in GFR calculated as $[M(0) \cdot \alpha_2]/B$ in equation 11.15 and also decreases with decreasing GFR. A more accurate way to measure ECF volume is therefore to use the transit time equation (Ladegaard-Pedersen 1972):

$$T = V_{ECF}/Z$$

or

$$V_{ECF} = Z \cdot T$$

where Z is plasma clearance of the tracer.

Transit time is the mean residence time of tracer in the ECF compartment (before being filtered at the glomerulus). The plasma clearance Z is equal to the GFR if the tracer is inulin and almost the same as GFR if the tracer is a filtration marker such as

chromium-51 EDTA or technetium-99m DTPA. The residence time of a tracer in a compartment from which it disappears mono-exponentially is simply the reciprocal of the rate constant of disappearance. However, for a multi-exponential disappearance, as obtained with filtration markers, the residence time is a more complex function and can be obtained from the first moment of the transit time (see Section 2.1). Thus

$$T = \frac{\int t \cdot C(t) \cdot dt}{C(t) \cdot dt} \qquad (13.2)$$

from which, for a bi-exponential disappearance where the two exponentials have intercepts and rate constants A, B, α_1, and α_2 respectively,

$$T = \frac{A/\alpha_1^2 + B/\alpha_2^2}{A/\alpha_1 + B/\alpha_2}. \qquad (13.3)$$

[†]Although a tracer like iodine-125 albumin is also lost from the plasma compartment, the principle of volume measurement, based on the dilution estimated from extrapolation of a falling time–concentration curve, is valid for plasma volume measurement because the mixing time within the compartment is virtually instantaneous relative to the rate of loss from the compartment.

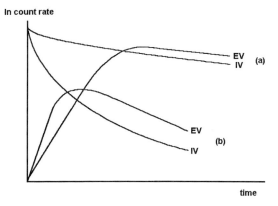

In count rate

EV
IV   (a)

EV
(b)
IV

time

▮ **Fig. 13.2** Relationship between intravascular and extravascular concentrations of solutes which exchange freely between plasma and interstitial fluid but are excluded from the intracellular space. The extravascular concentration rises and, if not protein bound in plasma, eventually exceeds the intravascular concentration. In the absence of protein binding in either space, the concentration difference between the two spaces is positively related to the plasma clearance of the tracer. If the tracer is not cleared at all, then the concentrations equalize.

In order to obtain A and α_1, as well as B and α_2 multiple samples must be taken, and from these an accurate measurement of plasma clearance Z can then also be made from the following equation (Section 11.14).

$$Z = \frac{M(0)}{A/\alpha_1 + B/\alpha_2} \qquad (13.4)$$

where ECF volume is then given by $V_{ECF} = T \cdot Z$.

Recalling that $C(0)$ in equation 13.1 is the same as B in equation 13.3, the overestimation made in ECF volume using equation 13.1 can be evaluated from equations 13.1, 13.3 and 13.4.

A third approach for measurement of ECF volume is based on the concept that the turnover of the ECF volume by GFR is equal to the terminal rate constant α_2; i.e.

$$V_{ECF} = GFR/\alpha_2. \qquad (13.5)$$

This assumes that the concentration of tracer is the same in the extravascular and intravascular spaces. However the extravascular concentration exceeds intravascular concentration (**Fig. 13.2**). This must be true otherwise the extravascular compartment would never be cleared of tracer. In order to accommodate

its tracer content at the same concentration as in the intravascular space, the extravascular volume would have to be larger than it is, so equation 13.5 overestimates ECF volume. The overestimation resulting from equation 13.1 is however larger. As in equating α_2 to GFR/V_{ECF}, the overestimations in ECF volume by equations 13.1 and 13.5 become less with decreasing GFR.

A fourth approach, analogous to the measurement of the sodium space (equation 13.17) is to divide the plasma concentration at any time following equilibration into the amount of filtration marker left in the body at this time. The latter amount is equal to the injected amount minus the amount in pooled urine collected up to the time of measurement. This again overestimates ECF volume because of the concentration gradient across the endothelium but only one plasma sample, and no clearance measurement, are required.

So far in this discussion only filtration markers like DTPA, EDTA, iothalamate and inulin have been considered for the measurement of ECF volume. Other, smaller molecular weight tracers have also been used, including bromium-77 and chlorine-36. These give larger ECF volumes than EDTA, inulin and DTPA, or more precisely, have larger distribution volumes. In fact, with these tracers, there is some intracellular uptake. In any event, the approximate inverse relationship between molecular size and the distribution volume emphasizes the fact that ECF is a functional rather than an anatomical space, with a volume that is partly dependent on the tracer used to measure it. As a result of tubular reabsorption, these smaller tracers have a much lower renal clearance than the filtration markers and so can be more accurately used in conjunction with equation 13.1.

13.1.1.2 Distribution of tracers between plasma and interstitial fluid

It is important to appreciate the existence of a concentration difference between the intravascular and extravascular spaces for these filtered tracers. The faster the plasma clearance, the greater the concentration difference. Indeed, by knowing the clearance, it is possible to calculate the extravascular to intravascular tracer concentration ratio (C_e/C_i) that exists once equilibration is established. Equilibrium is defined here as equality of rate constants of tracer disappearance. Thus, the extravascular concentration C_e is the total amount M_e of tracer in the extravascular space divided by extravascular volume. The quantity M_e is what remains of the injected dose $M(0)$ when the total amount cleared from plasma up to time t, and the amount, M_i, remaining in plasma are subtracted (Ladegaard-Pedersen 1972, Peters *et al.* 1994). That is

$$M_e = M(0) - M_i - Z \cdot \int_0^t C_i(t) \cdot dt. \qquad (13.6)$$

As shown in equation 13.6, the total amount of tracer cleared from plasma is given by the product of the integral of the plasma concentration curve up to time (t) and the clearance.

Since

$$M_e = C_e \cdot V_e \quad \text{and} \quad M_i = C_i \cdot V_i \qquad (13.7)$$

where V_i and V_e are the plasma and interstitial fluid (i.e. extravascular) volumes, respectively

$$C_e = \frac{M(0) - C_i \cdot V_i - Z \int_0^t C_i(t) \cdot dt}{V_e}. \qquad (13.8)$$

Dividing by C_i, followed by re-arrangement,

$$\frac{C_e}{C_i} = \frac{M(0) - Z \int_0^t C_i(t) \cdot dt}{C_i \cdot V_e} - \frac{V_i}{V_e}. \qquad (13.9)$$

Separating the total area under the plasma curve into (i) area up to time t and (ii) area after time t,

$$M(0) = Z \int_0^t C_i(t) \cdot dt + Z \int_t^\infty C_i(t) \cdot dt$$

so

$$M(0) - Z \int_0^t C_i(t) \cdot dt = Z \int_t^\infty C_i(t) \cdot dt$$

and after re-arrangement,

$$\frac{C_e}{C_i} = Z \frac{\int_t^\infty C_i(t) \cdot dt}{C_i \cdot V_e} - \frac{V_i}{V_e} \qquad (13.10)$$

where $\int_t^\infty C_i(t) \cdot dt$ is the area under the clearance curve *from* time t.

The area under a mono-exponential curve from any time t is the ratio of the y-axis value at t to the rate constant. For a bi-exponential curve,

$$C_i(t) = A \cdot e^{-\alpha_1 t} + B \cdot e^{-\alpha_2 t} \qquad (13.11)$$

so

$$\int_t^\infty C_i(t) \cdot dt = \frac{A \cdot e^{-\alpha_1 t}}{\alpha_1} + \frac{B \cdot e^{-\alpha_2 t}}{\alpha_2}. \qquad (13.12)$$

Equation 13.10 can be further simplified for equilibration of the tracer throughout its distribution volume when the area between t and infinity is given by $C_i(t)/\alpha_2$:

$$\frac{C_e(\text{equil})}{C_i(\text{equil})} = \frac{Z}{V_e \cdot \alpha_2} - \frac{V_i}{V_e}. \qquad (13.13)$$

The ratio C_e/C_i may be obtained by measuring plasma volume and V_e (or basing them on height and weight) and measuring Z from A, B, α_1 and α_2. Because of its heavy protein binding in plasma, MAG3, is thought not to enter the extravascular space to any significant extent. However, using equation 13.13, it can be seen that C_e/C_i normally becomes 0.75 at 1 hour after injection of MAG3 (Peters *et al.* 1994). As renal function deteriorates, this ratio drops sharply. DTPA on the other hand gives C_e/C_i ratios which, as one would expect from the absence of protein binding, are always greater than 1, approaching 1 as GFR approaches 0.

The time at which the extravascular concentration is maximal is given by $[\ln(\alpha_1/\alpha_2)]/(\alpha_2 - \alpha_2)$ as shown in Section 9.4.1.1 for the similar model describing the maximal intrahepatic concentration of IDA. The time at which the intravascular and extravascular concentrations of a filtration marker instantaneously equalise can be calculated from equation 13.10. Thus at this time $C_e/C_i = 1$

so

$$Z \frac{\int_t^\infty C_i(t) \cdot dt}{C_i \cdot V_e} = \frac{V_i}{V_e} + 1. \qquad (13.14)$$

By rearrangement

$$\frac{\int_t^\infty C_i(t) \cdot dt}{C_i} = \frac{V_i + V_e}{Z} = T. \qquad (13.15)$$

Substituting for $\int_t^\infty C_i(t) \cdot dt$ and C_i, in equation 13.15

$$\frac{\dfrac{A \cdot e^{-\alpha_1 t}}{\alpha_1} + \dfrac{B \cdot e^{-\alpha_2 t}}{\alpha_2}}{A \cdot e^{-\alpha_1 t} + B \cdot e^{-\alpha_2 t}} = T. \qquad (13.16)$$

It can be demonstrated graphically (see Question 14, Chapter 14) that the time at which $C_e = C_i$ is the time at which the left hand side of equation 13.16 is equal to T and also the time at which C_e is maximal. This intuitively makes sense since the time at which C_e is maximal corresponds to momentary steady state. At steady state, C_e must be equal to C_i.

On the basis of kinetic studies with filtration markers, the extravascular component of the ECF volume itself appears to consist of two volumes. It was pointed out in Section 6.2.2.4.4 that the plasma clearance of a filtration marker such as DTPA is in fact composed of three exponentials rather than two (Neilson 1985). Indeed, the first is the largest in terms of its zero-time intercept. However is not easily identified in plasma clearance curves based on antecubital venous sampling because it is obscured by exchange of the marker across the microvasculature of the vascular bed drained by the antecubital vein. Ignoring this fast exponential makes little impact on GFR measurement because, as a result of its high rate constant, the area it encloses is small. It is however easily identified on arterial sampling which, combined with venous sampling, allows an estimation to be made of net tracer extraction fraction as a function of time after intravenous injection. Dual solute studies with inulin (MW 6000 Da) and technetium-99m DTPA (MW 492 Da) show that whereas the respective rate constants of the first exponentials obtained from arterial sampling in the resting forearm are similar, the extraction fraction from plasma to extravascular space is 0.5 for DTPA compared with 0.2 for inulin. Furthermore, the respective arterio–venous concentration gradients disappear (and then reverse) at the same time, about 20 minutes (Cousins *et al.* 1998). This can be most readily explained by different volumes of the compartments into which the tracers diffuse from plasma. Since the two markers have similar final (equilibrium) distribution volumes, the interstitial space seems to consist of two compartments, the first of which, adjacent to the plasma compartment, has a higher functional volume when measured with DTPA compared with inulin. The notion of a model of distribution consisting of three compartments in series (**Fig. 13.3**) is consistent with a tri-exponential plasma clearance curve.

It is recognized that the interstitial space comprises a phase within which small solutes and proteins are dispersed and a less accessible gel meshwork, made up of huge molecules, which can be penetrated by small solutes but only very slowly by proteins (Katz 1980). The intermediate exponential in the plasma clearance curve is likely to represent diffusion of DTPA into the gel meshwork (third space). Inulin, by diffusing first into a volume (the second space) which is functionally smaller than that of DTPA would give a first exponential in its plasma clearance curve with a rate constant as fast as that of DTPA even though its diffusibility, on the basis of molecular weight, is only about half that of DTPA. This is consistent with the previous suggestion of a fast exponential even for albumin, so fast that it is 'hidden' in the phase of vascular dispersion following bolus injection. It has been suggested that the volume of the second space for albumin is 5–8% of plasma volume — about 200 ml (Bent-Hansen 1991). If whole body albumin clearance was typically about 70 ml/min total (corresponding to a unidirectional extraction fraction from plasma to interstitial fluid of 0.02) then, for a plasma volume of 3 liters, the rate constant of the first exponential for albumin would be [70/3000] + [70/200], or 0.37 min^{-1}, which, in turn, corresponds to 95% equilibration between first and second spaces in less

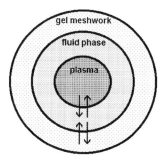

▮ **Fig. 13.3** Compartmental model representing the distribution of the ECF. The total volume is about 13 litres of which 3 litres is plasma. The volumes of the two extravascular compartments are 'functional volumes' and seem to depend on the size of the molecule used to measure them. With technetium-99m DTPA (MW 492) the fluid phase has a volume of about 5 litres. The gel meshwork is a space in which very large molecules (complex proteins with molecular weights exceeding one million) are crowded together and which solutes penetrate more slowly. The volume of the fluid phase measured with albumin (MW 66 000) is about 200 ml and with inulin (MW 6000) about 2 litres.

than 10 min.[†] So it could be speculated that if the volume of the second space is directly proportional to the size of the molecule used to measure it, then the rate constant of the exponential reflecting equilibration between plasma and second space may be relatively constant and rather independent of molecular size. The relative *amplitude* of the first exponential will be different from molecule to molecule and will vary inversely with the amplitude of the second exponential, which reflects penetration into the third space.

DTPA and inulin ultimately distribute throughout a similar volume. The similarity in times at which inulin and DTPA achieve complete dispersion throughout their respective distribution volumes may be the result of slower diffusion of technetium-99m DTPA within the remainder of the interstitial space, although it is not clear why this should be so for a smaller molecule. Perhaps the gel meshwork behaves like a sephadex column with relative hindrance of small molecules. This may facilitate diffusion of the larger inulin within the meshwork, thereby effectively increasing the rate constant of transfer of inulin from the third space back into the second space, and allowing it to 'keep up' with DTPA with respect to rate of final equilibration.

13.1.2 Total body water and intracellular fluid volumes

The tracers used for measuring total body water include tritiated water, radio-iodinated antipyrine, urea and ethanol, all of which distribute rapidly throughout total body water. The rapid distributions of antipyrine, urea and ethanol are to be expected from their lipophilicity and ability to cross cell membranes. As will be recalled from Sections 3.1.3.1 and 6.2.1.2, water also takes a predominantly transcellular route when equilibrating throughout its distribution volume, and this is the basis of measuring organ perfusion with oxygen-15 labelled water.

As a result of its high diffusibility, water equilibrates rapidly so when measuring the dilution factor for labelled water, the amount lost from its distribution volume from fluid loss between injection and sampling can be ignored, because as long as there is no fluid intake, the specific activity of tritium in blood samples remains constant. With the other three indicators however there are appreciable losses, e.g. ethanol into the liver, and it is necessary to take several plasma samples over several hours following injection and extrapolate the plasma disappearance curve to zero time. However, as equilibration is still relatively rapid, extrapolation does not introduce as great an error as in the measurement of ECF volume with filtration markers. Ethanol is cleared from blood in a linear fashion at a rate of 0.15 g/l/hr.

A difference between total body water and ECF volume or plasma volume is that in the case of the former it is water volume specicifcally that is measured in contrast to a fluid volume. So when measuring total body water by dilution it is necessary to take into account the water content of blood or plasma, depending which is sampled. The fractional water content of blood is 0.84 ml/ml and of plasma 0.95 ml/ml. So if the indicator concentration in blood, extrapolated to zero time, was x mg/ml following injection of y mg, then the total body water volume would be $(y/x) \times 0.84$. Another consideration for indicators other than water is partition between lipid and water; red cell membranes represent a significant lipid 'sink' in blood. Total body water in standard man decreases with age from a value of 60% of body weight in young men aged 20–30 to 50% of body weight in men over 60.

13.2 Electrolytes

13.2.1 The sodium space and exchangeable sodium

About one third of the total body sodium is present in the skeleton in a relatively non-exchangeable form. The remainder, present principally in the extracellular fluid, is much more rapidly exchangeable. The sodium space is the apparent volume of distribution within this exchangeable space, while

[†]According to the fibre matrix theory, the interendothelial junction gaps, through which solute diffusion takes place, have a high albumin concentration which promotes the permselective properties of the endothelium, rather like a plughole blocked with debris.
The matrix, rich in glycoproteins, is called the endothelial glycocalyx, and, by binding albumin, may effectively represent the volume of ~200 ml into which albumin apparently enters rapidly (Vink and Duling 1997).

the total exchangeable sodium is the quantity of sodium present in this space. Both can be measured with radio-sodium; sodium-22 (half-life 2.6 years) or sodium-24 (half-life 15 hours). Two methods are available, both based on the dilution principle.

Any technique based on the dilution principle requires a period of equilibration between tracer injection and the sampling time, during which the tracer mixes throughout its distribution volume. For sodium this is 24 hours. During this period, tracer is continuously being lost from the body, and this has to be subtracted from the administered dose before measuring the dilution factor. Traditionally, for radio-sodium studies, the amount lost is determined from a pooled 24-hour urine sample, plus a 24-hour faecal sample if the patient is losing sodium via the faeces, as in diarrhoea.

The apparent volume of distribution of sodium-24 at 24 hours, the sodium space, is then

$$V = \frac{\text{injected activity} - \text{pooled lost activity}}{\text{sodium-24 plasma concentration (24 hours)}}.$$

$$(13.17)$$

The exchangeable sodium is the product of V, the apparent volume of distribution and the native sodium concentration within it. Alternatively, using the γ-emitting sodium isotope, sodium-22, whole body counting can be employed to measure the amount of radio-sodium lost from the body. In this case, the amount lost is calculated as a fraction F of the injected activity by comparing the whole body count rate at any time after 24 hours with that recorded at about 2 hours after oral or immediately after intravenous administration of the tracer. This is analogous to the measurement by whole body counting of calcium absorption or whole body indium-111 labelled granulocyte loss. Then

$$V = \frac{\text{injected activity} - F \cdot \text{injected activity } (t)}{\text{sodium-22 plasma concentration } (t)}$$

$$(13.18)$$

where t is greater than 24 hours.

Exchangeable sodium (but not the sodium space) can be determined from a random urine sample by measuring the concentrations of urinary radio-sodium and native sodium (ie, the specific activity). Although V now has no real meaning, exchangeable sodium is obtained by substituting urinary concentration for plasma concentration in equations 13.17

and 13.18 and measuring specific activity (SA) in the urine. Exchangeable sodium, which is the product of SA and whole body activity and has units of meq, can be measured daily by this whole body technique for several weeks, the amount in the body being determined from whole body counting. It slowly rises as the radio-sodium gradually exchanges with native sodium in the more slowly exchanging skeletal space.

The sodium space is about 20 litres. This is appreciably higher than the ECF volume, as would be expected as a result of entry of radio-sodium into the intracellular compartment. Radio-sodium can be used for measuring ECF volume, but it is clear that for a more accurate estimate of the ECF volume, the extent of dilution needs to be measured before complete equilibration within the exchangeable pool. This can be based on the zero time value determined by extrapolation, but this tends to underestimate ECF volume (Veall and Vetter 1958). The same is true, although less so, for radio-bromine as a tracer for ECF volume. There are fewer losses by excretion of radio-bromine than is the case with sodium and the apparent volume of distribution does not change significantly for several hours after equilibration, which itself takes between 4 and 6 hours.

13.2.2 The potassium space and exchangeable potassium

Dilution techniques for measuring exchangeable potassium are essentially the same as for exchangeable sodium. The volume of distribution is a rather meaningless variable when applied to potassium because of its overwhelming predominance in the intracellular compartment. Apparent volumes of distribution are based on concentrations in plasma; i.e. the volume of distribution is expressed in terms of the volume occupied by the tracer if it were at the same concentration in this volume as it is in plasma. The potassium 'space' in contrast to that of sodium is therefore enormous. Total exchangeable potassium (meq/kg) is a useful variable since, due to the distribution of potassium, plasma concentrations of the electrolyte give a poor reflection of the total whole body potassium. Also, and in contrast to sodium, nearly all the body's potassium is in the rapidly exchanging pool, which equilibrates in about

20 hours compared with about 12 hours for rapidly exchanging sodium. More slowly exchanging pools (which equilibrate by about 60 hours) exist in red cells and in the brain. The timing for potassium equilibration is relevant to the use of potassium analogues, such as thallium-201, for cardiac imaging, wherein the distribution of tracer immediately after injection reflects blood flow, while the distribution after equilibration (three hours is usually allowed for in cardiac imaging) reflects the distribution of the potassium space. Nevertheless, the need for longer equilibration times for thallium-201, in the search for hibernating myocardium, is now well recognized and easy to appreciate from a knowledge of potassium kinetics.

13.2.3 Calcium turnover and gastro–intestinal calcium absorption

Approximately 99% of total body calcium, or 1 kg, is present in the skeleton, less than 1% of which is readily exchangeable with calcium in the ECF. In an average daily diet containing about 1 g of calcium, 300 mg is absorbed, although net gastrointestinal absorption is less than this as a result of faecal loss of calcium from intestinal secretions. This amounts to about 125 mg per day; the net calcium absorption of 175 mg per day is balanced by urinary losses. The extracellular calcium pool is about 1 g of which half exchanges with skeletal calcium per day. After intravenous injection, radiocalcium mixes throughout the extracellular calcium pool, the plasma level initially falling rapidly, then decreasing more slowly and reaching a terminal rate constant of about 0.1 day^{-1} at about 24 hr after injection.

The traditional method for measuring gastrointestinal calcium absorption is the dual calcium isotope technique. Calcium-45 is given by mouth and calcium-47 by intravenous injection (or vice versa) (Heaney and Recker 1985). The intravenous dose is given two hours after the oral dose, a time which is assumed to be the mid point of the period of the absorption of the oral dose. At the completion of absorption, the two isotopes are handled *in vivo* identically so that the ratio of their respective concentrations in body fluids (plasma or urine), expressed in relation to the corresponding injected activities, is not only constant with the passage of

time but also equal to the fraction F of the orally administered activity absorbed: i.e.

$$\frac{C_{\text{oral}}}{C_{\text{IV}}} = \frac{F \times \text{activity}_{\text{oral}}}{\text{activity}_{\text{IV}}} \qquad (13.19)$$

where C refers to calcium isotope concentration in urine or blood. A potential source of error is the timing of the two doses. Thus an individual with slow absorption would show, for the same value of F, a different plasma ratio compared with a fast absorber. It is important to administer the oral dose as part of a meal, since absorption of calcium may be different when the tracer is given on an empty stomach. If the concentration ratio is measured prior to 'equilibration' (i.e. the time at which the oral tracer 'catches up' with the intravenous tracer), then it will be underestimated. A simpler approach is to measure the specific activity of radio-calcium (usually calcium-45) in plasma at a specified time after a meal. It has been shown empirically that the time point which gives a fractional absorption value correlating best with the dual isotope method is 5 hours after the meal.

Another approach, which uses a single intravenous dose of radio-calcium, is to measure faecal native calcium under conditions of a stable oral calcium intake (Corey *et al.* 1964, Heaney and Recker 1985). A proportion of faecal calcium originates from the endogenous pool as a result of gastrointestinal secretions **(Fig. 13.4)**. The unabsorbed fraction ($1-F$ of the oral intake) is therefore

$$1 - F = \frac{\text{total faecal calcium} - \text{endogenous faecal calcium}}{\text{calcium intake}} \qquad (13.20)$$

with units of

$$\frac{\text{mg/day} - \text{mg/day}}{\text{mg/day}}.$$

Endogenous faecal calcium is measured from plasma and faecal counting following an intravenous dose of radiocalcium using an approach similar in principle to measurement of urinary tracer clearance (Section 2.2.1.4). Thus the radiocalcium 'cleared' into the faeces up to time t after intravenous injection of radiocalcium is given by

$$\frac{dM'_{\text{F}}}{dt} = \alpha \cdot C'_{\text{p}} \qquad (13.21)$$

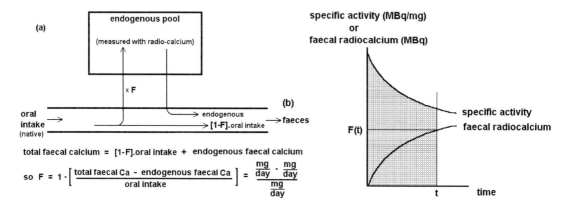

▮ **Fig. 13.4** Measurement of gastrointestinal calcium absorption by a combination of faecal native calcium estimation and an intravenous injection of radioactive calcium. (a) F is the fraction of ingested calcium that is absorbed (unitless). (b) Faecal calcium from the endogenous calcium pool can be measured from an intravenous injection of radiocalcium followed by sequential measurement of plasma radiocalcium and native calcium (to give specific activity) and the radiocalcium accumulating in the faeces, an approach analogous to the measurement of urinary clearance of a substance. Thus, endogenous faecal calcium (mg/day) is equal to accumulated faecal radiocalcium (MBq) up to time t divided by the area under the specific activity–time curve (MBq·mg^{-1}.days) up to time t.

where C'_p is plasma radiocalcium concentration and α is a constant of proportionality. A similar equation can be written for native calcium:

$$\frac{dM_F}{dt} = \alpha \cdot C_P. \tag{13.22}$$

Dividing equation 13.21 by 13.22 followed by rearrangement

$$\frac{dM'_F/dt}{dM_F/dt} = \frac{C'_p}{C_p} \tag{13.23}$$

where C'_p/C_p is the specific activity, spA, of radiocalcium with units of MBq/mg. dM_F/dt is the rate of excretion of endogenous native calcium and under stable dietary conditions is a constant. So integrating equation 13.23 followed by rearrangement

$$dM_F/dt = \frac{M'_F}{\int spA(t) \cdot dt} \tag{13.24}$$

with units

$$\frac{mg}{day} = \frac{MBq}{(MBq/mg) \cdot day}.$$

The value dM_F/dt can then be inserted into equation 13.20. The specific activity is the same in plasma and body fluids, so it may be measured in urine or even saliva instead of plasma. The longer faeces are collected the less the uncertainty in the correction for

the time lag between arrival of radiocalcium in the gut and collection in the faeces. Although cumbersome and technically demanding, the method using equation 13.20 is the gold standard for gastrointestinal calcium absorption.

A further approach is to use the whole-body counter, in a way analogous to its use for measuring iron absorption or bile acid loss (using SeHCAT) (Shipp *et al.* 1987). A confounding factor is the loss of secreted radio-calcium into the gut and consequently the technique is only of value for studying interventions when the patient is his/her own control. Endogenous gastrointestinal radio-calcium can however be accounted for if two sequential whole body studies are done. Thus an intravenous dose of radiocalcium is given about 5 days after an oral dose when it can be assumed that non-absorbed oral radio-calcium had been lost in the faeces. Sequential whole body counting is repeated after an interval of time equal to the interval between the oral dose and the first whole body count. The intravenous dose defines the fraction of absorbed radio calcium lost from the endogenous pool.

Then

$$F = \frac{WB \; count_1 \; (5 \; days)}{WB \; count_1 \; (0)} \times \frac{WB \; count_2 \; (0)}{WB \; count_2 \; (5 \; days)}. \tag{13.25}$$

Note that WB count$_2$(0) does not have to be corrected for the counts resulting from the preceding oral dose since by 5 days counts due to the oral dose will have been absorbed and included in the injected counts recorded as WB count$_2$(0).

13.3 Bone

In spite of all the calcium it contains, its rigidity and the impression it gives of being generally inert, bone is metabolically active and has a relatively substantial blood flow and metabolic turnover. The skeleton itself weighs about 10 kg in standard man and contains 99% of the whole body calcium. Bone is composed of mineralized organic matrix, of which about 30% is organic matrix (osteoid), and 70% is a mineral phase consisting mainly of a crystalline salt of calcium and phosphate called hydroxyapatite. It is the latter to which the bone-seeking agents technetium-99m methylene diphosphonate (MDP) and fluorine-18 fluoride ion bind extracellularly for the purpose of imaging bone. The rate of bone turnover determines the amount of the salt available for binding these radiopharmaceuticals.

13.3.1 Skeletal haemodynamics

Skeletal blood flow stretches the imagination. It varies from bone to bone, from region to region in the same bone and is approximately three times higher in trabecular bone compared with cortical bone. The vascular arrangements are different between long bones and flat bones and in the different segments of long bones. Estimates of bone blood flow vary widely but typical values are 10–15 ml/min/100 ml for trabecular bone in the spine and 5 ml/min/100 ml for cortical bone. Values for bone marrow flow measured in experimental animals are much higher than those for bone blood flow, possibly because of an almost exclusive use of labelled microspheres which would lodge first in bone marrow sinusoids, before arrival in bone capillaries, as a result of the vascular arrangement in long bones (see below). However, in man, in whom microspheres have not been used, recorded values for marrow are only modestly higher than those for bone. Conversely, this may be a distortion related to the difficulty of separating bone marrow

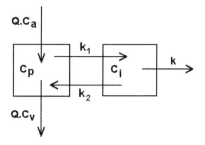

Q = blood flow
C_a = arterial concentration
C_v = venous concentration
C_p = capillary concentration
C_i = bone fluid concentration
k_1, k_2, k = transport constants (PS product)

∎ **Fig. 13.5** Model describing skeletal kinetics of technetium-99m MDP. This model is similar to the model (Fig. 13.7) for skeletal fluorine-18 uptake, except the concentrations are given as compartmental concentrations and the transfer constants are therefore *PS* products. Since the *PS* products governing transfer across bone capillaries have been measured experimentally, it is possible to examine bone blood flow and capillary permeability as determinants of skeletal technetium-99m MDP clearance.

from bone in human blood flow measurements. One way to separate them would be to use radio-pharmaceuticals which are exclusively bone or bone marrow-seeking; however bone-seeking tracers have extraction fractions that are difficult to define and there are no adequate bone marrow-seeking tracers. PET, on the other hand, while good for measuring regional perfusion, records tracer concentration within the whole region, including bone and bone marrow. This is analogous to quantitative contrast CT, which records tissue attenuation per unit volume of whole tissue or tracer concentration within a region, irrespective of precisely where the contrast medium or tracer is located in that region.

In long bones, blood vessels supplying the cortex arise mainly from within the marrow, wherein the control of bone blood flow is predominantly located. Consequently, increased marrow flow, such as occurs in myeloproliferative conditions, tends to be accompanied by increased cortical flow and increased bone tracer clearance, even in bones with pre-existing red (active) marrow. Venous return is via the periosteum, so bone blood flow tends to be centrifugal, i.e. moves from centre to periphery. On the other hand, at sites of muscle attachment, muscle arterioles enter bone to supply the cortex via the periosteum. The arrangement of bone blood flow changes with age; cortical flow itself declines with ageing, partly as a result of arteriosclerosis which involves arteries in marrow perhaps 10 years earlier than those supplying myocardium and brain. This results in an increasing proportion of cortical blood flow arriving via periosteal vessels. Venous drainage remains periosteal. This arrangement is reminiscent of the vascular supply of the liver in which a minor proportion is arterial and the majority via a portal venous system.

Like skeletal muscle and skin, bone capillaries possess continuous endothelium and the transport of small solutes between plasma and bone interstitial fluid is governed by similar transport constants. Bone marrow capillaries, in contrast, are fenestrated and have very high permeability. The *PS* product of bone capillaries for MDP is similar to that for EDTA in skin and muscle (McCarthy and Hughes 1989). In bone, bone crystal adds an additional compartment, into which the movement of MDP, and especially fluoride ion, is essentially unidirectional. These kinetics can be summarised in the model shown in Fig. 13.5. The bone transport constant k reflects bone metabolic activity and the surface area available for tracer uptake. Taking a *PS* product for MDP of 4 ml/min/100 ml, the determinants of skeletal MDP clearance and the distribution of uptake on a bone scan can be evaluated from this model (Peters 1993). Thus firstly clearance is minimally influenced by bone blood flow, especially at low levels of flow; secondly clearance is minimally influenced by bone capillary permeability, except at high levels of bone transport constant (k) and high blood flows; and thirdly clearance is influenced by the bone transport constant, especially at high levels of bone capillary permeability.

By exclusion of major tissues and organs for which blood flow in terms of fraction of cardiac output are reasonably well established, blood flow to the total human skeleton, including bone marrow, would not be expected to be higher than 10% of cardiac output. For a skeleton weighing 10 kg and a cardiac output of 5000 ml/min, 10% corresponds to a mean bone perfusion of 5 ml/100 g/min. Techniques for measuring bone blood flow are similar to those used in other organs.

13.3.1.1 Radiolabelled microspheres

Radiolabelled microspheres have been used extensively in the experimental animal but not in man. By measuring radioactivity in arterial samples encompassing microsphere injection and subsequent capillary impaction and in samples obtained either from marrow or bone, perfusion can be measured in ml/min/100 g tissue. The interpretation of the values obtained in long bones seems to be somewhat confounded by the portal arrangement which would be expected to result in fewer microspheres reaching cortical capillaries than expected from cortical blood flow.

13.3.1.2 Inert gas clearance

There are no descriptions in man of measurement of bone blood flow from intra-arterial injection of inert gas. Intravenous administration followed by counting over the greater trochanter yielded a bi-exponential clearance which was interpreted to reflect different perfusions in bone marrow and bone (Lahtinen *et al.* 1981). As a result of uncertainty relating to recirculation, the value obtained of 7.4 ml/min/100 g is likely to be an underestimation. Moreover, the volume of distribution achieved by xenon as a fraction of total bone volume and the partition coefficient of xenon between blood and heterogeneous skeletal tissues are also uncertain.

13.3.1.3 Plasma clearance

Bone displays a high extraction of fluoride ion, the clearance of which from plasma therefore provides a technique for measuring blood flow to the whole skeleton. Fluoride however also simultaneously enters the extracellular fluid space and undergoes renal clearance, the magnitude of which needs to be controlled by a second marker, specifically a filtration marker. One such method is based on chromium-51 EDTA (Wootton *et al.* 1976) and assumes a steady-state bone fluoride extraction efficiency of 100%. It gives skeletal blood flow in units of percent of total blood volume per minute, and a normal value of about 5%. This is approximately doubled in osteomalacia and Paget's disease but, surprisingly, normal in hyperparathyroidism.

The technique is based on deconvolution analysis applied to both fluoride and EDTA. Plasma radioactivity is used as the input function, while the output curve is the amount of tracer (M_e) in the

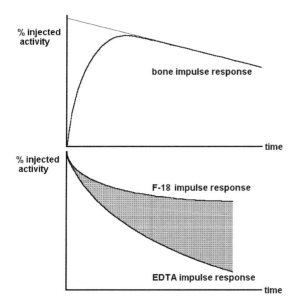

❚ **Fig. 13.6** Principle of measurement of global skeletal blood flow from plasma fluorine-18 clearance. Fluorine-18 enters interstitial fluid generally and undergoes renal clearance as well as skeletal uptake. Extraskeletal kinetics can be accounted for with a simultaneous injection of chromium-51 EDTA which does not undergo skeletal uptake but otherwise has similar kinetics to fluorine-18. The difference between the impulse response functions of the 2 tracers with respect to blood (lower panel) represents the impulse response function of fluorine-18 in bone (upper panel). Since the *y*-axis units are percent of administered dose, the units of skeletal blood flow are percent of total blood volume per min. The technique assumes that the extraction efficiency of fluorine-18 in bone is 100%. The slowly declining phase of the bone impulse response function reflects the slow rate of loss of fluorine-18 from bone (along the pathway k_4 in Fig. 13.7).

extravascular space, derived by subtracting the time-dependent amount of activity in plasma (M_i) and cumulative urinary excretion (M_u) from the injected dose (M_0) (analogous to the measurement of intravascular to extravascular concentration ratio for a diffusible solute — see Section 13.1.1.2); i.e.

$$M_e = M_0 - (M_i + M_u). \tag{13.26}$$

Whereas M_u for EDTA can be calculated as the product of GFR (measured with EDTA) and the integral of the plasma curve ($\int C_i(t) \cdot dt$), M_u for fluoride has to be obtained directly from urine collection because renal fluoride clearance is not equal to GFR. (However, by comparing urinary concentra-

tions and plasma concentrations of the two tracers, urine collection need not be complete.) Having obtained M_e deconvolution analysis is used to generate impulse retention curves for both tracers. The difference between the two retention functions yields the retention function of fluoride in bone (**Fig. 13.6**). Since this is the curve that represents instantaneous deposition of tracer into and retained by the skeleton and since the units of M_e are expressed as percentage of injected dose, the *y*-axis intercept of the bone retention function is the percentage of injected dose retained in bone. Bone blood flow is therefore expressed as the percentage of blood volume per min and refers to the whole skeleton.

The validity of the technique relies on the assumption that bone fluoride extraction efficiency is 100%. Although this may hold for cortical bone, where perfusion is low, it is unlikely to hold for regions of bone with much higher flow. It has been shown for example in canine long bone that whereas the steady-state extraction fraction of radiostrontium is 0.7 at 5 ml/min/100 g, it is only about 0.4 at 15 ml/min/100 g (corresponding to a *PS* product of about 7 ml/min/100 g). If overall extraction was significantly less than unity, blood flow would be underestimated. Since the normal value given by the technique is only about 250 ml/min, this seems to be the case. Furthermore, since EDTA enters bone interstitial fluid, the difference between the impulse response curves for EDTA and fluoride reflects steady-state fluoride extraction, in contrast to uni-directional extraction fraction from plasma to bone interstitial fluid, which for measurement of bone blood flow by positron emission tomography (PET) based on fluorine-18 is assumed to be unity (see below). Another uncomfortable assumption made in the plasma fluoride clearance technique, incompatible with a 100% fluoride bone extraction efficiency, is that the extravascular clearance kinetics of fluoride and EDTA are identical, even though their molecular sizes are different.

13.3.1.4 Regional bone tracer uptake measured by PET

Measurement of regional skeletal perfusion by PET has been based on quantification of tracer uptake using fluorine-18 as the fluoride ion (Nahmias *et al.* 1986, Hawkins *et al.* 1992) or oxygen-15 labelled water, given either as a continuous infusion (Martiat *et al.* 1987) or bolus injection (Ashcroft *et al.* 1992). Because PET measures the concentration of tissue radioactivity, perfusion is obtained as ml/min/ml of tissue and includes all skeletal elements (including marrow in trabecular bone) in the sectional region of interest. (Conversion to ml/min/g requires division by a factor for bone density, about 1.4, which can be determined from bone densitometry.) So although fluorine-18 is cleared by mineralized elements, perfusion is expressed as flow per unit volume of *global* skeletal tissue. On the other hand, although the distribution volume of oxygen-15 labelled water includes the unmineralised constituents of bone, such as the interstitial fluid, bone blood flow based on oxygen-15 is weighted towards marrow blood flow. When this tracer is used specifically to measure marrow blood flow by continuous inhalation of oxygen-15-labelled carbon dioxide and PET, a correction can be applied to account for the volume within the ROI occupied by bone (Martiat *et al.* 1987). In normal subjects, this technique gives a value of 10 ml/min/100 ml in posterior iliac crest, rising to between 25 and 35 ml/min/100 ml in patients with myeloproliferative disorders.

The kinetics of fluorine-18 may be based on a three-compartmental model consisting of bone plasma, bone interstitial fluid and bone crystal **(Fig. 13.7)** as described in Section 3.1.3.4 for myocardial FDG uptake or, considering plasma and interstitial fluid as one well-mixed compartment, on a two-compartmental model as for rubidium-82 in the myocardium (Section 3.1.3.2). Although the molecular size of fluoride is smaller than rubidium, consistent with even more rapid diffusion between plasma and interstitial fluid, PET data acquired from the lumbar spine appears to fit a three- better than a two-compartmental model (Hawkins *et al.* 1992). The transport constant, k_4 (three compartments) or k_2 (two compartments), representing back-diffusion from bone crystal to bone interstitial fluid, is considered to be zero in either model. Equating regional bone clearance to bone blood flow in a two-compartmental model requires that the steady state extraction efficiency of fluoride is 100%. On the other hand, equating k_1 (regional bone unidirectional fluoride clearance) to bone blood flow in the three-compartmental model depends on the assumption that an extraction efficiency of 100% exists for the

unidirectional transport of fluoride from plasma to bone interstitial fluid. Hawkins *et al.* obtained a value for k_1 of about 10 ml/min/100ml. Since fluoride ion exchanges very slowly with the hydroxyl ion of hydroxyapatite crystal, k_4 is negligible and so steady state fluoride clearance (K) into bone, which is equal to $[k_1 \cdot k_3]/[k_2 + k_3]$, can be measured from the slope of a Patlak–Rutland plot (Hawkins *et al.* 1992), similarly to the steady-state myocardial clearance of fluorine-18 FDG based on the same model.

Comparison of k_1 with K using PET gives an indication of the steady state fluoride extraction efficiency in bone. If they were similar, k_2 would be relatively low. Hawkins *et al.* (1992) however found k_2 to be substantial and K to be about 40% of k_1. Given the likely steady state PS product of fluoride in bone (~5 ml/min/100ml), this value of 0.4 implies that k_1 is close to bone perfusion (~10 ml/min/100 ml)[†] and that, in contrast, steady-state extraction fraction of fluoride is relatively low. In trabecular bone (lumbar vertebrae), which is relatively well perfused, a steady state extraction fraction of 0.4 is not unexpected and re-emphasizes that steady-state fluoride extraction fraction is likely to vary from one bone region to another. The parameter k_4 corresponds to a $t_{1/2}$ of bone fluoride release of about 5 hours, which is consistent with the rate of decline of the fluoride impulse response curve obtained from the technique based on deconvolution of extravascular fluoride described above.

Making comparison again with measurement of myocardial blood flow (Section 7.1.1.2), Nahmias *et al.* (1987) used the mass over area technique and assumed stable binding of fluoride to bone crystal. That is

$$\text{bone clearance } (Z) = \frac{\text{accumulated radioactivity}}{\text{area under plasma clearance curve}} \tag{13.27}$$

or, taking tissue volume into account

$$\frac{Z}{V} = \frac{C(t)}{\int C_a(t) \cdot dt}. \tag{13.28}$$

Assuming bone fluoride extraction fraction is unity,

$$Z/V = Q/V.$$

[†]Since $E = 1 - e^{-PS/Q}$

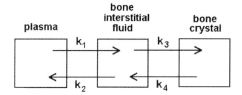

▌ Fig. 13.7 Model for fluorine-18 uptake in bone. In contrast to the model in figure 13.5, in which the transport constants are *PS* products, the transport constants in this model, with the exception of k_1 are fractional rate constants since PET measures the concentration in each compartment as if the tracer was dispersed throughout total regional bone volume. k_1 represents the clearance of fluorine-18 from plasma to bone interstitial fluid and is equal to bone blood flow if extraction fraction across this interface is unity (a less shaky assumption than the analogous assumption regarding *E* for fluorine-18 in Fig. 13.6).

13.3.2 Bone turnover

Skeletal turnover is synonymous with bone remodelling and is the result of the activity of microscopic bone remodelling units consisting of osteoclasts and osteoblasts. The osteoblast synthesizes osteoid and is the source of skeletal alkaline phosphatase, elevation of which in the blood is a marker of increased bone turnover. Osteoblasts possess receptors for parathyroid hormone and vitamin D, factors which are important in the control of bone turnover. Once encased in the bone which they have helped form, osteoblasts become metabolically inactive and are known as osteocytes. Bone resorption occurs concurrently with bone formation and is achieved through the action of osteoclasts. Although not possessing receptors for PTH or vitamin D, osteoclasts are nevertheless indirectly controlled by these hormones. Remodelling is not a haphazard process but instead the result, first, of a phase of new bone formation in which a row of osteblasts lay down an osteoid seam, followed by osteclast reabsorption on the opposite side of the bone trabecula. The newly formed osteoid is subsequently mineralized, and it is this recently mineralized osteoid that binds bone-seeking radiopharmaceuticals.

Bone turnover can be measured with any one of several bone-seeking radiotracers, including MDP, radiocalcium, radiostrontium or fluorine-18. A simple method is to measure the whole body retention of MDP with a whole body counter or uncollimated gamma camera 24 hr after intravenous injection, similarly to the measurement of whole body retention of indium-111 labelled granulocytes (Section 10.3.4) or selenium-75 labelled SeHCAT (Section 9.5.2). The count rate at 24 hr, at which time plasma MDP clearance is virtually complete, is corrected for physical decay of the isotope and compared with the count rate recorded 5 minutes after injection before any significant elimination of radioactivity from the body has taken place (Fogelman *et al.* 1978). Provided there is no urinary retention (as may occur in urological disease), normal subjects retain about 45% of the dose but this is elevated to levels as high as 90% in metabolic bone disease such as primary hyperparathyroidism and osteomalacia.

Whole body MDP retention is effectively a titration between skeletal MDP clearance and urinary MDP clearance. Skeletal MDP clearance is a specific, potentially more useful variable. Its measurement from whole body retention requires simultaneous measurement of renal clearance. Thus, assuming that renal MDP clearance is close to GFR, then

$$\frac{\text{WBR}}{1 - \text{WBR}} = \frac{Z_{\text{MDP}}(\text{skeleton})}{Z_{\text{EDTA}}} \tag{13.29}$$

where Z_{EDTA} is GFR measured separately with a filtration marker such as chromium-51 EDTA.

If whole-body retention is plotted as a function of time (Caniggia and Vattimo 1980), then a curve is obtained which exponentially approaches an asymptote (achieved at the completion of MDP clearance from plasma) with a rate constant α which is equal to the plasma MDP clearance per unit of its distribution volume (analogous to GFR/ECF volume). Although skeletal MDP clearance still requires a knowledge of GFR/ECF volume, both can be obtained at the same time with one tracer by regional probe counting without blood sampling (again, as in the measurement of GFR/ECF volume; Section 11.1.2.1).

Thus

$$\frac{Z_{\text{MDP}}(\text{skeleton})}{\text{ECF volume}} + \frac{Z_{\text{MDP}}(\text{urine})}{\text{ECF volume}} = \alpha \tag{13.30}$$

and

$$\frac{M_{\text{o}} - M_{\text{r}}}{M_{\text{r}}} = \frac{Z_{\text{MDP}}(\text{urine})/\text{ECF volume}}{Z_{\text{MDP}}(\text{skeleton})/\text{ECF volume}} \tag{13.31}$$

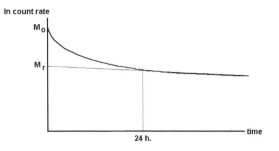

▌ Fig. 13.8 Principle of simultaneous measurement of urinary and skeletal technetium-99m-MDP clearance from a single intravenous bolus injection of technetium-99m MDP. The *y*-axis is whole body or regional count rate. At 24 hr, a fraction M_r of the initial count rate, M_0 is retained in the skeleton. The rate constant with which the curve approaches the asymptote M_r is equal to the sum of urinary and skeletal clearances (expressed as rates of turnover of ECF). M_r/M_0 based on whole body counting is the proportion of the sum which is skeletal clearance.

where M_o and M_r are the initial and asymptotic count rates, respectively **(Fig. 13.8)**, from which urinary and skeletal MDP clearance, per unit volume ECF, can be separately calculated.

An alternative approach is to co-inject MDP and chromium-51 EDTA and measure the plasma concentration ratio of the two tracers normalized for the injected doses (Nisbet *et al.* 1984). The ratio is essentially constant, about 1.4 (EDTA/MDP), up to about 6 hr after injection.

13.3.3 Bone mineral density

Measurement of bone mineral density (BMD) by dual X-ray absorptiometry has become widely practised for the assessment of patients at risk of fracture from osteoporosis. The principle of the measurement is to record the attenuation of a beam of x-ray photons by tissue, where attenuation differs for bone and soft tissue as a function of photon energy. The patient lies on a couch, underneath which a photon source is located. This is highly collimated to produce a narrow pencil beam which is counted by a detector placed above the patient on a gantry and in exact line with the pencil beam. The detection system is therefore highly efficient. The source and detector are mounted on a common gantry, which moves backwards and forwards across the patient, and gradually from head to toe, to eventually scan the whole body. The X-ray source produces photons in two discrete energy ranges

which, as the following demonstrates, enables the measurement of;

(a) the ratio of fat mass to water (or lean mass) in soft tissues;
(b) bone mineral density (in this context g/cm^2) in skeletal tissue;
(c) bone mineral content (in g).

13.3.3.1 Composition of soft tissue

First the machine determines the fat and water content in soft tissue along a path, one pixel in diameter, free of bone (the bone and non-bone pixel counts are separated by applying a threshold). If *D* is the total distance of the path and *d* the distance corresponding to the fat component then, imagining *d* to be represented by a length at the end of the path **(Fig. 13.9)**,

$$n = N_0.e^{-\mu_W \cdot (D-d)} \qquad (13.32)$$

where *n* is the count rate recorded at the imaginary interface between water and fat, and

$$\begin{aligned} N &= n.e^{-\mu_F \cdot d} & (13.33) \\ &= N_0 \cdot e^{-\mu_W \cdot (D-d)} \cdot e^{-\mu_F \cdot d} & (13.34) \\ &= N_0 \cdot e^{d(\mu_W - \mu_F) - D\mu_W} \end{aligned}$$

μ_W and μ_F are the linear attenuation coefficients for water and fat. Therefore

$$\ln(N/N_0) = d \cdot (\mu_W - \mu_F) - D\mu_W. \qquad (13.35)$$

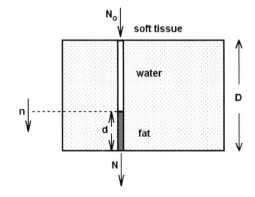

▌ Fig. 13.9 Principle of measurement of fat and water content and soft tissue (imagined, for convenience, to be discretely separated) from bone densitometry. N_0 is the incident photon flux and *N* the exiting flux. Water attenuates the signal to an imaginary value *n* through the distance *D* – *d*. Fat then further attenuates *n* to *N* through the distance *d*.

Equation 13.35 is formulated for both photon energies, low (L) and high (H), whereupon we have two equations, one for μ_{WH} and μ_{FH} and one for μ_{WL} and μ_{FL}. All four attenuation coefficients can be obtained from phantoms, i.e. are known, so the two unknowns, D and d, can be calculated. The depth of the tissue can therefore be measured for each pixel and the proportions of fat and water, which are d/D and $(D–d)/D$ (scaled for the density of fat) respectively, can be determined for each pixel.

13.3.3.2 Bone mineral density

The next stage in bone densitometry is similar and measures the bone attenuation coefficient, which depends on the amount of calcium present in it. In this operation, transmitted count rates are compared in two places, one where the path is composed only of soft tissue (subscript s; path 1) and one in which bone (subscript b) is present (path 2). Again equations can be developed for the transmitted count rates N_1 and N_2 corresponding to each photon energy range, using D to represent total tissue pixel-path length and d to represent bone pixel-path length:

$$N_1 = N_0 \cdot e^{-\mu_s \cdot D} \tag{13.36}$$
$$N_2 = N_0 \cdot e^{-\mu_s \cdot (D-d)} \cdot e^{-\mu_b \cdot d}. \tag{13.37}$$

This reduces to

$$N_1/N_2 = e^{d(\mu_b - \mu_s)} \tag{13.38}$$
$$\ln(N_1/N_2) = d(\mu_b - \mu_s) \tag{13.39}$$

and can be formulated for both photon energies, low (L) and high (H), so that

$$\frac{\ln(N_1/N_2)^H}{\ln(N_1/N_2)^L} = \frac{(\mu_b^H - \mu_s^H)}{(\mu_b^L - \mu_s^L)} \tag{13.40}$$

where μ_s^H and μ_s^L are known from the previous measurement of soft tissue attenuation over a non-osseous region, μ_s being based on the proportions of fat and water. The parameters D and d cancel and the value of μ_s indicates the bone mineral content, independent of the depth of the bone in the photon path. Bone mineral content in a region of interest is accordingly expressed as g per cm^2 of projected bone. The assumption has to be made that the proportions of water and fat in soft tissue are the same in paths 1 and 2; i.e. μ_s is the same for both positions.

From a whole body analysis, using standards with known fat to water ratios to calibrate the high and low energy attenuations, fat and water content of soft tissue and the mineral content of osseous tissue, total body water, fat/water ratio (i.e. adipose to lean body mass) and total and regional bone mineral content can be measured. DEXA scanning is becoming increasingly used to determine:

(1) lean body mass in patients with conditions such as muscular dystrophy;
(2) whether adipose tissue is predominantly central or peripheral (which is a prognostic factor for coronary heart disease);
(3) likelihood of fracture in patients at risk of osteoporosis;
(4) the condition of bone in the region of a prosthetic joint.

References

Bent-Hansen L. Whole body capillary exchange of albumin. *Acta Physiologica Scandinavica* 1991, **143** (Suppl 603): 5–10.

Caniggia A and Vattimo A. Kinetics of technetium-99m tin-methylene-diphosphonate in normal subjects and pathological conditions: a simple index of bone metabolism. *Calcific Tissue International* 1980, **30**: 5–13.

Corey KR, Weber D, Merlino M, Greenberg E, Kenny P and Laughlin JS. Calcium turnover in man. In: *Dynamic clinical studies with radioisotopes*. Eds Kniseley RM, Tauxe WN. US Atomic Energy Commision, Springfield, Virginia. 1964, 519–36.

Cousins C, Gunasekera RD, Mubashar M, Mohammadtaghi S, Strong R, Myers MJ and Peters AM. Comparative kinetics of microvascular inulin and Tc-99m-DTPA exchange. *Clinical Science* (in press).

Fogelman I, Bessent RG, Turner JG, Citrin DL, Boyle IT and Greig WR. The use of whole body retention of ^{99m}Tc-diphosphonate in the diagnosis of metabolic bone disease. *Journal of Nuclear Medicine* 1978, **19**: 270–5.

Hawkins RA, Choi Y, Huang S-C, Hoh CK, Dahlbom M, Schiepers C, Satyamurthy N, Barrio JR and Phelps ME. Evaluation of the skeletal kinetics of fluorine-18-fluoride ion with PET. *Journal of Nuclear Medicine* 1992, **33**: 633–42.

Heaney RP and Recker RR. Estimation of true calcium absorption. *Annals of Internal Medicine* 1985, **103**: 516–21.

Katz MA. Interstitial space — the forgotten organ. *Medical Hypotheses* 1980, **6**: 885–98.

Ladegaard-Pedersen J. Measurement of extracellular fluid volume and renal clearance by a single injection of inulin. *Scandinavian Journal of Clinical and Laboratory Investigation* 1972, **29**: 145–53.

Lahtinen R, Lahtinen T and Romppanen T. Bone and bone-marrow blood flow in chronic granulocytic leukemia and primary myelofibrosis. *Journal of Nuclear Medicine* 1982, **23**: 218–24.

Li G, Bronk JT and Kelly PJ. Canine bone blood flow estimated with microspheres. *Journal of Orthopedic Research* 1989, **7**: 61–7.

Martiat Ph, Ferrant A, Cogneau M, Bol A, Michel C, Rodhain J, Michaux JL and Sokal G. Assessment of bone marrow blood flow using positron emission tomography, no relationship with bone marrow cellularity. *British Journal of Haematology* 1987, **66**: 307–10.

McCarthy ID and Hughes SPF. Multiple tracer studies of bone uptake of ^{99m}Tc-MDP and ^{85}Sr. *American Journal of Physiology* 1989, **256**: H1261–5.

Nahmias C, Cockshott WP, Belbeck LW and Garnett ES. Measurement of absolute bone blood flow by positron emission tomography. *Skeletal Radiology* 1986; **15**: 198–200.

Neilsen OM. Extracelluar volume, renal clearance and whole body permeability-surface area product in man measured after a single injection of polyfructosan. *Scandinavian Journal of Clinical and Laboratory Investigation* 1985, **45**: 217–22.

Nisbet AP, Edwards S, Lazarus CR, Malamitsi J, Maisey MN, Mashiter GD and Winn PJ. Chromium-51 EDTA/

technetium-99m MDP plasma ratio to measure total skeletal function. *British Journal of Radiology* 1984, **57**: 677–80.

Peters AM. Bone turnover in osteoporosis. In: *Bone circulation and vascularization in normal and pathological conditions*. A Schoutens, J Arlet, JWM Gardeniers, SPF Hughes (eds). Plenum, New York, 1993, pp. 177–183.

Peters AM, Brown H and Cosgriff P. Measurement of the extravascular concentration of renal agents following intravenous bolus injection. *Nuclear Medicine Communications* 1994, **15**: 66–72.

Schiepers C. Skeletal fluoride kinetics of ^{18}F- and positron emission tomography (PET): in-vivo estimation of regional bone blood flow and influx rate in humans. In: *Bone circulation and vascularization in normal and pathological conditions*. A Schoutens, J Arlet, JWM Gardeniers, SPF Hughes (eds). Plenum, New York, 1993, pp 95–100.

Shipp CC, Maletskos CJ and Dawson-Hughes B. Measurement of ^{47}Ca retention with a whole body counter. *Calcified Tissue International* 1987, **41**: 307

Veall N and Vetter H. *Radioisotope techniques in clinical research and diagnosis*. Butterworth, London, 1958, 189–222.

Vink H and Duling BR. Identification of distinct luminal domains for macromolecules, erythrocytes and leukocytes within mammalian capillaries. *Circulation Research* 1997; **79**: 581–9.

Wootton R, Reave J, Veall N. The clinical measurement of skeletal blood flow. *Clinical Science and Molecular Medicine* 1976, **50**: 261–8.

14 Exercises

14.1 Questions

1. General questions

a) During continuous intravenous infusion of para-aminohippurate, the arterial concentration at steady state was 12 MBq/ml and the renal venous concentration was 4 MBq/ml. What was the steady-state extraction fraction?

b) During continuous infusion of bromosulphthalein (BSP) at a rate of 1200 mg/min, the steady-state arterial concentration was 1 mg/ml and the hepatic venous BSP concentration was 0.2 mg/ml; what was liver blood flow? (Assume no extrahepatic uptake of BSP).

c) A patient with a cardiac output of 5600 ml/min and a pulse rate of 70/min has a left ventricular ejection fraction of 0.64. What are the left ventricular end-diastolic and end-systolic volumes?

d) Following injection of a labelled intravascular tracer, cerebral blood volume was found to be 75 ml; if cerebral blood flow was 250 ml/min, what was the mean cerebral vascular transit time?

e) The area under an arterial fluorine-18 time–concentration curve, recorded in a cerebral region of interest up to 10 min after bolus intravenous injection of fluorine-18-fluorodeoxyglucose (FDG), was 15 MBq·ml^{-1}·min. If the cerebral tissue fluorine-18 concentration in the region of interest at this time was 5 MBq/ml, what was the regional cerebral FDG clearance? If the arterial glucose concentration was 90 mg/ml, what was the regional cerebral glucose utilization rate (CMR$_{glu}$)? What physiological assumption do you have to make for this calculation?

2. Whole body counting

a) A patient with inflammatory bowel disease was injected with 20 MBq of indium-111 labelled granulocytes. He stood 4 m away from an uncollimated gamma camera 1 hr after injection and again 5 days after injection. On each occasion an indium-111 standard was counted from the same distance.

Results (kilocounts/min):

	1 hr	5 days
anterior	1680	260
posterior	1800	300
standard	650	200
background	20	22

Estimate the fraction of circulating granulocytes excreted in the faeces, first using and then not using the standard. $t_{1/2}$ indium-111 = 67 hr.)

b) A patient was injected with technetium-99m methylene diphosphonate (MDP). A whole body count performed 5 min later and corrected for photon attenuation was 400 000 cpm. The following day, 24 hr after injection, the whole body count rate was 10 000 cpm. Creatinine clearance was known to be 100 ml/min. What is the approximate total skeletal MDP clearance? (Assume negligible soft tissue uptake of MDP.)

3. Measurement of cardiac output

Technetium-99m labelled albumin was given by bolus intravenous injection and a first-pass time–activity curve was recorded from a region of interest over the left ventricle. The area under this curve up to a time t just before recirculation was 5000 counts, and the count rate from the same ROI at time t was 78 cps. An exponential function fitted to the data points of the downslope of the curve, up to time t, had a rate constant of $k = 0.13$ sec^{-1}. The injected dose was 400 MBq. A blood sample of 1 ml, taken 5 min after injection and counted at 24 hr after injection, gave a count rate in a well counter of 200 000 cpm. The count rate over the ROI at this time was 50 cps.

Estimate:

(a) mean circulation time

(b) cardiac output

> (well-counter sensitivity $= 4 \times 10^7$ counts/min/MBq, $t_{1/2}$ technetium-99m $= 6$ hr).

4. Measurement of tissue perfusion with xenon-133

Xenon-133 in saline was selectively injected into the coronary artery and the following time–activity curve recorded over the myocardium.

time (sec)	counts/sec
10	280
20	205
30	150
40	110
50	80
60	58

Plot these values on semi-logarithmic graph paper and then determine the myocardial tissue perfusion in units of ml/min/100 g. (Assume a myocardial tissue density of 1.02 g/ml and a xenon partition coefficient of 0.7 between myocardium and blood.)

5. Cerebral perfusion

Xenon-133 was selectively injected into the internal carotid artery and the following time-activity curve was recorded over the cranium with a scintillation probe.

Time (min)	Counts/sec
1	609
2	386
3	268
4	199
5	163
6	137
7	119
8	105
9	94
10	84
11	75
12	68

Assume the following constants

λ (white) $= 1.5$; ρ (white) $= 0.8$;
λ (grey) $= 1$; ρ (grey) $= 1$;
λ — partition coefficient between blood and tissue;
ρ — density of cerebral tissue.

a) What proportion of total cerebral blood flow supplies

> (i)   the white matter;
> (ii) the grey matter?

b) What is grey matter perfusion?

c) What is white matter perfusion?

d) What is mean cerebral perfusion?

6. Tc-99m DTPA clearance

a) Estimate the plasma clearance of technetium-99m DTPA from the following data: patient injected at 12.00 noon on 1.11.90; injected dose 150 MBq at 11.00 am on 1.11.90; all samples were counted at 12.00 noon on 2.11.90.

Time from injection	Counts/min in 0.5 ml plasma
120 min	8000
180 min	4900
240 min	3000

A standard (containing 0.005 MBq) was counted at the same time, giving 200 000 counts/min. What further data would be required for the measurement of 'true' clearance? ($t_{1/2}$ of technetium-99m $= 6$ hr.) What assumptions are required to equate this clearance to GFR?

7. Measurement of mean platelet survival

a) The following data were obtained from whole blood and cell-free plasma samples of 1 ml each taken at the times indicated below and counted in a well counter 144 hr after injection of 12 MBq of indium-111 labelled platelets.

Time after injection	Whole blood (cpm)	Cell-free plasma (cpm)
5 min	25 000	3000
30 min	20 000	3333
24 hr	18 100	3500

Time after injection	Whole blood (cpm)	Cell-free plasma (cpm)
48 hr	15 800	3000
72 hr	14 160	3600
96 hr	11 920	3200
120 hr	9680	2800
144 hr	7620	2700

The well-counter sensitivity is 47 000 000 cpm/MBq indium-111; the total blood volume is 5000 ml and the haematocrit of each sample is 0.4.

(i)   What is mean platelet lifespan?

(ii) What is the labelled platelet recovery (i.e. fraction of injected labelled platelets) circulating at 30 min after injection?

(iii) Estimate the size of splenic platelet pool (as a percentage of the total platelet population)

b)   In another patient, the following data were obtained 5 days after injection of 10 MBq indium-111 labelled platelets. What is the mean platelet lifespan? ($t_{1/2}$ indium-111 = 67 hr.)

Time after injection	*cpm
30 min	20 000
24 hr	9 000
48 hr	4 400
72 hr	2 000
96 hr	900

*counts/min in whole blood after correction for free activity in plasma

8.   Measurement of right to left pulmonary vascular shunting

A patient with a right-to-left vascular shunt as a result of a pulmonary arterio–venous malformation was injected with technetium-99m labelled human albumin microspheres. A posterior gamma camera view taken at 2.00 pm gave 10 000 counts in 2 min in a region of interest over the right kidney. From lateral views taken at 2.05 pm, the left kidney was shown to have a mean depth of 6 cm and the right 7 cm. The activity in the injection syringe, calibrated at 1.00 pm, was 70 MBq. The residual activity in the

syringe and intravenous injection line at 2.15 pm was 30 MBq. What fraction of the cardiac output is flowing through the shunt. (Assume that the right kidney receives 10% of cardiac output. Attenuation co-efficient for technetium-99m in tissue = 0.12 cm^{-1}; camera sensitivity: 130 cps · MBq^{-1}; technetium-99m $t_{1/2}$: 6 hr.)

9.   Ventilation signal

A patient with a ventilatory turnover of 0.8 ml/min/ml breathed an inert gas with a half-life of 69 seconds, and then increased his ventilation by 100% (i.e. doubled) and his lung volume by 25%. By how much would the count rate from his lungs have increased? (Assume no changes in photon attenuation.)

10.   Gastrointestinal bleeding

A quantity of 100 MBq of technetium-99m sulphur colloid was injected intravenously into a patient with gastrointestinal bleeding. He had no porto-systemic shunting. His liver blood flow was 1500 ml/min. How much technetium-99m sulphur colloid would have accumulated at the bleeding site if the rate of bleeding was 0.5 ml/min? (Assume an hepatic sulphur colloid extraction efficiency of 80% and ignore bone marrow and splenic uptake.)

If the sulphur colloid had been injected directly into the superior mesenteric artery, the vascular territory from which the bleeding occurred, instead of intravenously, how much would have accumulated at the bleeding site? (Assume that the superior mesenteric artery supplies two thirds of the total mesenteric venous flow and that splenic blood flow is 300 ml/min.)

11.   Using one agent to quantify organ uptake of another

a)   The count rate in a region of interest over the periphery of the lung following the intravenous administration of 50 MBq of technetium-99m labelled macroaggregated albumin (MAA) was 2000/min. A few minutes after the MAA, 500 MBq of technetium-99m labelled red cells were injected. After allowing 5 min for complete mixing of these red cells in the circulation, a count rate of 3800/min was recorded from the same region of interest over the lung. Assuming negligible physical radionuclide decay between this sequence of events, calculate the pulmonary red cell volume as a fraction of total red cell volume. (Ignore red cell counts recorded from the blood volume of the chest wall.) What other physiological assumption do you need to make?

b) A patient with an arterio–venous vascular malformation in the vascular territory of the femoral artery was given a bolus injection of 40 MBq of xenon-133 in saline selectively into the femoral artery at the time of angiography. A portable scintillation probe positioned over the lung recorded a time–activity curve which reached a peak of 500 counts/sec 20 sec after injection while the patient held her breath. Thirty minutes later, 40 MBq of xenon-133 in saline was administered by bolus intravenous injection, giving a time–activity curve, recorded by the same probe, which reached a peak of 2000 counts/sec at 10 sec after injection, again during breath holding. What fraction of the femoral artery flow, *at the arterial catheter tip*, was undergoing arterio–venous shunting. What assumptions will you make in order to perform this calculation?

12. Measurement of perfusion from oxygen-15 labelled water

A patient continuously inhaled carbon dioxide labelled with oxygen-15 while undergoing positron emission tomography. In a slice penetrating the left ventricle, the count rate from the blood in the chamber of the left ventricle was 30 000 cpm/pixel and from the septum 20 000 cpm/pixel. What is myocardial septal perfusion in units of ml/min/ml? Assume the water content of myocardium is 0.7 ml/ml and of blood 0.9 ml/ml, and that the physical half life of oxygen-15 is 2 min.

13. Patlak–Rutland plot

The following counts/ml of tissue or blood ($\times 10^{-5}$) were recorded in intervals of one min duration from regions of interest in a PET slice following bolus intravenous injection of fluorine-18.

Time (min)	Left ventricle	Vertebral body
1	100	27
2	75	41
3	60	45
4	55	47
5	50	48
6	48	50
7	46	53
8	44	55
9	43	58
10	42	61
11	40	62
12	39	64

Use linear graph paper to determine the steady state clearance of fluorine-18 into the vertebral body. Why is the first part of the plot curved and what does the zero time intercept of the plot represent, first taking into account, and then *not* taking into account, the initial curved portion?

14. Tracer equilibration between plasma and interstitial fluid

The plasma clearance curve of chromium-51 EDTA following injection of 3 MBq was resolved into two exponentials with rate constants α_1 and α_2 and corresponding zero time intercepts A and B, with the following values: A = 0.0003 MBq/ml, B = 0.0002 MBq/ml, $\alpha_1 = 0.06$ min^{-1} and $\alpha_2 = 0.008$ min^{-1}.

a)   At what time after injection would the concentration in the interstitial fluid have been maximal?

b)   Prove that this time is the same time at which the intravascular and interstitial fluid concentrations momentarily equalise. Then

c)   calculate extra-cellular fluid volume.

(Note, the reader may find it easier to tackle (b) using a graphical approach.)

15. Instantaneous versus steady state clearance

Following injection of 120 MBq of a radiolabelled organic anion, a bi-exponential plasma clearance curve was recorded. The zero-time intercepts of the two exponentials were 0.015 MBq/ml and

0.005 MBq/ml, and the corresponding rate constants were 0.28 min^{-1} and 0.03 min^{-1}. What is the steady state plasma clearance of this organic anion? What assumptions would have to be made in order to calculate steady state hepatic extraction fraction? Having made these assumptions, what is the steady state hepatic extraction fraction? Calculate liver blood flow, first using steady-state extraction fraction and then not using it.

16. Permeability–surface area product and clearance

The steady state extraction fraction of thallium-201 in a normal region of myocardium was 0.4 and the regional perfusion was 250 ml/min/100 ml. What was the regional permeability–surface area (*PS*) product? In another, ischaemic region of myocardium, the perfusion was 90 ml/min/100 ml. What was the extraction fraction in this region if the steady state *PS* product was

a) 50% of the value in the normal region;

b) the same as the value in the normal region;

c) 150% of the value in the normal region?

What would the regional myocardial thallium clearances be in the normal and abnormal regions? What actually determines the image — regional clearance, regional perfusion or regional *PS* product?

17. 'Cross-talk' in sample counting

A sample containing a mixture of an iodine-123 labelled tracer (tracer 1) and a technetium-99m labelled tracer (tracer 2) gave a count rate of 9876 counts/min in a well counter on the technetium-99m photopeak. When counted again 6 hr later, the count rate was 6543 counts/min. What is the proportion of counts arising from iodine-123 at each counting time ($t_{1/2}$ technetium-99 and iodine-123 6 hr and 13 hr respectively).

18. Measurement of tissue perfusion using microspheres

Starting at exactly 11.00 am, an arterial blood sample was drawn at a constant rate. 10 sec after starting this withdrawal, 10 MBq of radiolabelled microspheres were injected as a bolus into the left

ventricle. At exactly 11.01 am the arterial withdrawal was terminated, having obtained 30 ml. A sample of renal tissue, weighing 3 gm, was obtained 15 min later and counted in a well counter with 1 ml of blood diluted with haemolysate to a total volume of 3 ml. The count rates obtained from renal tissue and blood were respectively 24 000 and 150 counts per sec. What is renal perfusion?

19. Double integration

a) Following injection as a bolus into the carotid artery, xenon-133 washed out of a region of brain with a $t_{1/2}$ of 1.54 min. Assuming a mean λ of 1.25, what is mean regional perfusion and how much xenon remained in the region after one minute as a percentage of the amount delivered to the region? If an image was continuously acquired during this period of one minute, how many counts would be acquired in the region as a percentage of the counts that would have accumulated if there had been no xenon washout? If the xenon was given as a continuous infusion (assuming that a constant arterial concentration was reached immediately), what would the count rate be after one minute as a percentage of what it would have been had there been no xenon washout? If an image was continuously acquired for one minute from the start of the infusion, how many counts would it contain, as a percentage of the counts that would have accumulated if there had been no washout? Another region of the brain had a $t_{1/2}$ of xenon-133 clearance of 2.2 min after bolus intra-carotid injection. Repeat the above exercise for this region. Create your own data from the $t_{1/2}$ values given and do the exercise on a simple graphics programme (using the command 'running sum' in order to integrate.)

b) For two minutes following injection of 250 MBq of technetium-99m DTPA, the following counts (in thousands) were recorded in 10 sec frames from a region of interest over the left ventricle: 95, 90, 86, 82, 78, 74, 70, 67, 64, 61, 58 and 55. A blood sample taken at 20 min after injection, when the count rate recorded from the left ventricle was 4000 per sec, contained 0.006 MBq. The left kidney, which was at a depth of 6 cm from the surface of the posterior abdominal wall, had a technetium-99m DTPA plasma clearance of 60 ml/min. An image of the left kidney was acquired continuously over the period of 2 min following injection and corrected for background: how many counts were in the image? (Linear attenuation coefficient for technetium-99m $= 0.12$ min^{-1}; blood sample haematocrit 0.4; assume that the left ventricular signal includes no extravascular counts.)

20. *PS* product and capillary tracer concentration

Following intravenous injection, 100 MBq of a tracer disappeared from blood exponentially with a clearance half-time of 10 min, as a result of uptake into two organs. After 15 min, arterial plasma tracer concentration was 0.005 MBq/ml, the tracer content of one organ (organ 1) was 23 MBq and of the other (organ 2) was 42 MBq. If the permeability surface (*PS*) product for the tracer in organ 1 was 350 ml/min (whole organ) and in organ 2, was 520 ml/min, what was the mean capillary tracer concentration in each organ at 15 min after injection?

21. Urinary clearance

Following the injection of 200 MBq of tracer X, 90 MBq had been recovered in the urine up to 60 min after injection. The plasma cleared bi-exponentially with the following curve parameters: zero-time intercept, $A = 15$ kBq/ml, zero-time intercept, $B = 20$ kBq/ml, rate constant $\alpha_1 = 0.08$ min^{-1}, rate constant $\alpha_2 = 0.009$ min^{-1}. What is the urinary clearance of tracer X in absolute terms (i.e. in units of ml/min) and as a fraction of plasma clearance. The same measurement was attempted in another patient who had difficulty emptying his bladder. In this case, 25 MBq were recovered in the urine and the plasma clearance curve parameters were $A = 20$ kBq/ml, $B = 15$ kBq/ml, $\alpha_1 = 0.045$ min^{-1} and $\alpha_2 = 0.002$ min^{-1}. Because difficulties were anticipated with bladder emptying, and therefore with achieving a complete urine collection, this patient was also given 3 MBq of chromium-51 EDTA, for which α_2 was 0.003 min^{-1} and GFR was calculated to be 35 ml/min. At 60 min after EDTA injection, 0.3 MBq of chromium-51 had been recovered in the urine. What is the urinary clearance of tracer X in this patient?

22. Blood clearance versus plasma clearance — effect of tracer binding to red cells

Following injection of 200 MBq of a tracer which was partially bound to red cells in the blood, but not to protein, and was cleared only by the liver, the area under the plasma time–concentration curve was 0.4 MBq.ml^{-1}. min while the area under the blood time–concentration curve was 0.3 MBq·ml^{-1}·min. The peripheral haematocrit (in samples on which the clearance measurements were based) was 0.4. The steady-state extraction fraction of the tracer by the liver was determined by hepatic venous catheterisation to be 0.65. What is the *PS* product of the tracer if the intrahepatic haematocrit was 0.8 that of peripheral haematocrit? (Assume liver weight is 1 kg.)

23. Outflow detection versus residue detection for measurement of transit time

The following histogram of transit times was obtained by sampling from the venous drainage of an organ following bolus injection of a radioactive tracer into the artery supplying the organ:

Time sec (t)	% administered activity/volume (C)
5	2
6	5
7	10
8	20
9	26
10	17
11	10
12	6
13	3
14	1

Calculate mean transit time using

a) the outflow curve;

b) the residue curve that would have been recorded by a detector placed over the organ.

24. Pulmonary alveoalar epithelial permeability

For a pulmonary DTPA aerosol clearance curve, 20 MBq of technetium-99m DTPA was first given intravenously and the following counts (in thousands) per 5 sec frames were recorded from regions of interest over the lung and liver.

Lung: 36, 30, 26, 25, 21.5, 21, 19, 18, 15.5, 15.
Liver: 18, 15, 13.5, 12.5, 11.5, 10, 9, 8.5, 8, 7.5.

Tc-99m DTPA aerosol was then inhaled after which the following counts (in thousands) were obtained from the same regions of interest in one-minute frames.

Lung: 2110, 2070, 2020, 1960, 1920, 1860, 1825, 1755, 1715, 1665.
Liver: 96, 108, 120, 132, 138, 144, 155, 157, 160, 162.

What was the DTPA clearance rate calculated:

a) with no background correction;
b) with background correction based on liver activity?

25. Biological versus physical half-time (= half-life)

a) Compare the effective half-lives of iodine-123 hippuran (plasma clearance 500 ml/min, protein binding in plasma 50%) and technetium-99m MAG3 (plasma clearance 350 ml/min, protein binding in plasma 80%), assuming red cell binding to be zero. (Assume plasma volume of 3 litres and extracellular fluid volume of 13 litres.)

b) What is the effective half-life of indium-111 labelled granulocytes in a patient with inflammatory bowel disease involving the colon who was excreting 50% of granulocytes into the inflamed colon. (Assume a biological half-time of indium-111 granulocytes of 69 days in subjects with no inflammation and that the patient has a mean intracolonic transit time of 6 hr and an intravascular granulocyte half time of 7 hr.)

c) The following count rates were externally recorded over the upper arm of a subject 120, 160, 200 and 240 min after intravenous injection of 200 MBq technetium-99m DTPA. Estimate the subject's renal function.

14.2 Answers

1. a) Extraction fraction is equal to the arterio–venous concentration difference divided by arterial concentration; i.e. $E = [C_a - C_v]/C_a = [12 - 4]/12 = 0.67$.

b) At steady state, infusion rate I of indicator is equal to excretion rate, which in turn is equal to blood flow Q multiplied by arterio–venous concentration difference (Fick principle). That is

$$I = Q(C_a - C_v)$$
$$1200 = Q(1 - 0.2)$$

So

$$Q = 1500 \text{ ml/min.}$$

c) Since cardiac output = stroke volume × pulse rate

$$5600 = SV \times 70$$

and

$$SV = 80 \text{ ml.}$$

Also

$$\text{ejection fraction} = \frac{EDV - ESV}{EDV}$$
$$= SV/EDV = 0.64$$

So

$$EDV \times 0.64 = 80$$

Therefore

$$EDV = 125 \text{ ml}$$

and

$$ESV = 45 \text{ ml}$$

d) This uses the transit time equation, i.e.

$$T = V/Q$$

so

$$T = 75/250 \text{ min} = 18 \text{ sec.}$$

e) This is an example of the general equation, clearance (Z) = mass (M) divided by area under curve (A). In this case, $A = \int C_\tau(t) \cdot dt = 15$, so

$$Z = \frac{5 \text{ MBq} \cdot \text{ml}^{-1}}{15 \text{ MBq} \cdot \text{ml}^{-1} \cdot \text{min}}$$

and

$$Z = 0.33 \text{ ml/min/ml.}$$

Assuming that the cerebral clearance of native glucose is the same as that of FDG, then

glucose utilization rate = glucose concentration × glucose clearance
$$CMR_{glu} = 90 \times 0.33$$
$$= 30 \text{ mg/min/ml}.$$

2. Since the distribution of indium-111 in the body changes with time, it is necessary to correct for photon attenuation. This can be performed by calculating the geometric mean (the square root of the product) of anterior and posterior counts.

a) The geometric means (background corrected) at 1 hr and 5 d are 1719 and 257 kilocounts per min, respectively, 2.73 and 1.45 times the standard. Using the standard, which decays at the same rate as indium-111 in the body, this represents 53% retention. Ignoring the standard and making a correction for physical decay of the radionuclide, the counts at 5 d would be, in the absence of physical decay, $257.e^{[0.693/67] \times 119}$ which represents 51% retention.

b) By assuming negligible soft tissue uptake, the counts cleared between 5 min and 24 hr will be partitioned between the skeleton and the kidney. Correcting the 24 hr counts for physical decay gives a skeletal uptake = 158378 cpm = 39.5% of the 5 min counts. Urinary clearance accounts for the remaining 60.5% cleared, so skeletal clearance = $[39.5/60.6] \times 100 = 67$ ml/min.

3 a) Cardiac output is inversely proportional to the area under the first pass curve. The 5 min count rate effectively calibrates the curve in relation to the injected dose. Mean circulation time is also inversely proportional to cardiac output. Using the transit time equation, $T = V/Q$,

$$\text{mean circulation time} = \frac{\text{area under first pass curve}}{\text{count rate in same ROI at 5 min}}$$

with units

$$\frac{\text{counts}}{\text{counts per sec}} = \text{sec}.$$

Area under curve up to time t is equal to 5000 counts.
Area under curve from t to ∞ = count rate × time

$$= 78 \text{ cps} \times \frac{1}{k \text{ sec}^{-1}}$$
$$= 78 \text{ cps} \times 7.7 \text{ sec}$$
$$= 600 \text{ counts}.$$

Therefore

$$\text{total area} = 5600 \text{ counts}$$

and

$$\text{mean transit time} = \frac{5600 \text{ counts}}{50 \text{ counts} \cdot \text{sec}^{-1}}$$
$$= 112 \text{ sec}.$$

b) There are two possible approaches, one from the circulation time (and the general equation for transit time), the other using the Stewart–Hamilton equation for cardiac output.

(i) We have

$$\text{circulation time} = \frac{\text{blood volume}}{\text{cardiac output}}$$

$$\text{blood volume} = \frac{\text{injected dose}}{\text{tracer concentration at 5 min}}.$$

Using the well-counter sensitivity and physical decay correction, the 5 min concentration is 0.079 MBq/ml, so blood volume = 400/0.079 = 5063 ml. Therefore cardiac output is Q = 5063/112 sec = 45.2 ml/sec = 2712 ml/min.

(ii) Also

$$\text{cardiac output} = \frac{\text{injected dose (MBq)}}{\text{area under first pass curve (min} \times \text{MBq/ml)}}.$$

The area under the first-pass curve is the more difficult part and needs to converted to absolute units from camera counts and well-counter counts. The way forward is to use all the information and arrange it into an expression in which the units reduce to those of the area under the first-pass curve; i.e. min × MBq/ml. It is usually fairly self-evident whether a term appears in the numerator (above the line) or denominator (below the line) in the equation defining the area under first-pass curve. Thus the area under the curve in counts is above the line so its calibration, the count rate in the ROI at 5 min, is below the line. The latter in turn is calibrated by the well counts recorded from the blood sample which therefore goes above the line. Lastly, the calibration for the blood sample; i.e. the standard in the well counter, goes below the line.
So

$$\text{area under first pass curve (min} \times \text{MBq/ml)}$$
$$= \frac{5600 \times 200\,000 \times \text{dcf}}{50 \times 60 \times 40\,000\,000}$$

$$\left(\text{units are } \frac{\text{counts} \times \text{min}}{\text{counts}} \times \frac{\text{min} \times \text{MBq}}{\text{counts}} \times \frac{\text{counts}}{\text{min} \times \text{ml}} \right)$$

[where dcf is decay correction factor $= e^{[0.693/6] \times 24} = 16] = 2679$ ml/min (not identical because of rounding up).

4. The xenon-133 is washed out of the myocardium as a single exponential with a rate constant of 0.031 sec^{-1}. In units of ml/sec/ml, the perfusion is therefore $0.031 \times 0.7 = 0.0217$, or taking density into account, 0.0213 ml/sec/g $= 128$ ml/min/100 g.

5. This cerebral xenon-133 washout curve can be resolved into two exponentials with zero-time intercepts of 825 and 240 counts per sec and corresponding rate constants of 0.73 and 0.106 min^{-1}. The proportion of total flow supplying the white matter is $240/1065 = 0.225$, and supplying grey matter, 0.775. Grey matter perfusion is 73 ml/min/100 g and white matter perfusion is $10.6 \times [1.5/0.8] = 20$ ml/min/100 g.

Mean cerebral perfusion can be calculated in several ways:

(a) as height/area (where area is $[825/0.73] + [240/0.106]$ and mean λ and ρ are taken as the averages for grey and white matter) $= 1065/[1130 + 2264] \times [1.25/0.9] = 44$ ml/min/100 g;

(b) initial slope, which, based on the first 3 points, is 57 ml/min/100 g;

(c) taking individual values for λ and ρ into account as follows:

Grey matter mass $= 0.775Q/73$ g;
white matter mass $= 0.225Q/20$ g.

Therefore

$$Q/V = \text{total flow/total mass}$$
$$= Q/[0.0106.Q + 0.01125.Q]$$
$$= 46 \text{ ml/min/100 g.}$$

6. Technetium-99m DTPA clearance is equal to GFR provided there is no extra-renal uptake or plasma protein binding of the tracer, and all the radioactivity remains associated with the ligand. It is also assumed that there is no tubular secretion. The calculation should be approached using the general equation for clearance Z which is $Z =$ injected activity/area under plasma time–concentration curve. All counts should be calibrated to the time of dose

calibration, so dose $= 150$ MBq. The area under the plasma curve is equal to the zero-time intercept (B) of the terminal exponential divided by the rate constant (α_2), which is 0.00817 min^{-1}. From the raw data, B is 42 670 counts/min/ml of plasma. This needs to be corrected for 25 hr of technetium-99m decay, which gives 765 851 counts/min/ml. From the standard we know that the well-counter sensitivity is 4×10^7 counts/min/MBq. The value of B is therefore $765\,851/4 \times 10^7$ MBq/ml and so GFR $= 64$ ml/min. To obtain 'true' clearance, more data, before 2 hr, would be required for the true area under the plasma time-concentration curve.

7 a) When a cell-survival curve of this type is performed, the cell-bound activity in blood samples is required and assumed to be associated only with platelets. Cell-free plasma is counted to determine the level of non-cell-bound indium-111. The volume of plasma in the whole blood samples is calculated from the sample haematocrit. The cell-free sample counts are therefore multiplied by 0.6 and then subtracted from whole blood counts to give cell-bound counts. From 30 min, when the labelled platelets have equilibrated with the splenic platelet pool, the disappearance profile is clearly linear and cuts the time axis at 216 hr, which is platelet life span (**Fig. 14.1**). The recovery is the fraction of the injected platelets in blood (excluding splenic pool) at 30 min. The cell-bound blood counts at 30 min are 18 000 per ml; total blood volume is 5000 ml so total blood platelet activity counts are 9×10^7. Correcting this for isotope decay and dividing by well-counter sensitivity in counts/min/MBq gives the total circulating platelet-associated indium-111, which is 8.5 MBq. The recovery is therefore 8.5/14 or 60%. Since the great majority of 'un-recovered' platelets are in the splenic pool, the latter represents about 40% of the total circulating platelet population.

b) This is obviously an abnormal platelet survival curve, clearly exponential (**Fig. 14.1**), with a rate constant of clearance of 0.032 hr^{-1}. Mean platelet life span in this case is the reciprocal of the rate constant, i.e. 31 hr.

8. The fraction of the cardiac output flowing through the right-to-left shunt is equal to the fraction of the injected dose reaching the systemic circulation, of which 10% is delivered to the right kidney. Count rates can be calibrated to imaging time. The

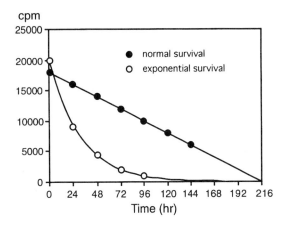

∎ **Fig. 14.1** Platelet survival profiles from Question 7. The normal profile is linear, cutting the time axis at 216 hr, which, for a linear survival, is platelet life-span. Note that since the profile is linear, there is no spread of platelet survival times — all platelets have the same life span. The abnormal exponential survival profile, in contrast, represents a wide range of life spans as the platelets are removed from the circulation at random. The half-time of the curve is 21.7 hr, corresponding to a rate constant of disappearance of 0.032 hr^{-1}, the reciprocal of which, for an exponential survival, is mean platelet life-span — 31 hr.

residual activity in the syringe requires 'up-correction' by 15 min to 31 MBq. The activity in the injection syringe requires down-correction by 60 min, to 62 MBq. The administered activity is therefore 31 MBq. After depth correction, counts over the right kidney are 193 counts per sec. Divided by camera sensitivity, this represents 1.48 MBq so 14.8 MBq reached the systemic circulation, a shunt of 48%.

9. The count rate over the lung N_1 is proportional to $\dot{V}/[(\dot{V}/V) + \delta]$; i.e. $\dot{V}/1.4$. Under the conditions of increased ventilation the count rate N_2 is proportional to,

$$\frac{2\dot{V}}{[(2\dot{V})/(1.25V)] + 0.6}$$

therefore

$$\frac{N_2}{N_1} = \frac{2.8}{[(2/1.25) \times 0.8] + 0.6}$$
$$= 1.49$$

10. The 'clearance' of tracer into the gut lumen at the bleeding site compared with clearance into the liver determines the fraction of the dose which is extravasated. The hepatic clearance is 0.8×1500 ml/min = 1200 ml/min. The amount of technetium-99m accumulated at the bleeding site is therefore $[0.5/1200] \times 100$ MBq = 0.042 MBq. Mesenteric venous flow is 1500 – 300 ml/min = 1200 ml/min, two thirds of which is coming from the vascular territory of the mesenteric artery, i.e. 800 ml. Therefore $[0.5/800] \times 100$ MBq = 0.0625 MBq will accumulate at the bleeding site. Essentially 99.9 MBq will then be exposed to the hepatic vascular bed, of which 20%, i.e. 20 MBq will recirculate and behave as though it had been injected intravenously. *In addition* therefore a further $[0.5/1200] \times 20$ MBq = 0.0083 MBq will accumulate at the bleeding site as a result of subsequent passes, giving a total of 0.071 MBq.

11. The entire dose of MAA, 50 MBq, will be retained in the lung on first pass. The value 2000 counts/min is therefore equivalent to 50 MBq. After red cell equilibration the count rate increased by 1800 counts/min, which is equivalent to 45 MBq. The fraction of injected red cell-associated activity in the lungs is therefore 45/500 = 9%, so the pulmonary blood volume as a fraction of total blood volume is 0.09. The physiological assumption is made that the regional distribution of pulmonary blood flow is matched by the regional distribution of pulmonary blood volume; i.e. that mean intravascular pulmonary transit time is homogeneous. This is not quite true, there being a vertical gradient of intravascular transit times in the lung.

12. This is the straightforward use of equation 3.30. The value for λ is 7/9 so $Q/V = 162$ ml/min/100 ml.

13. The linear phase of the Patlak–Rutland plot has a slope of 0.072 min^{-1}, corresponding to a steady-state fluorine-18 clearance of 7.2 ml/min/100 ml. The non-linearity of the first part of the curve has been exaggerated in order to bring out the fact that fluorine-18 first exchanges between plasma and the interstitial fluid of bone (**Fig. 14.2**). Some of this curvature will also be due to vascular dispersion in the bone capillaries and bone marrow sinusoids. The zero-time intercept of the extrapolated linear portion, 0.47 ml/ml in this case, represents the extracellular

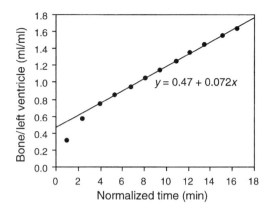

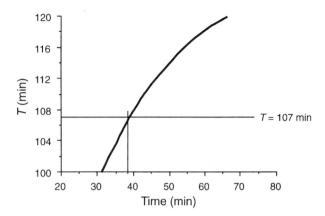

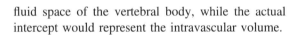

▌ Fig. 14.2 A Patlak–Rutland plot based on the data of Question 13. The gradient, with exclusion of the first 3 data points, is 0.072 ml/min/ml or 7.2 ml/min/100 ml. The regression line, extrapolated to zero time, lies above the first two points because the initial part of the curve reflects (a) vascular dispersion and (b) transfer between plasma and interstitial fluid, which is bi-directional, in addition to (c) unidirectional uptake into bone crystal. The plot becomes a straight line after complete vascular mixing and equilibration of tracer between plasma and interstitial fluid.

▌ Fig. 14.3 The left-hand side of equation 14.1 (Question 14) has been plotted against time. Although T is shown here as a variable, it is in fact a discrete value which for technetium-99m DTPA is equal to ECF volume (i.e. $V_i + V_e$) divided by GFR and, from the parameters of the bi-exponential plasma clearance curve, can be calculated to be 107 min. The value of t at which $T = 107$ min is 38.7 min, identical to the value given by $[\ln(\alpha_1/\alpha_2)]/(\alpha_1 - \alpha_2)$.

fluid space of the vertebral body, while the actual intercept would represent the intravascular volume.

14. Concentration in the extravascular space C_e is given by the difference of two exponentials, the rate constants of which are the same as those in the plasma clearance curve. The equation describing the time course of C_e is the same as that describing the time course of hepatic activity after intravenous injection of IDA (Section 9.4.1.1). The time of maximal concentration in the extravascular space is the time at which $dC_e/dt = 0$ and is equal to $[\ln(\alpha_1/\alpha_2)]/(\alpha_1 - \alpha_2) = 38.7$ min.

The time at which the intravascular (C_i) and interstitial fluid (C_e) concentrations become equal can be obtained from equation 13.14. At this time, $C_e = C_i$, so

$$\frac{Z \int_t^\infty C_i(t) \cdot dt}{C_i \cdot V_e} = 1 + \frac{V_i}{V_e}.$$

By rearrangement

$$\frac{\int_t^\infty C_i(t) \cdot dt}{C_i} = \frac{V_e + V_i}{Z} = T$$

where T is mean residence time of tracer in the extracellular fluid (ECF). Substituting for $\int_t^\infty C_i(t) \cdot dt / C_i$ as in equation 13.16

$$\frac{(Ae^{-\alpha_1 t})/\alpha_1 + (Be^{-\alpha_2 t})/\alpha_2}{Ae^{-\alpha_1 t} + Be^{-\alpha_2 t}} = T. \quad (14.1)$$

Note that T can be measured from the parameters of the bi-exponential clearance curve and is 107 min. By plotting the left-hand side of equation 14.1 against time t it will be seen that it gives a value of T of 107 min when t is 38.7 min **(Fig. 14.3)**. ECF volume is the product of steady state clearance and T, and is 10 690 ml.

15. The steady-state plasma clearance is given by the ratio of injected activity and total area under the plasma concentration–time curve, and is equal to 545 ml/min. Provided the unidirectional extraction fraction of organic ion from plasma to hepatocyte is unity, the steady-state extraction fraction is equal to $k/(k_2 + k)$, where k and k_2 are the fractional rate constants in Fig. 9.3 and which can be calculated from the parameters of the bi-exponential plasma clearance using equations 9.1 to 9.3. Thus k is 0.039 min^{-1}, k_2 is 0.054 min^{-1}, and so steady-state extraction fraction is 0.417. Combining clearance

and extraction fraction gives a liver blood flow (LBF) of 545/0.417 = 1307 ml/min. The alternative approach is to use k_1 which, in the absence of significant distribution of the tracer in the whole body interstitial space, is the fraction of total blood volume (TBV) serving the liver per unit time. Otherwise it is tracer distribution volume, higher than TBV. Distribution volume is dose divided by zero-time concentration which is the sum, $A + B$. The fractional rate constant defining unidirectional transfer of tracer from plasma to hepatocyte k_1 is 0.2175 min^{-1}, so LBF by this approach is 6000 × 0.2175 = 1305 ml/min. (They are not exactly the same because of rounding up.)

16. Permeability surface area (*PS*) product can be obtained from perfusion (*Q*) and extraction fraction (*E*) using the equation: $PS = -Q \cdot \ln(1 - E)$, and in the normal region is 128 ml/min/100 ml. The clearance $(= Q \cdot E)$ is 100 ml/min/100 ml. This equation can be rearranged: $E = 1 - e^{-PS/Q}$, giving *E* values for (a), (b) and (c) of 0.51, 0.76 and 0.88, and corresponding clearance values of 46, 68 and 79 ml/min/100 ml. Regional clearance determines the initial thallium image; i.e. before redistribution commences. It is unlikely therefore that ischaemia results in an increase in *PS* product, even though endothelium might be expected to become more leaky, otherwise no regional defect would become apparent.

17. Over 6 hr, iodine-123 will have decayed to 0.73 and technetium-99m to 0.5 of their respective contributions to the first count rate. Therefore

$$N_1 + N_2 = 9876$$

and

$$0.73N_1 + 0.5N_2 = 6543.$$

The solution to these equations is $N_1 = 6978$, i.e. iodine-123 contributes 71% of total count rate. At the second counting time, iodine's contribution is 78%.

18. The rate of arterial withdrawal was 0.5 ml/min. This flow rate corresponds to the total activity in the withdrawn blood which is given by 150 × 30 = 4500 counts/sec. One gram of renal tissue accumulated activity giving 8000 counts per sec. Tissue perfusion is therefore (8000/4500)× 0.5 ml/min/g = 89 ml/min/100 g.

19 a) With a $t_{1/2}$ of 1.54 min and λ of 1.25, regional cerebral perfusion is 56 ml/min/100 ml;

$e^{-0.45} = 64\%$ of activity remains at 1 min. A continuously acquired image over one minute represents an integration of the washout curve, and would contain 80% of the counts if there was no washout. The activity at the end of one minute of continuous infusion represents the same integration. An image continuously acquired in the brain region during a continuous infusion represents a second integration, and would contain 85% of the counts acquired if there had been no washout (**Fig. 14.4**). The corresponding values for a clearance $t_{1/2}$ of 2.2 min are 39 ml/min/100 ml, 73%, 85% and 90%.

b) The blood sample at 20 min contained 0.006 MBq/ml, which is equivalent to 0.01 MBq/ml plasma and corresponds to 40K in a 10-sec frame over the cardiac blood pool region of interest. During the first 10 sec therefore 95K counts in the cardiac region corresponded to a plasma DTPA concentration of 0.02375 MBq/ml. With a clearance of 60 ml/min, the kidney would accumulate 1.425 MBq during this time. The amounts accumulated in each 10 sec-frame can be calculated similarly. Summation of these amounts gives the activity accumulated at 2 min — 13.2 MBq. With a camera sensitivity of 145 counts/sec/MBq, this would give a count rate from the kidney of 1914/sec. This is attenuated to 932 counts/sec, or 9320 for the frame. The counts recorded from all frames can be calculated similarly. The total number of counts accumulated over 2 min is the summation of all the frame counts — 66 131. Note that two integrations have been performed — one by the kidney and one by the gamma camera.

20. Plasma clearance is injected dose divided by area under time concentration curve. From the clearance half-time, the zero-time plasma concentration was 0.0141 MBq/ml. The rate constant of disappearance is 0.0693 min^{-1}. The area under the plasma time concentration curve is therefore 0.0141/0.0693 = 0.2 (MBq/ml × min) and plasma clearance 100/0.2 = 500 ml/min. Of this plasma clearance 23/65 enters organ 1 and 42/65 enters organ 2, so the steady state organ clearances are 177 and 323 ml/min. The product of *PS* product and mean capillary concentration C_p is the rate of tracer uptake by the organ which is also equal to the product of arterial concentration and organ clearance: i.e. $C_p = (177/350) \times 0.005 = 0.0025$ and $(323/520) \times 0.005 = 0.003$ MBq/ml.

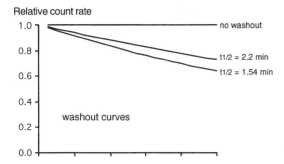

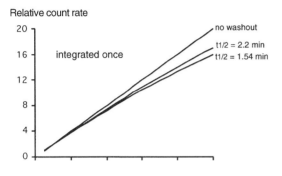

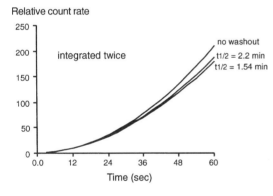

❚ **Fig. 14.4** Effect of integration and double integration on cerebral xenon-133 washout curves (a) when there is washout and (b) in the hypothetical situation of no washout (Question 19.a). Each panel contains three lines, one corresponding to no washout and the other corresponding to washout half-times of 1.54 min and 2.2 min.

21. Measurement of urinary clearance is similar to measurement of organ clearance. Thus the amount of tracer cleared into the urine at time t is compared with the area under the plasma clearance curve up to the same time. In the case of organ clearance, the denominator is the same, namely the area under the plasma curve, whilst the numerator is the amount of

activity accumulated by the organ over the same time. The area under a mono-exponential function up to the time t is the difference between (i) the zero time intercept divided by the rate constant and (ii) the y-axis value at time t divided by the rate constant. The area under the plasma curve to 60 min is therefore given by

$$\text{area} = \frac{A(1 - e^{-\alpha_1 60})}{\alpha_1} + \frac{B(1 - e^{-\alpha_2 60})}{\alpha_2} \quad (14.2)$$

$$= 1.11 \text{ MBq} \cdot \text{ml}^{-1} \cdot \text{min}.$$

Urinary clearance is therefore 81 ml/min and plasma clearance 83 ml/min.

For the second patient GFR, or more specifically α_2, is so low that any area under the plasma clearance curve up to infinity will not be significantly influenced by the area under the first exponential of the EDTA plasma clearance curve. The zero-time intercept B of the EDTA clearance curve is therefore given by

$$B = \frac{\alpha_2}{\text{GFR}} \times \text{injected dose}$$

$$= \frac{0.003 \times 3}{35}$$

$$= 0.257 \text{ kBq/ml}.$$

The area under the EDTA clearance curve up to one hour is therefore

$$\frac{0.257 - 0.215}{0.003} \text{ kBq} \cdot \text{ml}^{-1} \cdot \text{min}$$

$$= 0.014 \text{ MBq} \cdot \text{ml}^{-1} \cdot \text{min}.$$

For EDTA,

$$\text{urinary clearance } (Z_u) = \text{plasma clearance } (Z_p)$$
$$= 35 \text{ ml/min}$$

Therefore

$$M_u = 35 \times 0.014 = 0.49 \text{ MBq}.$$

In other words, 0.49 MBq should have been recovered in the urine at 1 hour instead of 0.3, indicating a recovery of 61% of urine activity. Also 25 MBq tracer X was recovered which should have been $25/0.61 = 41$ MBq. From equation 14.2 therefore Z_u for tracer X is 32 ml/min.

22. Plasma concentration of the tracer was higher than that of whole blood, giving a larger area under the clearance curve than whole blood. Plasma and

blood clearances were 500 and 667 ml/min, respectively. The concentration ratio of tracer in whole blood to plasma was therefore 0.75. From equation 2.17, the partition coefficient of tracer between red cells and plasma was 0.375. The fraction of tracer in blood that is bound to red cells is equal to $(H \cdot \lambda)/[(H \cdot \lambda) + (1 - H)]$; this was 0.2 in peripheral blood and 0.15 in hepatic sinusoidal blood. Focusing on the latter value, 85% of tracer was present in plasma, corresponding to a clearance of 500 ml/min, and 15% was bound to red cells, corresponding to an additional effective clearance of $(15/85) \times 500 = 88$ ml/min. Total effective liver clearance is therefore 588 ml/min, insertion of which into equation 6.18 gives a PS product of 95 ml/min/ 100 g.

23. Mean transit time from the outflow curve is given by

$$T = \frac{\int t \cdot C(t) \cdot \mathrm{d}t}{\int C(t) \cdot \mathrm{d}t}$$

where the numerator is the sum of the products $t \cdot C$ and the denominator is the sum of the second-to-second concentrations C.

Time sec (t)	% administered activity (C)	$t \cdot C$
5	2	10
6	5	30
7	10	70
8	20	160
9	26	234
10	17	170
11	10	110
12	6	72
13	3	39
14	1	14
	100	909 = sum

That is

$$t = \frac{909}{100} = 9.09 \text{ sec}$$

The residue curve is obtained by integration towards zero time.

Mean transit time from the residue curve is equal to area divided by initial height. The area under the residue curve is the sum of all the values in the curve, i.e. 909. Therefore $T = 909/100 = 9.09$ sec.

Time sec	Outflow curve	Residue curve
14	1	1
13	3	4
12	6	10
11	10	20
10	17	37
9	26	63
8	20	83
7	10	93
6	5	98
5	2	100
4	0	100
3	0	100
2	0	100
1	0	100 = initial height
		909 = sum

24. Following intravenous injection of technetium-99m DTPA, the count rate from the lung was twice that from the liver and the ratio of their count rates was clearly not changing with time. Following inhalation of the aerosol, liver count rate increased as a result of DTPA in the lung alveoli diffusing across the alveolar epithelium into blood. The counts recorded in the lung region of interest from DTPA in pulmonary blood would therefore have been twice the liver count rate. So multiplication of the liver count rate by two followed by subtraction from the recorded lung counts gives the background corrected lung curve (**Fig. 14.5**). With correction, the rate constant of DTPA aerosol clearance was 0.04 min^{-1} (a typical value for a habitual cigarette smoker), but without correction it was only 0.027 min^{-1}. Note that, before applying this background correction, there is no need to subtract the counts resulting from the preceding intravenous injection as this subtraction is incorporated in the background correction after inhalation.

25a) Protein binding of 50% for hippuran corresponds to a volume of distribution of 8 litres and for MAG3, 5 litres. With their corresponding clearances of 500 ml/min and 350 ml/min, the transit time equation can be used to calculate mean residence times in the whole body of 8000/500 = 16 min and 5000/350 = 14.3 min, respectively. Iodine-123 half-life is 13 hr. To find effective half-life it is perhaps easier to think of biological half-life in terms of a rate constant, which is the reciprocal of mean

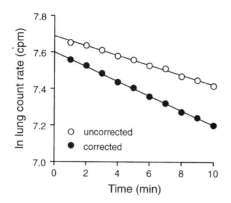

▌ Fig. 14.5 Logarithm alveolar technetium-99m DTPA aerosol clearance curves from question 24 based on (a) the pulmonary time–activity curve not corrected for vascular background and (b) the pulmonary time–activity curve corrected for vascular background (taken to be equal to twice the count rate from the region of interest over the liver). The rate constants for curves respectively not corrected and corrected are 0.027 min^{-1} and 0.04 min^{-1}.

residence time, so the effective rate constant is the sum of physical decay rate constant and whole body disappearance rate constant (i.e. the biological rate constant). For iodine-123 hippuran, biological and physical decay rate constants are 3.75 hr^{-1} and 0.053 hr^{-1} respectively, giving a sum of 3.8 hr^{-1}, which corresponds to an effective half-time of 10.9 min. The biological rate constant for technetium-99m MAG3 is 1/14.3 = 0.07 min^{-1} and the physical decay rate constant is 0.001925 min^{-1}, giving a total of 0.072 min^{-1}. This corresponds to an effective half time of 9.6 min. Note that biological half time is equal to 0.693 (i.e. the natural logarithm of 2) of biological residence time.

b) The biological half-life in this patient is biphasic with 50% of the labelled granulocytes undergoing faecal excretion with a half-time related to the intravascular half time and intracolonic half time and 50% having a long, normal biological half-time. Mean residence time in blood is 10 hr (corresponding to a half time in blood of 7 hr) and mean residence time in colon is 6 hr, a total mean whole body residence time of 16 hr, corresponding to a rate constant of 0.0625 hr^{-1}. The biological rate constant of indium-111 not gaining access to bowel lumen is 0.00042 hr^{-1}. There are therefore two phases of indium-111 loss or, in other words, a biexponential whole-body loss, with a mean residence time equal to total area (0.5/0.0625 plus 0.5/0.00042 hr) divided by initial height (unity); this is 8 + 1190 = 1198 hr, a rate constant of 0.02 day^{-1}. Indium-111 decays with a half-time of 2.8 days, which corresponds to a rate constant of 0.25 day^{-1}. The effective rate constant is therefore 0.02 + 0.25 = 0.27 day^{-1} or, in terms of half-time, 2.57 days.

c) The externally recorded values give a rate constant of 0.0075 min^{-1}. This is the effective half-time and includes the physical decay constant of technetium-99m, which is 0.001925 min^{-1}. Biological half time is therefore 0.0075 – 0.001925 = 0.0056 min^{-1}. With appropriate scaling (Section 11.1.2.1), this corresponds to a GFR/ECF volume of 6.1 ml/min/litre or, for a standard ECF volume of 13 litres, 80 ml/min.

Index